NURSING CARE OF THE EYE

NURSING CARE OF THE EYE

Heather Boyd-Monk, S.R.N., R.N., B.S.N.
Assistant Director of Nursing
for Education Programs
Wills Eye Hospital

Clinical Instructor
Department of Baccalaureate Nursing
Thomas Jefferson University
Philadelphia, Pennsylvania

Charles G. Steinmetz III, M.D.
Attending Surgeon
Consultant, Pathology Department
Wills Eye Hospital

Clinical Associate Professor, Ophthalmology
Thomas Jefferson University
Philadelphia, Pennsylvania

 APPLETON & LANGE

Norwalk, Connecticut/Los Altos, California

0-8385-7018-6

Notice: Our knowledge in clinical sciences is constantly changing. As new information becomes available, changes in treatment and in the use of drugs become necessary. The author(s) and the publisher of this volume have taken care to make certain that the doses of drugs and schedules of treatment are correct and compatible with the standards generally accepted at the time of publication. The reader is advised to consult carefully the instruction and information material included in the package insert of each drug or therapeutic agent before administration. This advice is especially important when using new or infrequently used drugs.

88 89 90 91 / 10 9 8 7 6 5 4 3 2

Prentice-Hall of Australia, Pty. Ltd., Sydney
Prentice-Hall Canada, Inc.
Prentice-Hall Hispanoamericana, S.A, Mexico
Prentice-Hall of India Private Limited, New Delhi
Prentice-Hall International (UK) Limited, London
Prentice-Hall of Japan, Inc., Tokyo
Prentice-Hall of Southeast Asia (Pte.) Ltd., Singapore
Whitehall Books Ltd., Wellington, New Zealand
Editora Prentice-Hall do Brasil Ltda., Rio de Janeiro

Library of Congress Cataloging-in-Publication Data

Boyd-Monk, Heather.
  Nursing care of the eye.

  Includes index.
  1. Ophthalmic nursing.   I. Steinmetz, Charles G.
II. Title. [DNLM: 1. Eye Diseases—nursing.
2. Ophthalmology—nurses' instruction. WY 158 B789n]
RE88.B69   1987   610.73′677   87-11366
ISBN 0-8385-7018-6

Design: Kathleen E. Peters

PRINTED IN THE UNITED STATES OF AMERICA

To my friends, the nurses of Wills Eye Hospital, who inspired me

Heather Boyd-Monk

To my daughter, Nancy Lowry Steinmetz, a dedicated nurse

Charles Gordon Steinmetz III

Contents

Preface

Nursing care of patients with eye disorders has changed considerably in the last few years. The specialty of ophthalmology has changed its emphasis from inpatient medical and surgical intervention to one that emphasizes outpatient care. Nurses in general nursing practice are required to asssess the whole patient and identify early symptoms so that they may preempt disorders from advancing and help maintain the patient in a state of wellness. Ophthalmic health care professionals must be cognizant of all these changes, including a technical explosion in the equipment field, in order to render the best care to their patients.

The vast amounts of ophthalmology literature make this specialty difficult for the general nursing practitioner to keep up with. This book serves as a foundation for ophthalmologic terminology and provides methods and procedures related to general eye care. It discusses each of the eye's structures and how each functions in relation to the whole eye. Congenital and acquired eye disorders and diseases have been identified, and guidelines for nursing intervention have been included wherever they are appropriate. Topics have been illustrated with numerous graphics and photographs.

The chapters have been reviewed by both ophthalmic nurses and ophthalmologists for accuracy. We wish to thank Maggie Easterlin, R.N., B.S.N., who contributed the information relating to the operating room; Karen Akoff, whose exquisite drawings most certainly enhance this presentation; Gloria Parker and Fleur Weinberg, without whose patient help in the library we could not have managed; and photographers Dave Silva and Jack Scully for their expertise. A special thanks goes to the Wills Eye Hospital nurses for their support in the project, the pharmacists who helped update drug information, and the ophthalmologists who so freely gave us copies of their photographs, who reviewed specific areas of the material for accuracy, and who recognize that the value of knowledge develops only when it is shared. Our thanks also go to Kathleen O'Brien of Appleton & Lange, for the care she took as our editor to ensure that this work would reflect up-to-date integrated information.

Heather Boyd-Monk, S.R.N., R.N., B.S.N.

Charles G. Steinmetz III, M.D.
Philadelphia

I

OPHTHALMOLOGY FUNDAMENTALS

1

Anatomy of the Eye, Anatomic Terminology, and Other Ophthalmologic Terminology

Ophthalmology, like a foreign language, has a selection of words which when learned will help unveil the secrets of the "window of the soul," as the eye is sometimes referred to. The reader who takes a little time to review and digest these key words prior to reading the information will find that the following terms are used in a variety of ways, describing nouns as embellishing adjectives. Anyone involved in nursing care of eye patients will see the terms used as admitting diagnoses, surgical procedures, or treatment modalities. Awareness of the significance of a term makes the text much easier to read and will enable the health care professional to form a picture in the mind's eye of what patients' needs will be.

To keep this new vocabulary in its true perspective one should remember that for each term presented, a lecture, symposium, or chapter in a book has been written about the subject. In this chapter the words are merely defined in order to use them as building blocks for subsequent material.

ANATOMY TERMS RELATING TO THE EYEBALL (Fig. 1–1)

The *cornea* is the clear, transparent portion of the outer coat of the eyeball forming the front of the aqueous chamber. It is continuous with the *sclera* (the white part of the eye) which forms the external, protective coat of the eye. The landmark corneoscleral junction is referred to as the *limbus,* and the fibrous sheath, *Tenon's capsule,* which envelops the eyeball, is part of the sclera.

The *iris,* the colored, circular membrane, can be seen behind the cornea, and is in front of the lens. The iris regulates the amount of light entering the eye by changing the size of the *pupil,* a contractile opening in the center of the iris. The *anterior chamber* (behind the cornea and in front of the iris) and the *posterior chamber* (between the back of the iris and the front of the lens) are spaces filled with *aqueous humor,* a plasma-like substance responsible for maintaining the hydrostatic pressure of the eye. After aqueous has circulated between the lens and iris it filters through the *trabecular meshwork* into the *Canal of Schlemm,* a circular canal situated at the juncture (angle) of the internal cornea and iris.

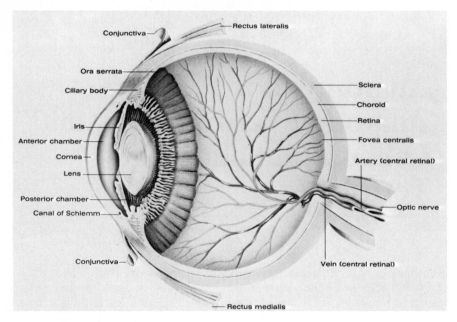

Figure 1–1. Anatomical structure of the eyeball. *(From Burroughs Wellcome Co. Research Triangle Park, N.C., 1979.)*

The *ciliary body* consists of ciliary processes (which are tufts of tissue projecting into the posterior chamber) and the ciliary muscle, and is the portion of the vascular coat between the iris and *choroid* (the intermediate, vascular coat of the eye which furnishes nourishment to the other parts of the eyeball). The iris, ciliary body, and choroid make up the *uveal tract.*

The *retina,* the innermost coat of the eye, is a collection of sensitive nerve fibers and axions from its ganglionic cell layer make up the *optic nerve* which carries messages from retina to brain. The head of the optic nerve is referred to as the *optic disc.* The optic disc is responsible for the physiological *blind spot* in the field of vision. The *macula lutea* a small, but important area of the retina, surrounds the *fovea centralis* and together they comprise the area of distinct vision. *Vitreous* (humor), a transparent, colorless mass of soft, gelatinous material fills the eyeball behind the clear, crystalline *lens.* *Zonules* (suspensory ligaments) suspend the lens from the ciliary processes between the aqueous filled posterior chamber and the vitreous. This posterior portion of the eye, visible with an ophthalmoscope, consists of the retina which includes the macula and the optic nerve, is referred to as the *fundus.*

ANATOMY TERMS RELATING TO THE ADNEXA (Fig. 1–2)

The opening between the eyelids is referred to as the *palpebral fissure,* while the angle at the junction of each side is called the *canthus,* (inner and outer). *Conjunctiva,* the thin, transparent mucous membrane lines the anterior sclera up to the

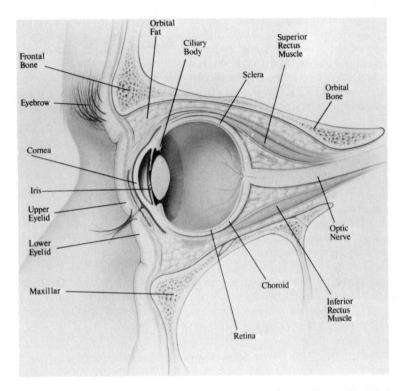

Figure 1–2. Anatomical relationship of the eyeball and the adnexa. *(Modified from Friedman AH, et al.: Optyl Atlas of the Human Eye. Norwood, N.J.: Optyl, 1979.)*

limbus (bulbar conjunctiva) and the posterior surface of the lids (palpebral conjunctiva). The upper and lower folds are referred to as *fornicies*. A synonym for the lower fornix is the *cul-de-sac*. *Eyelashes* are found at the lid margin. The *tarsal plates*, a framework of connective tissue gives shape to the eyelids. The *Meibomian glands* are long, sebaceous glands found in the tarsal plates of upper and lower eyelids. Upper and lower *lacrimal puncta*, found in the inner canthus, are the inlets to the *lacrimal canaliculi* through which tears drain.

The *orbits* are the bony sockets which contain the eyeball, and are composed of seven bones.

PHYSIOLOGICAL ACTIONS OF THE EYE

Accommodation is the ability of the eye to adapt to near vision by increasing the lens convexity. *Convergence* is said to occur when there is an inclination of the eyes toward a common point. *Divergence,* a spreading or tending apart of the eyes, occurs as the eyes return to their normal position from convergence. *Fusion* is the coordination of the separate images of the same object in the two eyes into one, which gives the dimension of depth perception. *Diplopia,* or double vision, occurs when fusion is broken and the two images are seen. *Amblyopia,* the uncorrectable blurred vision in one eye is due to disuse of the eye with no organic defect. The *refractive media* of the eye is composed of the cornea, aqueous, lens, and vitreous. *Refraction* is the deviation of light rays by the refractive media of the eye to bring the rays to proper focus on the retina. However, the term is also used to describe the determination of refractive errors and their correction by glasses.

ERRORS OF REFRACTION

Ametropia is an imperfection in the refractive powers of the eye, and results when light does not focus on the retina. *Astigmatism,* on the other hand, is the refractive error which prevents light rays from coming to a single focus on the retina because of corneal irregularity. (Occasionally, this can also be due to lens changes.) *Emmetropia* describes perfect visual refraction. Three other terms are frequently used in ophthalmology. *Myopia,* or nearsightedness, is imperfect vision caused by the focus of light rays in front of and not on the retina. *Hyperopia,* or farsightedness, is imperfect vision caused by the focus of the light rays behind rather than on the retina. The mechanism of *presbyopia* is a little different, for the impairment of eyesight is due to loss of elasticity of the lens in middle age.·

Terms Relating to the Extraocular Muscles

Orthophoria is the normal adjustment and equilibrium of eye muscles. *Strabismus,* (squint or heterotropia) is a deviation of one or both eyes from the proper direction. The deviations are referred to depending upon their direction or frequency: for example, *esotropia,* convergent strabismus (or crossed-eyes), is a definite abnormal turning inward of one or both eyes. *Esophoria* is a tendency of the eyes to turn inward. On the other hand, *exotropia,* divergent strabismus (or wall-eye), is a definite abnormal turning outward of one or both eyes, while *exophoria* is a tendency of the eyes to turn outward. Since the eyes can deviate in any direction, *hypertropia,* an actual deviation of the eye upward can occur, while in some cases only a tendency or *hyperphoria* is evident. By the same token there might be an actual deviation of the eye downward or a *hypotropia* or just a suggestion of a tendency of a deviation called *hypophoria.*

Terms Relating to Disorders of the Ocular Structures

The Greek root word for the lids is "blepharo". Inflammation of the eyelids, or *blepharitis,* may be observed at the eyelid margins. *Blepharospasm* is a spasm of the orbicularis muscle of the eyelids, the flutter one sees when flirting, or the defense mechanism one sees when trying to touch the eye. The lower lid can develop an eversion or turning out called *ectropion.* It can also turn in or develop an inversion referred to as *entropion.* There are many meibomian glands in both the upper and lower eyelids, a granulomatous inflammation in one of these is called a *chalazion.* When superficial lid glands of Zeis or Moll become infected this is called a *hordeolum* or sty. *Ptosis* is the drooping of the upper lid.

The Greek root word for the lacrimal system is "*dacryo*". A *dacryoadenitis* is an inflammation of the lacrimal gland, while *dacryocystitis* is an inflammation of the lacrimal sac. *Epiphora,* or tearing, may be due to lacrimal duct obstruction.

The conjuctiva is the mucous membrane which lines the inside of the eyelids (palpebral conjunctiva), and the exposed surface of the globe up to the cornea (bulbar conjunctivita). *Conjunctivitis* is an inflammation of the conjunctiva, either bulbar and/or palpebral conjunctiva may be involved. The usually clear conjunctiva looks red instead of transparent, as *injection*—congestion of ciliary and/or conjunctival vessels—occurs. This looks very different from a *subconjunctival hemorrhage* which occurs beneath the bulbar conjunctiva. A *pterygium* may be seen on the nasal side as a triangular fold (wing) of conjunctiva which extends from the conjunctiva over the cornea. Adhesions of the conjunctiva are called *symblepharon.*

Many changes can be observed in the cornea; the Greek root word for the cornea is *"kerato".* *Keratitis* is an inflammation of the cornea. *Keratoconus* is a cone-shaped deformity of the cornea. A milky-white opacity of the cornea is described as a *leukoma,* while a light corneal opacity might be described as *nebula*—it rather reminds one of the Milky Way if one has seen it. Sometimes one can see a circular corneal opacity (at the limbus); this is referred to as *arcus senilis* when it occurs in older patients. When the normally clear, transparent cornea becomes infiltrated with blood vessels, *pannus* is said to have occurred. *Xerosis* is abnormal keratoconjunctival dryness. Intraocular adhesions of the iris to the cornea or lens are called *synechia.*

When a half-moon of pus or cells is seen (through the cornea) in the anterior chamber, it is called a *hypopion.* Blood in the anterior chamber is termed *hyphema;* this often occurs as a result of blunt trauma and other structures may become inflamed as well. *Iritis* is an inflammation of the iris. *Cyclitis* is an inflammation of the ciliary body. Usually both structures are involved simultaneously and this is referred to as *iridocyclitis.* When the structures of the pigmentary layer of the eye or uveal tract become inflamed, the patient is said to have *uveitis. Sympathetic ophthalmia,* an iridocyclitis of the eye following disease or injury to the fellow eye, is a very serious kind of uveitis.

Aphakia refers to absence of the lens of the eye. This state is present after the patient has undergone removal of a *cataract,* which is an opacity of the lens.

When the fundus is viewed using an ophthalmoscope, an abnormality of the optic disc that can be observed is a *choked disc,* or *papilledema,* which is a congestion and inflamed state of the optic disc seen when there is increased intracranial pressure. *Glaucoma,* on the other hand, is intraocular pressure which damages optic neurons. Both of these entities may produce a *scotoma,* a blind or partially blind area in the visual field.

Endophthalmitis is an inflammation, or infection or both of the internal structures of the eye. *Panophthalmitis* is said to occur when all the structures surrounding and including the eye become inflamed or infected.

The eyeballs can be displaced outward for a variety of reasons, and when this occurs it is referred to as *exophthalmos;* a synonym for this is *proptosis.* The eyeball can also appear as if it has sunken into the orbit and this is termed *enophthalmus.* Care must be exercised not to confuse enophthalmus with exophthalmos; endophthalmitis stands for an intraocular infection, and the infectious patient should be cared for with isolation precautions. When only a portion of the eyeball is thinned and bulging, it is termed *staphyloma.* Normally the eyes move together in a coordinated, smooth manner; *nystagmus* is an involuntary rapid movement of the eyeballs over which the patient has little or no control.

Diagnostic Agents

Many instruments and different methods of examination are used in ophthalmology in order to facilitate identification of ocular function as well as problems. *Visual acuity* (VA), the acuteness or clearness of vision, is probably the most important test that can be performed on the eye patient, for it identifies how much a person can see. The Snellen chart of figures or numbers is used and central vision is tested. The *perimeter* is an instrument used for measuring the field of vision, or "visual fields," which is a way of measuring the extent of vision and visual acuity of the periphery of the eye. Visual fields are measured by size of the stimulating test objects and their limits are called *isopters*. The *tonometer* is used for measuring the intraocular pressure (IOP) of the eye, or "tension" as it is sometimes referred to. With the *Slitlamp,* a biomicroscope from which a brilliant slit-like beam of light can be projected into the anterior part of the eye, the ophthalmologist can study these structures in microscopic detail with binocular vision, on Slitlamp examination (SLE).

Direct and indirect *ophthalmoscopes* are instruments with special illumination and lenses used for viewing the fundus (inner eye), particularly the retina and associated structures.

Drug Terms

A *cycloplegic* is a drug that temporarily puts the ciliary muscle at rest, paralyzes accommodation, and dilates the pupil. On the other hand, a *mydriatic* is a drug that merely dilates the pupil, without affecting accommodation. These drugs are used to facilitate examination of the fundus as well as for treatment of inflammations.

Miotics are a group of drugs that cause the pupil to constrict when a drop is placed in the eye. *Carbonic Anhydrase Inhibitors* (CAI) decrease the secretion of aqueous by inhibiting the production of carbonic anhydrase in the ciliary body. *Osmotic agents* are used to reduce the intraocular pressure by making the plasma hypertonic to aqueous. These three categories of drugs are all used when it becomes necessary to reduce the intraocular pressure of the eye.

Surgical Procedures

As in all other specialties there are procedures in ophthalmology devised by surgeons who have lent their names to their particular procedure. Though there are many surgical procedures with many names, it is sometimes to the health care professionals' advantage to know just how to break the word down in order to understand just what has been done to or for the patient. Here are a few examples: *Dacryocystorhinostomy,* when broken down to its component parts is dacryo = lacrimal, cysto = sac, rhino = nose, ostomy = a hole into. Therefore, a DCR is the formation of a communication between the lacrimal sac and the nose, usually because of a blocked lacrimal duct.

Enucleation of an eye is the complete surgical removal of the eye. A less frequently performed procedure is *evisceration* of the eye; this procedure is the surgical removal of the contents of the eye, but the sclera is left intact. The most devastating procedure is *exenteration,* which is the surgical removal of the orbital contents. Each of these procedures requires special feeling, tact, and caring when dealing with patients who have undergone them. The *prosthesis,* an artificial eye, is almost exclusively made of plastic today.

Portions of the eye can be removed surgically, for example an *iridectomy* is the surgical removal of part of the iris. *Iridotomy,* on the other hand, is a small hole through the iris, and may be done surgically, or with a laser. *Vitrectomy* is removal of the vitreous. A paracentesis can also be done, but in the case of the eye it is referred to as an *anterior chamber tap.* A *vitreous tap* may also be done to remove a small quantity of vitreous. All surgical procedures should be done under strict aseptic (sterile) technique.

Photographs of most of the italicized words in this chapter will be presented in the appropriate chapters which deal with the subject matter. Just having a new knowledge base as a starting point will make the following material more intriguing to read.

BIBLIOGRAPHY

Gylys B, Wedding ME: Medical Terminology—A Systemic Approach. Philadelphia: Davis, 1983

Nolte J: The Human Brain—An Introduction to Its Functional Anatomy. St. Louis: Mosby, 1981

Weinreb EL: Anatomy and Physiology. Reading, Mass.: Addison Wesley, 1984

2

Embryology of the Eye

The human fetus develops from two cells in an orderly manner with the rapid multiplication of, and interaction between cells as they differentiate and grow at their different rates. In the forebrain these changes are dramatic with many different growth patterns occurring at the same time, and by the 3rd week the cells which form the eye have been determined. By the 4th week the pigmented, round optic vesicle can be seen. The *mesoderm* surrounding this vesicle will develop into the orbit. During the 2nd month of development the tissues move to form the definitive eyeball and orbit. From the 3rd month extending to the time of birth, differentiation of the immature cells which are in their final location continues. In the last 3 months the fetal blood vessels and excess embryonic mesoderm will atrophy. The individual structures will now be discussed in detail.

The development of the orbit is quite important since it will hold and protect the eye. Early in human development the orbits are derived from mesoderm which appears during the neural plate stage (Fig. 2–1). Around the 15th day, a streak (referred to as the primitive streak), develops in the neural plate and will become the notocord. The streak is composed of primitive cells which differentiate and form a thin layer under the *ectoderm*. These are mesodermal cells and will further differentiate into *paraxial mesoderm* and *visceral mesoderm*.

Growing at a disproportionate rate, the paraxial mesoderm extends forward and around the brain. As the forward portion of the embryo flexes downward, the forebrain and the optic vesicle are brought in close contact with the visceral mesoderm which will become the *maxillary process*. As embryo development progresses, the orbits are formed out of the paraxial mesoderm superiorly and nasally, while visceral mesoderm of the maxillary processes forms the inferior and outer walls. This occurs when the lateral nasal process (paraxial mesoderm) and the maxillary process (visceral mesoderm) meet at about the 12-mm stage, or during the latter part of the 5th week of development. In this union, which is called the naso-optic furrow, there is a burying of a cord of epithelial cells which will be the future *nasolacrimal duct* (Fig. 2–2). The continued uneven or disproportionate growth of the maxillary processes causes the axis of the orbits to rotate forward. This moves the visual axes from a lateral to a forward looking position. Still greater change in the orbital axis comes between the 2nd and 3rd fetal month, when the angles change from 180 to 105 degrees. At birth they average 75 degrees, and later in the adult they will measure 68 degrees (Fig. 2–3).

At the $3\frac{1}{2}$-month embryological state of development, the orbits are easily identified but still incompletely formed. Orbital shape is molded by its contents, the developing globe, lacrimal apparatus, and the superior and inferior oblique (extraocular) muscles.

Neural Plate   Neural Groove   Ectoderm

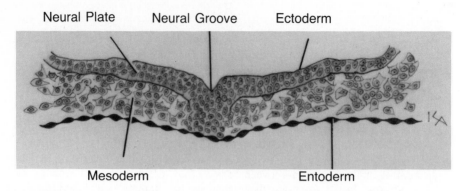

Mesoderm   Entoderm

Figure 2–1. The orbits are derived from mesoderm which appears during the neural plate stage. *(Modified from Arey L: Developmental Anatomy. Philadelphia: Saunders, 1943, p. 515.)*

At birth the height and width of the orbits are approximately equal, and this is maintained until puberty. At this time a major change occurs in the relative height of the orbit to the height of the face. At birth the orbit's height is about half the height of the face, while in the adult it is about one-third of this height.

The formation of the skull bones does not go completely through a cartilagenous stage before the osseous stage is reached. Most of the cranial vault, which includes the *frontal, zygoma, sphenoid, ethmoid, lacrimal and palatine*

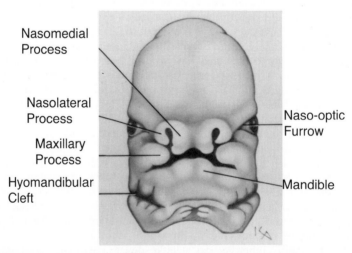

Nasomedial Process

Nasolateral Process

Maxillary Process

Hyomandibular Cleft

Naso-optic Furrow

Mandible

Figure 2–2. There is a burying of a cord of epithelial cells in the naso-optic furrow which will be the future nasolacrimal duct. *(Modified from Schaeffer JP: Morris' Human Anatomy, 10th ed. Philadelphia: Blakiston, 1944, p. 27.)*

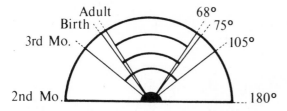

Figure 2–3. At birth the visual axes average 75 degrees, and later in the adult will measure 68 degrees. *(Modified from Duke-Elder S: Systems of Ophthalmology: Normal and Abnormal Development, Part I. St. Louis: Mosby, 1963, p. 215.)*

bones, as well as portions of the base of the skull, is ossified in membrane without the preformed cartilage.

ORBITAL CONTENTS

The contents of the orbit are formed from the loose matrix of stellate, undifferentiated paraxial mesoderm, into which the *optic vesicle* invaginates. Hematopoiesis is first noticed at the 3- to 4-mm stage. Shortly after this, mesodermal condensation (clumping and rapid cell growth) appears and will develop into *extrinsic ocular muscles.* The cranial nerves which innervate these muscles are formed at different times: the *oculomotor* (III CN) at the 7- to 8-mm stage; the *abducens* (VI CN) at the 8- to 9-mm stage; and the *trochlear* (IV CN) at the 10- to 12-mm stage. By the 6th week (13.5-mm stage), the muscles are quite obvious. The recti muscles blend with scleral mesodermal cells which are condensing and forming at the same time. The last muscles to appear are the *levator palpebrae superioris* (of the upper lids), which appear between the 22- to 30-mm stage in the 7th to 8th week of embryological development.

The primative *ventral ophthalmic artery* (which leads to the orbit then globe), is derived from the internal carotid artery at about the 9-mm stage. After many changes and variations, the final vasculature is present at birth. The vasculature of the veins resembles that of the arteries.

EMBRYOLOGY OF THE EYE

The first sign of the eye occurs in the differentiation on the embryonic plate where there is a thickening of *neuroectoderm* on either side of the anterior neural groove, at the 2.5-mm stage or at 2 weeks gestation. This area recesses and becomes a pit when the open end of the anterior neural tube closes and is surrounded by mesoderm (Fig. 2–4). At about the 4-mm stage this optic outgrowth constricts to form a hollow optic stalk connecting the optic vesicle with the embryonic forebrain.

The neural tube is undergoing rapid change and differentiation into the forebrain (*prosencephalon*), midbrain (*mesencephalon*), and hindbrain (*rhomben-*

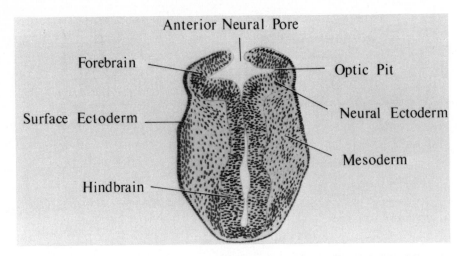

Figure 2–4. Optic pits arise from the thickening of neural ectoderm, and by disproportionate growth produce invagination. *(Modified from Wolff E, Last RJ: Anatomy of the Eye and Orbit, 5th ed. Philadelphia: Saunders, 1961, p. 392.)*

cephalon). The optic stalk can now be identified as the junction between the *telencephalon* (forebrain) and *diencephalon* (posterior portion of the prosencephalon).

At this 4-mm stage there is a chemical liberation by the distal curving optic vesicle which causes the surface ectoderm to thicken forming a plate (*placode*) which will later become the *lens* (Fig. 2–5).

The lens plate, growing in an uneven manner, will begin to invaginate and will form a small hollow ball which is known as the *lens vesicle*. While this lens vesicle is being formed the optic vesicle is also undergoing invagination and differentiation into an inner neuroectodermal cup (5-mm stage), and an outer neuroectodermal layer with an ever diminishing space between these two layers (Fig. 2–6). Both inner and outer layers are changing; with the inner layers becoming thicker, they will eventually become the ten layers of the neurosensory *retina,* and the outer layer will be the pigmented epithelial layer of the retina. These layers, referred to as the inner neurosensory layer and the outer pigmented layer are separated by a potential space which may accept fluid, and thereby cause retinal separation or detachment.

The lens vesicle is a hollow sphere with a single layer of cuboidal cells forming its wall (Fig. 2–7). At the 9-mm stage the lens vesicle has detached from the surface ectoderm by atrophy of the stalk and lies in the optic cup.

Continuing changes are taking place in the lens vesicle, i.e., cells of the posterior wall of the lens vesicle grow quite large. The central hollow is compressed to a small concave gap between the anterior wall cells, and the enlarging lens cells, which will form the fetal nucleus.

Only the posterior portion of the cells grow very rapidly and elongate, forming an arc in the anterior portion of the vesicle. This bowed line extends forward to completely close the cavity (Fig. 2–6). The anterior cells migrate to the equator, the widest portion of the lens vesicle, where they become secondary lens fibers by sending out anterior and posterior protoplasmic processes. In this way the lens

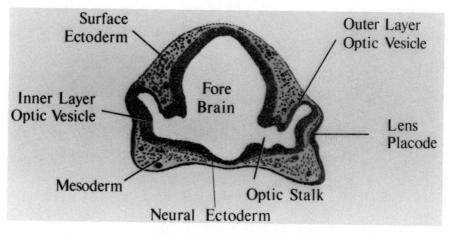

Figure 2–5. The distal curving optic vesicle causes the surface ectoderm to thicken forming a lens plate (placode). *(Modified from Wolff E, Last RJ: Anatomy of the Eye and Orbit, 5th ed. Philadelphia: Saunders, 1961, p. 393.)*

grows layer upon layer around the fetal nucleus and the cortex of the crystalline lens. A capsule is then secreted by the lens epithelium.

The optic vesicle, still growing in an uneven manner, permits vascular mesoderm from the surrounding tissue to enter the cup, through the fetal fissure of the optic stalk. This forms the vascular *hyaloid* system with its meshwork around the

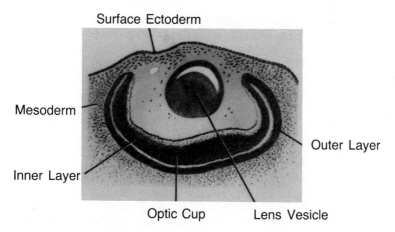

Figure 2–6. While the lens vesicle is being formed the optic vesicle is undergoing invagination and differentiation into an outer and inner neural (optic) cup. *(Modified from Barber AN: Embryology of the Human Eye. St. Louis: Mosby, 1955, p. 43.)*

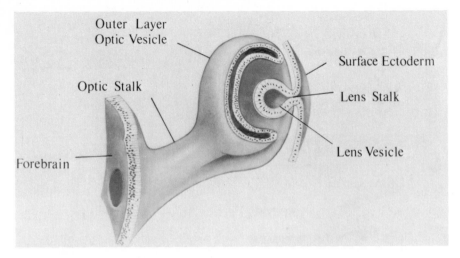

Figure 2–7. Diagram showing relationship of lens vesicle, lens stalk, and optic cup (vesicle). *(Modified from Wolff E, Last RJ: Anatomy of the Eye and Orbit, 5th ed. Philadelphia: Saunders, 1961, p. 395.)*

lens and its branches which extend throughout the *primary vitreous.* Occurring at the 13-mm stage, this is completed by the 18-mm stage, or by the end of the 6th week of fetal life (Fig. 2–8). By this time the fetal fissure has closed, and vascularity of a network of capillaries called the *choroidal capillary net* is present on the outer surface of the optic vesicle, with drainage into the superior and inferior network of veins called the *venous plexus.*

At the same time (starting at the posterior pole and progressing toward the periphery), the *neuroretina* is also growing and differentiating. At first there are two primitive layers of nuclei. The timing of the development is such that the cells move from the outer layer toward the inner nucleated layer, but the neurological development and maturity is from inner to outer layers. The importance of this is that when the rods and cones are finally developed and ready to function, the receptors and transmittors of the stimuli are also ready to function. As the optic vesicle enlarges the anterior portion and the portion immediately posterior to the optic cup's rim become the posterior or epithelial portion of the *iris* and the *ciliary body,* and further back, the epithelium covering the *ciliary processes, pars plana* and *choroid.*

Differentiation of the retina continues until birth except for the *macula* area which needs the stimuli of light to complete development. The *ganglion cells,* found in the inner layer of the retina, are the first to differentiate and send axons posterior toward the optic stalk where they penetrate the stalk and travel to the brain in a well-delineated pattern. Later these fibers become medulated, starting at the brain and travelling down to the globe where the medulation usually stops at the time of birth.

As *neuroectoderm* of the vesicle develops, a mesodermal component, which differentiates into collagen fibers that are felted together, forms the white, opaque shell responsible for maintaining the shape and protecting the fragile neuroectoder-

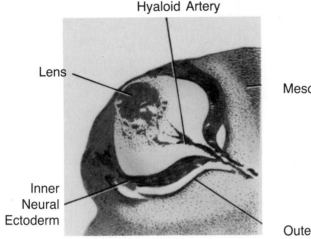

Figure 2–8. The vascular hyaloid system with its meshwork around the lens and its branches which extend throughout the primary vitreous. *(Modified from Barber AN: Embryology of the Human Eye. St. Louis: Mosby, 1955, p. 158.)*

mal cup. This is called the *sclera*. The anterior one-fifth of this structure has a different type of pattern. Instead of being felted, it is layered. Instead of being white and opaque it is crystal clear; this is known as the *cornea*.

The neuroectodermal cup, as it continues growing in an irregular and uneven fashion forms a notch in the rim which develops into a cleft that eventually extends to the optic stalk. This is known as the *optic fissure*. The mesodermal tissue that streams through this fetal fissure brings vascular tissue into the neuroectodermal cup, and it also brings cells to form the anterior layers of the iris and the layers of the choroid.

Mesodermal fibrils found around the primitive lens vesicle mix with fibrils from the inner surface of the small neuroectoderm cup. These fibrils form a matrix filling the space between the lens and the inner layers of the cup. Now another mesenchymal element is added; the vascular tissue, which comes through the fetal fissure and develops into the *hyloid artery*. This vascularized fibrillar tissue is called *primary vitreous*, which continues to develop until about the 6th week or the 13- to 14-mm stage.

Secondary vitreous formation begins at the 6th week and continues to form as long as the eye develops and increases in size. Later, however, its rate of development is much less. This secondary vitreous which fills the neuroectodermal cup is avascular. Primary vitreous now atrophies. The *tertiary* vitreous is also formed by the neuroectodermal cup cells, and can be seen as fibres which extend from the epithelium of the *pars plana* to the lens capsule. These are the *zonular fibers* which support the lens.

At the time of birth the eye is fully developed and functioning except for the macular area, but within several months this too has developed.

BIBLIOGRAPHY

Biagin J, Melloni PM, Gilbert M, Eisner MD: Melloni's Illustrative Dictionary, 2nd ed. Baltimore: Williams & Wilkins, 1984

Moore K: The Developing Human, 3rd ed. Philadelphia: Saunders, 1982

Smith JW, Murphy TR, Blair JSG, Lowe KG: Regional Anatomy Illustrations. Edinburgh: Churchill Livingstone, 1983

II

GENERAL EYE CARE

3

Ophthalmic Nursing Procedures

There are many ophthalmic nursing procedures which when learned and performed correctly, ensure that eye patients are made aware that gentle, concerned, and knowledgeable care is being given. At the same time, the patient can be helped to better understand his or her eye problem through *patient teaching*. The methods of care to be taught to the patient must first be learned by the health care provider. *Good handwashing technique is imperative for prevention of cross-contamination.* Extreme gentleness in technique is also of utmost importance, for patients who have ocular disease often fear that they are going to be made more uncomfortable if treatment is administered. If their concerns are confirmed, then they will flinch or recoil the moment they know anything is to be done to their eye.

The following procedures are usually performed in combination with one another to achieve the greatest comfort level for the patient, but each may be performed by itself.

LID HYGIENE

Lid hygiene is performed when exudate crusts the lid margins and causes the lashes to clump together. Frequent administration of eye drops or inflammation and infections of the lid margins can be the cause of the exudate. Cleansing the eyelashes with cotton-tipped applicator sticks (similar to a Q-Tip) is a useful procedure to use when the lashes are stuck together, and the nurse needs to cleanse them prior to administering eye drops.

Use of Applicator Sticks

1. Moisten the tip of the cotton-covered applicator with a drop of sterile basic salt solution or a commercially-prepared solution such as Eyestream or Irrigate and shake excess solution free; hold the stick horizontal to the eye.
2. Have the patient look down, and with a gentle rolling movement twist the applicator against the upper lid margin. Always twist away from the eye (toward the brow).
3. Have the patient look up in order to cleanse the lower lid margin. Start at the lid margin, and twist the applicator away (toward the cheek).

Many people suffer from blepharitis (inflammation of the lid margins), and one method of self-care is to have the patient perform his or her own "lid hygiene" in order to keep the problem under control.[1] For this a baby shampoo is probably best, because it will not burn the eyes.

1. A cotton-tipped swab, dipped into the shampoo, with the excess shaken free should be used.
2. The patient then closes his or her eyes, places the shampoo-moistened swab along the lashes, and gently rubs downward from lid margin to the tip of the lashes (on the upper lid).
3. When doing this procedure to the lower lid, the patient will gently rub from the lower lid margin to tip of the lower eyelashes.
4. Rinse the shampoo off with a warm washcloth and repeat the procedure at least twice a day.

CLEANSING THE EYE

During sleep, the eyelids are sealed shut by secretion from the Meibomian glands. Most people rub their eyes in the morning to open them, or wash them when they wash their face. This is not practical after a surgical procedure or if there is an eye infection, in which case the exudate needs to be cleansed prior to instillation of medication. For this procedure:

1. Moisten a cotton ball with sterile ophthalmic solution, such as Irrigate, Eyestream, or a sterile physiological normal saline solution.
2. Ask the patient to close both eyes, then gently cleanse the lids from the *inner to outer canthus*. Repeat this until the patient is exudate free and the eyes can be opened easily.
3. Separate pieces of cotton should be used for each eye. Unwetted cotton tends to cause filaments to cling to the lashes. These sometimes even poke the patient in the eye and cause persistent discomfort until the thread is removed. Gauze swabs can be used, but these are expensive. Tissues are clean but are nonsterile and are not practical when wet.

EYE IRRIGATIONS

Often it is necessary to irrigate the eyes in order to free them from mucous threads and exudate. This method of cleansing may be used prior to eyedrop instillation or to clean away particulate matter.

Old fashioned "undines" have long since disappeared from hospital equipment shelves; a sterilized bulb syringe in a bottle containing sterile normal saline is still occasionally to be found. In the United States these are being replaced by sterile, basic salt solutions contained in plastic bottles, such as Irrigate and Eyestream. When squeezed, these commercially-prepared bottles have a tip which allows the solution to flow out in a steady, gentle stream that is easily directed over the surface of the eyelids and eye.

Eye Irrigation Technique

It is easier to irrigate the eye when the patient is lying down, but if this is not practical have the patient sit up with his or her head tilted back and propped against the back of a chair or against the wall. Now you are ready to irrigate.

1. Position the patient's head toward the side being irrigated. This will prevent cross-contamination of the other eye if only one eye is involved.
2. Hold a piece, or several pieces of cotton or gauze at the outer canthus to catch the excess water so that the water does not run down the patient's neck.
3. Irrigate the closed eyelid by directing the stream of the solution toward the nose, permitting it to flow over the eyelid's surface toward the outer canthus. Once the lids have been cleansed, the cul-de-sac secretions can be washed out (Fig. 3–1).
4. Ask the patient to open his or her eyes and look up.
5. Direct the stream toward the inner canthus of the conjunctival cul-de-sac and have it flow over the conjunctival surface, catching the solution with a cotton ball.
6. Gently wipe the closed eye dry with the cotton, always stroking the lid from inner to outer aspect.

Irrigation for Chemical Burns

This type of irrigation needs to be copious and more aggressively persued by the nurse attempting to prevent damage by chemicals which have splashed into the

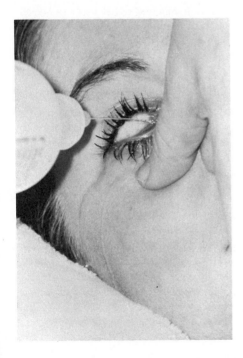

Figure 3–1. Irrigating the cul-de-sac.

eyes. The most important emergency measure is to irrigate the eyes with water as soon as the incident occurs. Showers are provided in laboratories for this purpose. Holding the eyes open under a water faucet is another method of irrigating chemicals from the ocular area. No time should be lost trying to accomplish this.

When a patient reaches an emergency room or dispensary setting stating that chemicals have splashed in his or her eye(s), it is always appropriate to inquire what prior emergency treatment was done. Whether or not the eye(s) has been washed out, the contaminated eye(s) should be copiously irrigated and the following equipment should be available for immediate use in this true ocular emergency:

- 1000 cc of sterile normal saline solution (a bag or bottle of intravenous solution is perfect for this)
- Intravenous tubing
- Towels
- Lid retractors
- Cotton-tipped applicators
- Local (topical) anesthetic drops such as proparacaine. These should be prescribed by a physician but can be given as part of a protocol.

When irrigating an eye for chemical burns, it is often necessary to obtain the assistance of a second person to hold the eyelids open, and retract the eyelids with the lid retractor. The patient experiences terrible pain and often cannot hold his or her eyes open and fights the irrigation.

1. Place the patient in a reclining position remembering to strap him or her on a stretcher for safety. The patient might be asked to hold the towels beside the eye which is being irrigated. This will keep his or her hands occupied. Having the eye irrigated is so uncomfortable that the patient often makes an attempt to stop the procedure.
2. Instill one or two drops of proparacaine anesthetic in the affected eye prior to irrigating.
3. Using IV tubing to guide the stream of the normal saline solution, direct it from the inner canthus and permit it to flow over the surface of the cornea to the outer canthus. Care should be taken not to direct the stream directly onto the cornea, because if the epithelium has been damaged the force of the stream on the cornea could increase the size of the abraded area.
4. Make sure that the fornices are well irrigated using a lid retractor to facilitate irrigation of the upper fornix (Fig. 3–2). If both eyes are involved, irrigate them alternatively. In this case a second liter (1000 cc) of sterile normal saline will be used.
5. After the initial irrigation examine the everted lid for retained particulate matter. Using an applicator stick, gently remove particles from the fornices.

Litmus paper may be used to determine the type of chemical causing the injury if the injured person does not know whether the chemical was alkali or acid. Alkali burns are usually more damaging than acid burns.

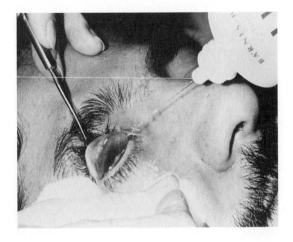

Figure 3–2. Using a Desmares lid retractor to facilitate irrigation of the upper fornix.

EVERTING THE LIDS

1. In order to evert the lower lid, merely pull down on inferior bony orbital rim and this will expose the cul-de-sac adequately (Fig. 3–3).
2. The upper lid can be everted using an applicator stick. For this method, grasp the lashes between the finger and thumb, and then use the applicator stick (on the skin surface of the lid) to "fold" the lid on itself. Remove the applicator stick and place it against the conjunctiva once the lid has been flipped (Figs. 3–4A and B).
3. To double evert the upper lid it is necessary to use a lid retractor. This is done by flipping the eyelid over the lid retractor (exposing the conjunctiva) and pulling the palpebral conjunctiva away from the bulbar conjunctiva. In

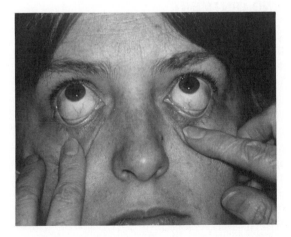

Figure 3–3. Examining the lower cul-de-sac.

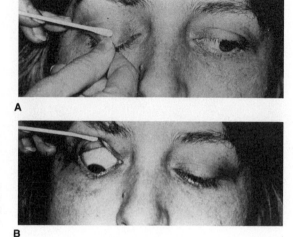

A

Figure 3–4. A. To evert the upper lid, grasp the lashes between the finger and thumb. **B.** Fold the lid on itself, holding it in place with an applicator.

B

the case of chemical burns the upper fornix will now be adequately exposed for thorough irrigation.

RETRACTING THE EYELIDS

Retractors may be required to open the lids in order to visualize the eyeball. Gently place the curved part of the retractor at the upper lid margin, then place a second retractor at the lower lid margin. Using both hands, gently pull the retractors in opposite directions, thereby exposing the widened palpebral fissure, so that the eye can be seen (Fig. 3–5).

INSTILLING EYEDROPS AND OINTMENT

As with all eye care, the hands should be washed prior to rendering an eyedrop or instilling ointment. Remember the eye is a very delicate structure, even though it is so well protected by the bony orbit and lids, so touch the area as little and as gently as possible.

Eyedrops

To instill an eyedrop:

1. Gently place a finger on the bony orbital rim under the lower eyelid.
2. Ask the patient to look up with both eyes. This will reduce blepharospasm, which tends to occur when the person receiving the eyedrops tries to see what is going to be done.
3. Pull the lid down exposing the cul-de-sac and with the opposite hand holding the bottle, squeeze one drop into the cul-de-sac (Fig. 3–6).
4. Ensure that the lashes do not contaminate the tip of the bottle or tube.

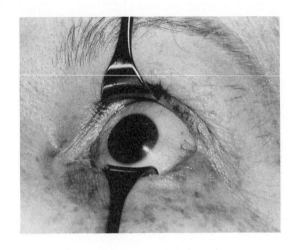

Figure 3–5. Retracting the eyelids using two retractors.

5. Ask the patient to close both eyes gently, so as not to squeeze the drop straight out of the eye.
6. Only one drop is necessary; if more than one is ordered, a short period should elapse before instilling the second.
7. Take a piece of cotton or tissue and gently dab the external canthus. No pressure should be placed on the eyeball itself.

Eye Ointments

Ointments are used for their lubricant property and/or to increase contact time of medication to the external ocular surface. Warn the patient that ointment blurs vision because it smears the cornea. Because of this blurring effect, ointments are most often used at bedtime.

Often the ointment strip tends to curl on itself, so holding the tube in the hand for a few minutes will warm the lubricant slightly and help to avoid this.

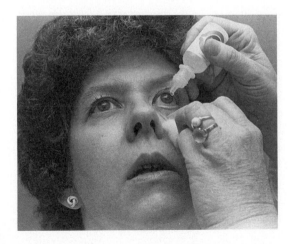

Figure 3–6. Instillation of eye drops.

1. To instill the ointment, have the patient look up with both eyes; pull down the lower lid exposing the cul-de-sac (Fig. 3–7).
2. Place a ½-inch strip of ointment in the cul-de-sac. Have the patient gently close his or her eyes.

Sometimes for oculoplastic surgical (lid) procedures, the ointment is placed on the external eyelid, either on the lid margin itself, or on the suture line. The nurse should be cognizant of the surgical procedure to ensure accurate placement of the ointment. For example, if the lid margins have been sutured together (a procedure called a tarsorrhaphy), the ointment will go on the suture line. However, if the procedure has been a partial tarsorrhaphy, then the physician might want the ointment to actually lubricate the eye through the small opening (see Chap. 13).

Alternatives to topical administration by drop or ointment include membrane release systems (Ocusert) and dissolvable ocular inserts (Lacrisert).[2] These are prescribed by the physician and are then inserted on a weekly or daily basis by the patient.

Self-Medication. If the patient is to be taught to self-medicate, after handwashing ask him or her to hold the bottle of eyedrops in the hand opposite the eye which is to receive the drop. The bottle should be held between the thumb and forefinger.

1. Have the patient rest the thumb on the bridge of the nose, and the forefinger on the forehead (the bottle is between); the tip should be over the center of the eye.
2. With the other hand, pull down on the lower eyelid.
3. Tilt the head back and look up.
4. Squeeze the bottle, and one drop will fall very easily into the eye. The eyes should be closed gently, then blotted if necessary.
5. Care should be taken never to contaminate the tip of the bottle with the lashes.

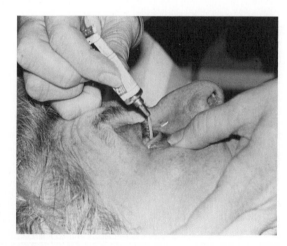

Figure 3–7. Instillation of eye ointment; place a ½-inch strip of ointment in the cul-de-sac.

If more than one medication is to be given, there should be a brief pause between the drops in order to permit absorption.

Occluding the Puncta. To prevent systemic absorption of an ocular drug, it is expedient to occlude the puncta, the openings to the lacrimal canaliculus through which the tears drain.

1. Instill the eyedrop, then press the index finger against the inner canthus until the bone can be felt beneath the skin.
2. Hold this position for a moment or two; either the patient or nurse can do this.

SUBCONJUNCTIVAL INJECTIONS

When adequate drug levels cannot be attained in the external anterior segment of the eye through the administration of topical medication, subconjunctival injection offers another route. Sub-Tenon's injections are deeper and are given under the episclera or Tenon's capsule; therefore, they are given by the physician.

1. A topical anesthetic drop such as proparacaine must be instilled prior to the subconjunctival injection.
2. The injection solution, usually not more than 0.5 cc, is drawn up into a Tuberculin syringe with a #27G needle.
3. The patient is asked to look up, and the tip of the needle with the beveled edge up, is slipped under the conjunctiva (Fig. 3–8).
4. As the drug solution is injected a small bleb (bubble) should appear in the mucous membrane (conjunctiva). This will gradually be absorbed in the next few hours.

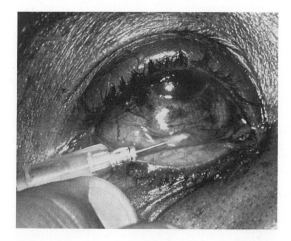

Figure 3–8. Subconjunctival injection. *(From Jeglum EL: Ocular therapeutics, in Boyd-Monk H., Ed.): Nursing Clinics of North America, Philadelphia: Saunders, 1981, p. 459, with permission.)*

COMPRESSES

Compresses, both hot and cold, have a therapeutic as well as a comforting action; both are prescribed for the eye patient. Self-administration helps the patient to feel as if he or she is contributing to his or her improved well-being.

Cold Compresses

Cold or ice compresses are used to vasoconstrict the blood vessels in the orbital region and also to decrease or numb sensitivity of the pain fibers in this area. A small amount of crushed ice placed in a "sandwich baggy" is just enough to last for about the 15 to 20 minutes the compress is prescribed. Commercially-prepared ice containers are available, but are expensive. Gloves can be used but are often uncomfortable, so the following method is recommended:

1. Moisten a 3″ × 4″ gauze with sterile eye solution—just in the center— leaving the surrounding portion dry.
2. Fill a plastic "sandwich baggy" with enough ice to fit in the palm of the hand and tie a knot in the open end.
3. Ask the patient to turn his or her head slightly to the side away from the eye receiving the compress.
4. Place the gauze over the closed eye; then place the "baggy" on top of the gauze. Tape the knotted end and the corner of the "baggy" to the forehead.
5. As the ice melts, the condensation on the "baggy" surface will be caught by the dry gauze[3] (Fig. 3–9).

Occasionally a person will have an adverse reaction to an ice compress and will get a headache from it rather than the agreeable relief that most often accompanies its use. If this happens, the cold compress should be discontinued.

Warm Compresses

Warm compresses are used to dilate the blood vessels in the periorbital region and thereby increase the blood supply and ultimately the number of leukocytes to the

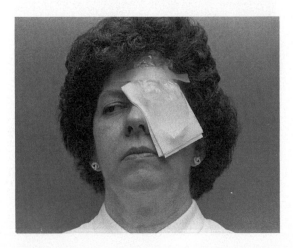

Figure 3–9. Ocular cold compress.

affected area. A warm compress is not usually a sterile procedure but it is a "clean" procedure. In order to accomplish this the person who needs to perform this procedure at home is requested to obtain a clean washcloth and run warm water from the faucet into a clean bowl. After ringing the cloth out, it should be placed against the eye until it cools down, then the process should be repeated for the next 15 to 20 minutes. Most often, warm compresses are ordered at least three or four times a day.

When a person is in a hospital setting, however, warm compresses are prescribed when there is an inflammatory response or an infection present. Having the patient do the compresses without assistance usually gives him or her the feeling of helping him- or herself, and making a contribution to the favorable outcome of the disease process. The patient can be "set up" as follows:

1. Seat the patient at the wash basin (Fig. 3–10).
2. Run warm faucet water into a sterile bowl containing sterile gauze.
3. Cover the patient's clothes with a towel.
4. Wring out the gauze and place it against the closed eye until the gauze cools, then discard it. Repeat the process again and again for the next 20 minutes. This will be prescribed two to four times daily.

PATCHING AND SHIELDING

The eye is patched and shielded for protection following surgery or trauma, as well as for comfort. However, a loose patch can be hazardous because an open eye under

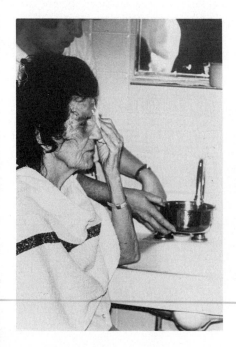

Figure 3–10. Patient performing warm compresses.

a patch can quite possibly develop a corneal abrasion if the patch rubs on the cornea. Tape placed thoughtlessly in the hairline, in the corner of the mouth, or so that it displaces the corner of the mouth upward can be quite distressing to the patient.

Light Patch

A light patch is placed on a traumatized eye to close the eye gently. It acts much as a bandage. Usually there is a little lid swelling, and it gives comfort and a reminder that the eye should be kept shut; however it does not actually securely close the lids.

1. Commercially-prepared eye patches are usually oval in shape and should be placed diagonally across the orbital area.
2. In order to hold the patch in place, take two pieces of tape and place them from the forehead to the cheek about one-half-inch apart.

A good way to ensure that you touch the eye as little as possible can be accomplished as follows:

1. Place the tape diagonally across the patch.
2. Then holding only the ends of the tape, place one end on the forehead, and the other end on the cheek; this way there need never be any pressure placed on the eyeball itself (Fig. 3–11).
3. The second piece of tape, also placed diagonally, is merely to secure the patch.
4. Either one-half-inch or one-inch tape is used.

Eye Shield

It may be expedient to shield the postsurgical or traumatized eye when injuries such as corneal laceration, hyphema, or perforated globe have been sustained. In order to protect the eye still further from an accidental bump or bang a plastic or metal shield is placed over the eye patch, or over the eye (without a patch) as follows:

1. Place the shield so that the edge is resting on the bony orbital rim of the eyebrow.

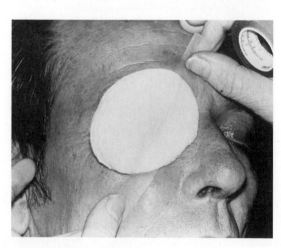

Figure 3–11. Light eye patch. Place patch on eye, applying pressure to forehead and cheek only.

2. The shield is taped diagonally. Make sure that the hairline is avoided, and that the mouth is not displaced upward (Fig. 3–12).

Pressure Patch

A pressure patch is placed on the eye to prevent lid swelling, to absolutely prevent the eye from opening, to stop bleeding, and to seal a wound leak in the ocular surgical site. Before applying this patch, take a look at the setting of the eyes. Some people have deeply set eyes, while others have eyes that almost appear to protrude. The latter have shallow orbits. From this observation you will be able to decide on the number of eye patches you will need to place on the eye.

1. Fold an oval eye patch in half and place it against the closed eye.
2. Place a second patch diagonally over the top of the first one.
3. Tape these patches from the forehead to the cheek with the first piece of one-inch tape.
4. Place the second piece of tape on the forehead (on the same place as the first), but cover the initial tape by two-thirds on the nasal side. Pull the lower end away from the mouth so that it ends on the same place as the first piece of tape.
5. The third piece of tape starts on the forehead but covers the first piece by two-thirds laterally.
6. A fourth piece of tape is once again directed from forehead, to the nasal side of the patch, and then on to the cheek.
7. The fifth piece is placed on the lateral side.

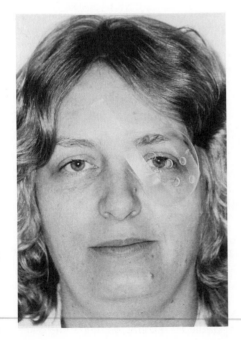

Figure 3–12. Shielding the eye.

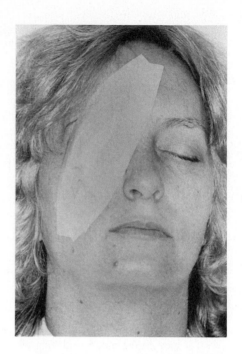

Figure 3–13. To pressure patch the eye, fold an oval patch in half and place it over the closed eye. Place a second patch over the first, then alternate five pieces of tape applying pressure from forehead to cheek over the patches.

8. The ends of the five pieces of tape should all come together on the lower cheek (Fig. 3–13).

The bearded man might offer a challenge, and one might have to shave the area in order to get the tape to stick properly. The sweaty person might require tincture of benzoin applied to the skin before the tape will stick.

The patient should not be able to open the lids underneath the patch. If the person acknowledges the ability to open the eye under the patch when asked to do so, the patch should be removed and replaced with a new one.

TRIMMING EYELASHES

Eyelashes may be clipped when the patient is to have intraocular or retinal surgery, or where there is a possibility that they might enter the surgical site during the operative procedure. In order to clip eyelashes successfully and easily the following steps should be taken:

1. Place a small amount of sterile vaseline petroleum jelly on a piece of gauze; then run (blunt-tipped) lash scissors through the jelly so that they are lightly coated on each side.
2. The patient may be seated or lying down. Ask him or her to close both eyes gently.
3. Elevate the eyelid so that the lashes are pulled slightly outward.
4. Cut the lashes to within 2 to 3 mm of the lid margin, starting at the outer

canthus and working inward. The cut lashes will adhere to the vaseline on the scissors.

5. The lower lashes may also need to be trimmed if they are long.

FACIAL SCRUB

Facial scrubs are also ordered preoperatively by the physician. The face may be washed with a cleansing agent such as a baby shampoo. The motion to be used is from the inner aspect to the outer aspect of the closed eyelid, the brow, and then the cheek. The area should be rinsed well and patted dry with a clean towel.

CONJUNCTIVAL EYE CULTURES

To facilitate identification of pathological microorganisms which cause eye disease, a small scraping is taken from the infected area. The specimen of the infected area can, through the laboratory techniques of culture, produce colonies of the infecting organisms when grown on suitable media. These organisms are then identified microscopically. The next stage of the procedure is to find out which antibiotics the pathogenic microorganisms are sensitive or resistant to, so that the correct antibiotic may be prescribed for the patient. This stage takes at least 48 hours, sometimes longer. Therefore, in order to get preliminary bacterial identification, a "smear" is obtained. For this, a second scraping from the infected area is taken and the specimen is smeared onto a glass slide, which is then stained using either the Geimsa or the Gram procedure. The specimen may contain a single microorganism or none at all. Identification of even one organism is helpful to the physician in prescribing antibiotic medication, for many antibiotics are specifically effective against Gram-positive organisms, while others work best against Gram-negative organisms. However, the true identity of the invading organism may only become apparent when it grows a colony on the culture plate.

An eye culture is done when an infection is suspected and should be taken before antibiotic eyedrops are initiated. The procedure is performed in the following manner:

1. The patient receives a topical anesthetic drop in the eye to be cultured.
2. A platinum wire ring or spatula is heated over a flame until it glows red. It is then cooled to room temperature.
3. The patient is asked to look up with both eyes; the lower lid of one eye is pulled down gently to expose the cul-de-sac.
4. The platinum spatula is passed over the surface of the conjunctiva from the inner to the outer canthus.
5. The specimen obtained is plated out (placed in a C-configuration) on blood-agar.
6. Remember to mark from which eye the culture was obtained; include the patient's name and the date on the culture plate and lab slip.

A preliminary bacterial culture report is usually available after 24 hours, with the definitive culture and sensitivity report forthcoming in 48 hours.

Commercially-prepared, sterile culture applicator sticks are also available and can be used satisfactorily for the eye culture procedure. However, the specimen obtained should be placed on culture media immediately; otherwise the swab tends to dry out and any potential bacterial culture is lost.

Corneal scrapings are most often performed by the physician or occasionally by a skilled and experienced microbiology laboratory technician.

Smears

A smear offers the possibility of quick identification of a bacterial intruder; however, it must be remembered that in order to obtain a smear and a culture, a separate swabbing procedure must be done each time.

To obtain a smear, follow Steps 1 through 4 given in the eye culture procedure, then:

5. Place the specimen on two separate glass slides. Different stains (Gram or Giemsa) will be used on each slide to try to identify whether the microorganism is a Gram-negative or Gram-positive bacteria, and whether it is rod-shaped or round, or whether it is a fungus.
6. Draw a circle around the area of the specimen to be stained for easy identification, since it only covers a minute part of the slide.
7. Mark each slide with the patient's name, the date, and the eye from which the specimen was taken.

PSYCHOSOCIAL ASPECTS OF CARE

Sensory Deprivation and Patient Safety

In any institution, the white-coated or uniformed health care professional is the one person who is sure to be asked where places are to be found by people visiting. Remember the visitors' safe arrival at a destination depends upon explicit directions. Should the situation be one in which the visitor is a patient and his or her major problem is poor vision, it is a good idea to describe a landmark close to the patient as a starting point and ask if he or she sees it. The answer should indicate how much the patient can see and thus allow the professional to tailor directions to the person's needs. Be sure to describe landmarks and give detailed directions using the terms right and left. Try this by having a colleague close his or her eyes, and directing him or her through a doorway.

Look down a corridor with obstacles on both sides; stop and consider for a moment what a wonder it is that there are not more accidents. On inpatient floors, all articles such as litters, janitorial carts, linen billies, etc. should be placed on one wall, leaving the wall closest to the patient's doorway free to enable poorly-sighted patients to travel in relative safety when exiting through doorways of the rooms. Even a poorly positioned briefcase left in the middle of a nurses' station or a chair that has been left out of place is a hazard; anything that can be tripped over should be moved.

If a patient with poor vision has been oriented to the room setting, remember that he or she has a "picture" in the mind's eye as to just where the furniture has been placed. This picture enables the patient to navigate safely around a hospital room. Do not move things without reorienting the person.

Some other useful points to remember when dealing with blind or poorly-sighted persons are the following:

1. When guiding a patient with poor vision, ask him or her to grasp your arm. This will permit the patient to be one-half step behind you. There is no need to push and tug; the motion of your body will be enough to guide the person as you safely navigate to a destination.
2. If a blind patient is to be offered a chair, place his or her hands on the back of the chair, and permit him or her to explore the back, the arms, and the seat. The patient will then be able to seat him- or herself.
3. Carpeted floors make it very difficult for the patient to hear someone approaching, so remember in the hospital setting to stop before getting right up to the bedside, address the patient by name, then identify yourself. This will let the individual know to whom you are speaking and who you are. Include the time of day by adding a "Good morning" etc., which helps to keep people oriented to the time of day. Many times a patient will respond by asking "What time is it?"
4. Remember that visually-poor patients often have excellent hearing, so do not shout; but do talk directly to them and when you address a patient, state his or her name. Do not talk to the patient through a third party.
5. When meal times approach, read the menu aloud. Set up a meal tray as if it were a clock; then describe where the food and utensils are placed. Two other methods of helping the patient become adjusted to the placement of food on a hospital tray may also be considered. One might hold the patient's hand and help him or her explore the things on the tray, thus giving tactile information while giving a verbal description. Secondly, one might describe a particular landmark, for example, "Your water glass is in the top righthand corner, the coffee cup is next to it, on the left, and your bread and butter is on the plate just below."

Office Etiquette

When relating to a visually-impaired patient in a medical office, keep in mind the variable degrees of vision loss among blind people. Some have adjusted to the visual handicap well, others not as well, so find out the best way to be helpful.

If the patient is to be invited into an examining room or an office, give clear instructions and, if necessary, offer an arm for guidance. When you are showing a patient into the examining room and find you have to leave for a moment, do not leave the patient lost in space. Show him or her to a chair or put him or her in touch with a wall or piece of furniture and say that you are leaving, thus avoiding leaving the patient talking to an empty room and becoming embarrassed when he or she discovers that he or she is alone.[4]

Explain procedures you are about to perform on the blind patient and indicate when you are about to start. Remember these patients cannot see the instruments and may jump when touched if they have not been forewarned.[4]

ACTIVITY LEVELS

Patient activity levels on admission depend upon the pathological state of the eye. Since most patients walk into the hospital, it often surprises them when they are suddenly placed in bed at rest after being seen by the physician. The activity levels are ordered by the physician, and the meaning of these activity levels should be clearly defined so that the nursing staff know just what limitations the patient may be subjected to. If abbreviations are used to designate these activity levels, these terms should be consistent and should be on an approved hospital list, which is available in each area. The following are some types of activity orders:

1. *Complete bedrest* indicates that the patient should be confined to bed, and may lie on either the back or uninjured or nonsurgical side. The patient is bathed in bed and should be given a bedpan or urinal when needed. The patient may have to be helped with meals. Unless otherwise stated, the patient may have the head of the bed up or down.
2. *Bedrest with bathroom privileges (BR c̄ BRP)* means that the patient is confined to his or her bed but may get up to use the bathroom. Unless otherwise stated, this patient has no restrictions as to whether the head of the bed may be up or down and also has no restrictions regarding which side may be slept on. This patient may also feed him- or herself.
3. *Head of bed up 30 to 40 degrees (HOB ↑ # °)* usually indicates that there has been some intraocular bleeding. The patient is placed in this position with the hope that gravity will help the blood particles settle into the inferior portion of the eye.
4. *Out of bed ad lib (OOB ad lib)* means that the patient may be up and about as much as he or she wants to be. The health care professional should interpret this order in light of the patient's current status. The statement encourages the elderly patient to try to assume the tasks of active daily living as soon as possible. However, it does not differentiate the amount of activity that the young healthy individual might expend when suddenly given the liberty to be up as much as desired. A happy medium must be left to the judgment of the person rendering the care.
5. *Out of bed with assistance (OOB c̄ help)*. This statement should apply to every patient who has undergone surgery. No patient should be permitted to get out of bed after surgery unless helped out for the first time. This way the health care professional can assess the state of the patient as he or she recovers from anesthesia. Many patients require constant assistance because of age or infirmity so this care should be individualized. Patients should be encouraged to ring the call bell and ask for this assistance at the time of the initial assessment. Remember, too, that the short-term memory in elderly patients is often poor, so these patients often need to be reminded again and again of this simple request for cooperation.

The hospitalized eye patient's care is considered to be ambulatory care, for by and large the hospital stay is very short and except for very special circumstances when positioning becomes important, the patient is not confined to bed for a long period of time. Today, more and more surgery is performed as a "same day surgical" or outpatient procedure.

METHODS OF DECREASING STRESS

One needs to keep in mind that people with poor vision tend to rely on information received through stimulation of the auditory and tactile senses to a much greater degree than persons with normal vision.

Fear of total loss of vision is often the most important consideration and concern that patients have as they enter a hospital setting, knowing they are about to have surgery on an eye. Anxiety about the surgical procedure may be verbalized or it may be internalized. In the latter case, anxiety may be manifested as a systemic symptom or symptoms. Examples of symptoms of internalized anxiety are the hypertensive individual who has an increased admission blood pressure or a diabetic who has an increased blood sugar level due to the stress of hospitalization. Allaying fear by patient teaching and by encouraging verbalization of the concern can be one of the most rewarding aspects of the nursing care of the eye patient.

Patients with poor visual acuity or a patched eye should have a thorough orientation to the surroundings. Descriptive language should be used. This should include such information as "the chair is six steps in front of you; the telephone is on the bedside cabinet on your left, and the call bell has been attached to the left-hand bed rail. When you get out on the left side of the bed and walk toward the foot of the bed, the bathroom door is three paces ahead of you." The opportunity to touch objects around the hospital room will help newly-admitted eye patients to feel much more comfortable with their surroundings.

Today, the public is generally much better informed about health care and medical problems than in the past. They receive their information from newspapers, magazine articles, and radio and television programs, so it is incumbent upon the health care professional to be able to answer questions that are uppermost in the patient's mind at the time he or she first becomes aware of an eye problem. The patient who requires eye surgery is especially in need of detailed information about the procedure from the nurse and physician. With an understanding of what is to happen prior to surgery, during surgery, and after surgery, patients will have a much smoother passage through their hospitalization.

Preoperative Care and Patient Instructions

1. *Patients should be told if they are to have eye medications prior to surgery.* Systemic medications might be given, and the effects of these medications should also be relayed to the patient. In our hospital setting, inpatients are premedicated successfully with one 10 mg Valium (diazepam) tablet or a 25 mg Visteral (hydroxyzine hydrochloride) tablet taken by mouth, and washed down with one ounce of water. This calms the patient but does not usually cause drowsiness. Further medication is given intravenously in the preoperative room. It is important to *emphasize that nothing by mouth in the form of food or drink should be taken for 6 hours prior to any type of*

anesthesia, no matter whether it is local or general anesthesia. It might be worthwhile to state that this is a precaution taken to prevent aspiration of the stomach contents into the lungs, while the person is undergoing the surgical procedure.

2. *Check that the patient's dentures are removed,* a precaution to ensure *general anesthesia* safety. This may cause the patient's concern, for many times the patient has family members who have never seen him or her without their dentures. A little understanding with respect to this concern will enable the nurse premedicating the patient to ensure that the teeth will be replaced as soon as he or she has recovered from anesthesia.

3. *Each patient should be encouraged to completely empty the bladder* prior to

TABLE 3-1. PATIENT INFORMATION PAMPHLETS

American Academy of Ophthalmology
655 Beach Street
P.O. Box 7424
San Francisco, Calif. 94120-7424

Amblyopia; Cataract; Contact Lenses; Detached and Torn Retina; Diabetic Retinopathy; Dry Eye; Eye Drops; Eye Injuries; Floaters and Flashes; Facts and Myths; Glaucoma; Headache; Laser Surgery of the Eye; Learning Disabilities; Low Vision; Macular Degeneration; Refractive Errors; Seeing Well As You Grow Older; Strabismus; Total Eye Care; Uveitis.

Krames Communications
312 90th Street
Daly City, Calif. 94015-2621
(Patient Information Library Series)

The Cataract Book*; Comunikit; Contact Lenses; Eye Safety; I Care*; Intraocular Lenses (IOL'S); The Retina Book; Strabismus and Amblyopia; Understanding Glaucoma, A Guide To Saving Your Sight.

Channing L. Bete Co., Inc.
South Deerfield, Mass. 01373
(A Scriptographic Booklet)

About Cataracts.

National Society to Prevent Blindness
79 Madison Avenue
New York, N.Y. 10016

Adult Eyes: *Cataract; Diabetic Retinopathy; Glaucoma—Sneak Thief of Sight; Glaucoma Patient Guide; Macular Degeneration; The Aging Eye: Facts on Eye Care for Older Persons; Home Eye Tests for Adults.*

Eye Safety: *Eyes in Industry; Eye Safety and Health: An Off-the-Job Program; Eye Safety is No Accident; What's Your Game; 21 Questions on Eye Safety; The Wise Owl Club of America; A Guide for Controlling Eye Injuries in Industry.*

Wills Eye Hospital
9th and Walnut Streets
Philadelphia, Penn. 19107

Age Related Macular Disease; Cataracts; Contact Lenses; Contact Lenses for Pediatric Patients; Community Resources for Visually Impaired; Corneal Diseases and Transplant; Day Surgery; Enucleation; Glaucoma; Low Vision Service; Pediatric Ophthalmology; Oculoplastic Surgery; Signs of Eye Problems; Radioactive Plaque Therapy of Eye Tumors; Radial Keratotomy; Retinal Detachment and Vitreous Surgery; Uveitis.

*Also in Spanish

premedication. Osmotic agents given prior to surgery often fill the bladder in the recovery period and make the patient need to empty it again. Catheterization is not recommended, for it exposes the patient to unnecessary potential of infection.

4. *Hard and soft contact lenses should be removed* from the eyes. Extended wear lenses should be removed by the ophthalmologist before surgery and replaced after the procedure.

There are a variety of patient information pamphlets (Table 3–1) that can be of assistance in the hospital setting, in a doctor's office, or a clinic. It is important to ensure that patients are familiar with such things as how to instill their own eyedrops properly (see discussion on self-medication on p. 28), so that the anxiety of how they will cope with this aspect of their care can be decreased after discharge. Specific postoperative measures will be discussed where they are appropriate in the following chapters. The eye patient's stay in the hospital is generally so short that it is a good idea to try to start any necessary teaching before the surgical procedure occurs. With this in mind, the best place is in the doctor's office, so that patient compliance with postoperative instruction will meet expectations.

In spite of the availability of the information aids, there is nothing that can replace the person-to-person contact between the patient and the health care worker. The ability to impart information and allay patient anxiety comes with practice and knowledge.

REFERENCES

1. Boyd-Monk H: Eye, ear and nose care, in Procedures. Springhouse, Penn.: Intermed Communications, 1983, pp. 708–714
2. Jeglum EL: Ocular therapeutics, in Boyd-Monk H., (Ed.), Nursing Clinics of North America. Philadelphia: Saunders, 1981, pp. 453–477
3. Luchmann J, Sorensen K: Medical–Surgical Nursing: A Psycho-physiologic Approach. Philadelphia: Saunders, 1980, pp. 1948–2040
4. Nevil Institute for Rehabilitation and Service: Relating to a Visually Impaired Patient in a Medical Office. Philadelphia: Nevil Institute for Rehabilitation and Service, 1983, pp. 1–2

BIBLIOGRAPHY

Smith JF, Nachazel DP: Ophthalmologic Nursing. Boston: Little, Brown, 1980
Smith S: Standards of Ophthalmic Nursing. San Francisco: American Academy of Ophthalmology, 1985

4

History Taking

NEW TERMS

Aphakic: without a lens.
Anisocoria: unequal pupils.
Anophthalmic: without an eye.
Limbus: corneo-scleral junction.
Photophobia: light sensitivity.

When a patient with an ophthalmic complaint presents at the doctor's office, clinic, emergency room, or for inpatient admission to a hospital, it is appropriate for the health care professional to request pertinent information in order to facilitate the future care to be given. Nonverbal clues will be observed long before there is a verbal encounter. These can be noted as the patient walks into the ophthalmology department seeking attention. The majority of people seeking attention for their eyes do so because there has been a change in their vision.

The eyes and visual system are limited in the manner in which they can react to disease. The retina and optic pathways can react only with defective visual sensations such as blurred image, defective color perception, monocular or binocular blindness, or visual field defects. Other sensory phenomena may be due to hyperactivity (e.g., the scintillating scotoma or migrane), or misinterpretation of image size. The ocular motor system becomes symptomatic when the images from the two eyes are not superimposed and diplopia results. This can occur where there is inadequate stabilization of fixation (oscillopsia—apparent movement of objects in the environment), with or without actual nystagmus; and when there is inability to turn both eyes in some direction, the defect is interpreted by the patient as a defect in "seeing" in that field of gaze, or the patient becomes aware that the head, rather than the eyes, must be turned to see.

Other than "seeing" and "moving," the eye can only "feel," i.e., perceive discomfort and pain or, conversely, be unable to perceive (hypersthesia, anesthesia).[1] These changes because of their unknown implications cause patients varying degrees of anxiety. Anxiety is expressed in various ways, which include being passive and sitting and waiting patiently with hands clenched to being aggressive, abrupt, and rude. Decrease in vision associated with acute pain can often be associated with the latter state.

Body language gives many clues as to where discomfort may be. A patient experiencing great pain may be observed holding a hand over the eye to shield it. If

43

the pain radiates to the head, the person may hold the head. Dark glasses will be worn by the light-sensitive or photophobic person as well as someone who has an unsightly, discolored eye and wants to cover it up.

A person with *itching and burning* eyes will "rub" them, while the person who has an *ocular discharge* will often "mop" the eyes profusely. Someone who has recently sustained an acute accident may be led into the emergency clinic area. A child who has a *painful eye* will be seen to rub it, shut it tightly, and if the child is nonverbal, he or she may just make a constant grizzling sound.

These patients must first be assessed or triaged to determine if their condition is truly an emergency. Remember every patient who seeks help for an ocular condition believes that at this time their condition needs attention and is more important than any other person who might also be waiting. *Every patient who seeks attention for their eyes should have their visual acuity taken and documented for medical and legal purposes.*

GENERAL CONSIDERATIONS FOR HISTORY TAKING

The *age* of the person is important, for some symptoms occur in people at one age group and not in another. For example, myopia (nearsightedness) tends to increase up to the third decade and then levels off. Presbyopia (an inability to focus at near which is caused by lens changes) begins to affect people about the age of 40.

Occupation should also be questioned, for the eye problem may be related to an occupational hazard. For example, the person who has a refractive error and wears glasses for close work may complain of "eyestrain" much sooner than the laborer with the same refractive error, who does not need to use his or her eyes for such detail.

Someone who does not wear safety glasses while working with metal may declare that he or she has something in his or her eye. This statement should caution the examiner to discover if there is a history of "steel on steel," for a sliver of steel may have flown into the eye, and the "something" would then be an *intraocular foreign body* (IOFB). Another person might make the same statement, but state that he was walking down the street when the incident occurred, and examination may reveal a *corneal foreign body* to be the cause of acute discomfort. True emergency patients are those who sustain *chemical burns,* for the eyes must immediately be lavaged, and patients who complain of experiencing sudden loss of vision in one or both eyes, for whatever reason. In an industrial accident a careful note should be made of the time and date that the injury occurred, and what was done before coming for emergency treatment.

Ocular History

Taking an ocular history requires some open-ended questions which can be asked as the external assessment of the eye is taking place.

"What specifically is bothering you?" and *"How long ago did it occur?"* should identify the *chief complaint* and its *duration.*

In the case of injury or accident inquire *when and how the injury occurred, and what was done prior to seeking attention or treatment.* The patient should then be questioned about any previous eye problems or surgery.

To assess the general health status of the patient include such specific questions as, *"Do you have hypertension, cardiac disease, diabetes, arthritis?" Do you have any allergies? Are you taking any medications?* Blurred vision can be associated with severe high blood pressure and high blood sugar. Medications can also have ocular side effects. Allergies can cause itching and medications can be the cause of the allergy. Inquiry should be made about a family history of glaucoma.

Assessing the External Eye. Observe the open and closed eyelids. *The open eyelid should fall half way between the limbus and the pupil.* The margins should be clear of crusting, scaling, discharge, lumps, bumps, growths, swelling, or drooping. Note any complaints of itching, pain, discomfort, or tearing. *The eyebrows and eyelashes should be the same color.* Note if any patches are missing. If tearing is a symptom, *gently palpate over the nasolacrimal sac area,* and ascertain if it is tender or if any exudate extrudes through the puncta.

"*Have you noticed any discharge from your eyes?*" and "*Were your lids stuck together this morning?*" may elicit a clue to an infection of the lids or the nasolacrimal system, or conjunctiva.

The *bulbar conjunctiva should be clear* so that the white or eggshell hue of the sclera can be seen through it. In the young person relatively few blood vessels are seen, but as a person becomes a little older it is normal for a few conjunctival blood vessels to become evident. Examination of *the palpebral conjunctiva should reveal a glistening pink surface,* much the same as can be seen when one looks at the mucous membrane of the mouth. Pale conjunctiva may be caused by anemia. Hyperemic conjunctiva may occur as a result of infection, and icteric conjunctiva can be seen in jaundice. Circumcorneal injection is associated with anterior uveitis (inflammation of the iris and ciliary body) and glaucoma, while peripheral injection of the conjunctiva is usually present in conjunctivitis. If a virus is suspected to be the cause, check the preauricular area to see if a node is present. A foreign body sensation is sometimes the chief complaint as is itching, which may be a symptom of allergy.

The cornea should be clear, and all the structures of the iris and pupil should be seen through it. Damage to the cornea will produce pain and photophobia, and if the damage has occurred in the pupillary region, there will be a decrease in vision. Corneal edema can cause a patient to see rings around lights, a symptom usually associated with glaucoma.

The *anterior chamber should be deep and formed* and can be examined at the same time that the pupils are checked. Hyphemia (blood in the anterior chamber) or hypopion (pus or cells in the anterior chamber) will cause a decrease in vision if it fills the whole anterior chamber.

The pupils should be equal, round, and react to light and accommodation (PERRLA). A history of trauma might reveal unequal pupils; however, 20 to 25 percent of the population normally has unequal pupils (anisocoria). In acute glaucoma the pupil will be mid-dilated but it will be constricted if anterior uveitis is present. Both of these entities will have the associated symptom of pain. If miotic pupils are observed, question the patient about the use of miotic drugs used for glaucoma and/or other drug use. Patients with dilated pupils should be questioned about cycloplegic drugs having been placed in the eye.

Once the examiner has observed the external eye and asked the appropriate questions, the next step is to *assess the visual acuity. "Have you noticed a change in your vision?"* followed by *"When did you first notice this change?"* are appropriate questions. If the visual loss is the chief complaint, ask *"Is this the first time it has happened?"* and *"Has this ever happened before?"* Inquire how the change in vision was discovered. All these questions will give clues to the current visual status. The disturbances in vision may include a chief complaint of *spots* before the eyes. Question whether these spots float, are stationary, or are in showers. Two other causes for blurred vision may be astigmatism or a macular lesion.

Vision is checked with and without correction, which may be achieved with either glasses or contact lenses. However, a presbyope who wears glasses for reading will not be able to see the chart which is set at a distance of 20 feet, using these glasses, so inquire of the patient whether the glasses are worn for distance. If the response is affirmative, request that they be worn, so that the best corrected visual acuity can be obtained.

The *extraocular muscles* (EOM) are assessed by asking the patient to look in each cardinal direction of gaze. This is important when there is a history of diplopia, for the double vision may only be present in one direction of gaze. Swelling and displacement of the globe can also produce diplopia.

Visual acuity might be excellent, but the patient may feel loss of vision and actually have a peripheral field defect. The confrontation or finger mimicking method can be used to *check each quadrant of the visual field.*

To complete the examination the fundus of the eye should be observed using an ophthalmoscope (see Chap. 17). In an ophthalmologist's office this will be accomplished by the physician after slitlamp examination of the anterior structures, and after the pupils have been well dilated.

Nursing Assessment
A nursing assessment should be performed on any patient who comes into the hospital and who is going to stay over night. Most eye patients are scheduled admissions, unless the situation is an emergency. Most institutions have specific forms designed to facilitate appropriate documentation. The following pointers are offered to help the nurse with history taking (Fig. 4–1).

The historian should be the patient: if there is a talkative relative present the nurse can end up assessing the relative and not the patient. The historian is the person who gives the most information, and if it is at all possible one really wants the historian to be the patient. However, *if the patient is a child then the historian will be the parent,* and this should be noted in the medical record.

The *admitting diagnosis* may differ from the *surgical procedure* which the patient is to undergo. For example, the patient's medical diagnosis is aphakic bullous keratopathy, left eye, but the surgical procedure for which the patient is being admitted may be a penetrating keratoplasty. By the same token the patient may already have had cataract surgery and therefore is aphakic, but is now being admitted for a secondary implant of an intraocular lens in the aphakic eye.

Tentative date of surgery: because of the new government regulations most eye surgery is done the same day as the admission, unless the patient is first to receive medical treatment for the eye complaint.

Patient states reason for admission: this statement gives the nurse a clue that the patient knows the reason he or she is being admitted. But if the patient says

"I've come here because of my eyes," the nurse must interpret this as a lack of understanding of the disease entity, and should recognize that patient teaching is required. By and large ophthalmic surgery is elective surgery, meaning that the patient has had an explanation from the physician and has chosen to have surgery in an attempt to correct the eye problem. Although most patients have some idea as to why they are coming to the hospital or surgicenter, many patients are anxious at the time they receive this information. Patient teaching will help to allay this anxiety.

Discharge planning starts the moment that the patient enters the hospital, if not before. It is necessary to identify how the patient is going home and who will care for him or her. The nurse should keep in mind the fact that many times patients have functioned with poor vision for a considerable time prior to the hospital treatment. They may not have an immediate improvement in their vision and when they go home they may be functioning with exactly the same vision that they had prior to admission, therefore, their lifestyle is not going to change in the immediate postoperative period.

There are relatively few restrictions that are imposed on the patient initially, but the nurse should ensure that if eyedrops are prescribed by the physician, the patient is able to instill these eye drops properly and also be able to cleanse the postoperative eye appropriately. A demonstration and a return demonstration enforces this patient teaching. Many times patients are very nervous about doing something a little bit out of their normal routine. Once the patient has been assessed, the nurse might find that this patient is truly a candidate for a visit from a public health nurse, and the social service department may need to be involved.

Listen to the patient's accent, since America is made up of people of so many different nationalities it is not inappropriate to *identify the "native" language.* Sometimes when a patient is coming out of anesthesia he or she may relapse into that native language.

Assess the mental status as questions are being asked throughout the interview, so that by the end of the assessment there is documentation that the patient is oriented to person, time, and place, or disoriented and/or confused. *The patient's level of comprehension can be assessed* at the same time. Does he or she understand the implication of being in a hospital or being in a strange place, or does he or she have no idea of what is going on. Occasionally one meets a patient who really does not know where they are or why they are there. A relative or an institution has made the decision for this patient to be hospitalized. At the other end of the spectrum there are those wonderfully bright, elderly people who will just amaze one with the information that they have.

Identifying the patient's occupation is important. In the younger person still actively involved with a job and working to maintain a lifestyle, a decrease in vision can present a devastating threat to their livelihood. Watch out for depression. On the other hand, the retired person who hopes to read a little bit more, has something to look forward to once cataract removal restores vision.

Who does the patient live with? This really is not such a personal question, for the spouse or friend can be used as a resource person and can give the patient some support with following instructions and assisting with care after hospital discharge.

Identify the smoker: how much and how long has he or she participated in this habit. Smoking should be prohibited in bed. If this rule is to be effective, a place should be provided where the smoker can smoke.

WILLS EYE HOSPITAL
HEALTH ASSESSMENT

DSU _____

AM ADM _____

PROCEDURE _____ ANESTHESIA   G   L

SURGEON _____ HOME PHONE _____

INFORMANT _____ OFFICE PHONE _____

INTERVIEW DATE _____ AGE _____ SEX ____ ALLERGIES _____

CHIEF COMPLAINT _____

PAST MEDICAL HISTORY

CV	RESPIRATORY	NEURO/PSYCH	MISCELLANEOUS
CAD	COPD	SEIZURES	DIABETES
CHF	ASTHMA	CVA	CANCER
ANGINA	TB	DEPRESSION/	BPH
BLEEDING	ECZEMA	ANXIOUS	RENAL
DISORDER		HARD OF HEARING	FAILURE
PACEMAKER			HEPATITIS
HYPERTENSION			ULCERS
MI			HSV/HZV

PREMATURE BIRTH ____ AGE OF GESTATION ____ WT ____ RECENT URI _____

PAST SURGICAL HISTORY	CURRENT MEDICATIONS	SOCIAL HISTORY
_____	_____	_____
_____	_____	_____
_____	_____	_____
_____	_____	_____
_____	_____	_____

Smokes   Y   N   Abnormal Lab Results _____

Alcohol   Y   N   Reported To _____

Diet _____

Signature _____R.N.

Admission Date _____ Vital Signs   T   P   R   BP   HT   WT

Mental Status _____ Level of Comprehension _____

Dentures: Full   Partial   None   /   Glasses   Contacts   Prosthesis

Last Oral Intake: Food   What _____   Valuables

When _____   _____

Fluid   What _____   _____

When _____   _____

Transfer to Room   _____   _____

Discharge Home   _____   _____

Signature _____R.N.

Figure 4–1. Nursing Assessment Form. Front. *(From Wills Eye Hospital, Nursing Department, Philadelphia, with permission.)*

DATE	PATIENT NEEDS/PROBLEMS	NURSING INTERVENTION	IMPLEMENTATION/ EVALUATION/ OUTCOME
	GENERAL CARE PLAN 1) Potential for anxiety due to hospitalization, unfamiliar surroundings and pending eye surgery. 2) Potential for harm to self due to decreased vision. 3) Discharge Plan	Explain tests and procedures. Encourage verbalization and questions. Demonstrate interest, empathy and understanding. Orient patient to room and hospital routines. Minimally keep one-half (top) siderail up at all times. Two (top) siderails up at H.S.; full siderails post-op. Call bell within reach. Keep environment free from obstacles. Assist with ADL prn. Assess patient's home situation and arrange assistance as needed. Stress good handwashing technique and compliance with return follow-up visits.	

POST-OP PROGRESS NOTES

_____

_____

_____

_____

Signature _____

Figure 4–1. Nursing Assessment Form. Back.

Identify the amount of alcohol consumed and the length of time the patient has imbibed. Alcoholics are not going to be cured during the time they are in the hospital for an ophthalmologic complaint, but the medical and nursing staff certainly wants to keep them from going into delirium tremors, which might lead to harm.

The patient's functional vision may be decreased when one eye is patched and the glasses do not fit properly because of the eye patch. The nurse will need to assess the vision in the nonsurgical eye so that the patient may be given appropriate assistance during the time that the glasses cannot be worn. Another example is the aphakic patient who wears an extended wear contact lens on the nonsurgical aphakic eye, and who is now coming in for a surgical procedure on the other eye. This lens needs to be identified prior to surgery; documentation should alert the operating room nurse to its presence, so that the physician may remove it before the surgery and replace it afterwards. If the patient does wear glasses, check if they are with the patient. Many people will confirm the wearing of glasses, but confide they do not improve vision, and when the visual acuity is assessed the glasses do not make much difference, because a new prescription is what is really needed.

If the patient is *anophthalmic and wears a prosthesis,* it should be identified. If the reason for admission is for reconstructive surgery, make sure that the prosthesis is with the patient when he or she goes to surgery.

Past ocular history: if a patient is going to have surgery, there must be some past ocular history unless it is an ocular emergency. Even the cataract patient has been losing vision for a period of time. If the patient has glaucoma maybe he or she does not really know how long the glaucoma has been evident, however, most glaucoma patients have been treated medically for quite an extended period of time prior to coming to have a surgical procedure. And if a patient has undergone laser or surgical treatments, document where and when it was done.

Current eye medications should be identified, and patients are asked to bring these eyedrops and any oral medications with them when they are admitted. Some of the intraoperative medications will be calculated on the patient's weight, so that this should also be recorded.

A medical history should reveal the name of the family physician who has prescribed the medications. So many patients describe their prescriptions as a white pill and a yellow pill and they cannot remember the names of them. Question the patient about any history of *high blood pressure (hypertension), seizure disorders,* or *diabetes.*

Many ophthalmology patients have diabetes. It is important to find out how long they have had the disease and to ask if there is a recent blood sugar result available. Identify what medication is being taken and whether the patient is insulin dependent or noninsulin dependent. The hypertensive patient may also be aware of how their blood pressure runs and of the medication they take for it. People will take a lot more care of their blood pressure if they know what it is. Question the patient about seizure disorders. Most people know whether they have any seizures or blackouts, and what medication they take for it. Inquire if there is a history of *cardiac problems.* Has there been an episode of chest pain in the last 2 to 6 weeks? Ask the patient if he or she has had an electrocardiogram (ECG) prior to being admitted. Sometimes patients will deny a medical problem and then produce a pill that is for a particular disorder. It is really a pretty logical thing to do, for the pill is supposed to cure the disease. When the nurse gets the list of medications, it is appropriate to go back and correlate their use with disease entities.

Patients who have *pulmonary disorders* often present with obvious symptoms such as coughing, wheezing, and shortness of breath. Note such signs as pursed-lip breathing, blue-rimmed lips, and clubbing of the fingertips. Find out when the last chest x-ray was performed, for there certainly will be a need for a recent one if the patient is to undergo anesthesia.

Assess the *gastrointestinal tract. Check diet preferences and identify elimination patterns.* The hospitalization is usually so short that there need not be any disruption in G.I. routines. However, it is important at this point to *check if the patient wears upper, lower, or partial dentures.* Dentures will be removed if the surgery is to be performed under general anesthesia, but may remain in the mouth if local anesthesia is to be administered. Children may have loose teeth.

Question the elderly male patient about any *genitourinary* problems which might be experienced. Many ophthalmology patients receive an osmotic agent to reduce the intraocular pressure and occasionally this precipitates a distended bladder in someone who has a hypertrophic prostate gland.

Depression is assessed throughout the interview. The nurse should closely observe the manner in which the patient answers questions and should look for signs of emotional distress. Ask if there have been any changes in sleeping habits i.e., insomnia, or if there has been a recent loss of appetite, for each of these entities can be associated with depression.

Previous surgical procedures should be identified, for if they recently occurred, they could affect the type of anesthesia to be used for the ophthalmic surgical procedure. They also need to be taken into account when placing the patient on the operating room table.

Assess the skin, identify any bruises, ulcers, rashes, and any recent injury which might have been incurred in a fall. Note any associated disabilities.

Ascertain if the patient has a hearing problem. Identify the better ear and if a hearing aid is used. Often patients who wear a hearing aid will be requested to leave it in when they go to the operating room so that they can hear the instructions given to them by the physician.

Finally, *assess the patient's functional vision.* Can the patient see well enough with the eye which is not to have surgery to be able to function with elements of active daily living. Does the patient wear a contact lens? What kind is it? Was it taken out prior to hospitalization, or is it in the eye now? Does the patient wear glasses?

The history-taking process enables the nurse to get to know the patient, set his or her mind at rest, and should be the beginning of a rapport of mutual trust for future interactions.

REFERENCES

1. Glaser JS: History taking, in Duane TD, (Ed.), Clinical Ophthalmology. Hagerstown, Md.: Harper & Row, 1984

BIBLIOGRAPHY

Luckman J, Sorensen KC: Medical–Surgical Nursing: A Psychophysiologic Approach, 2nd
    ed. Philadelphia: Saunders, 1980

5

Methods of Visual Screening

In order to establish what can be seen by a person, various methods of testing visual function have been developed. The visual acuity test should be part of a routine examination because it is designed as a method of measuring just how much a person sees using the most acutely seeing portion of the eye, namely the foveal region. Peripheral and central visual field tests are done when pathology of the retina, optic nerve, and optic pathways is suspected. Peripheral field examination is useful in detecting disorders that cause constriction of peripheral vision such as retinal detachment, retinitis pigmentosa, and chiasmal lesions. Central field examination is useful in detecting disorders causing loss of a portion of the central visual field, particularly in glaucoma, optic neuritis, macular disease, or malingering. Both peripheral and central field examinations are indicated when intracranial disease is suspected.[1] Tests to determine a person's ability to perceive primary colors and shades may be part of the physical examination required by the military or for persons whose occupations require good color perception.

A pertinent history is always elicited from the patient before proceeding with an examination of the eye and testing the visual acuity. The patient's complaints, their duration, and any other ocular information are reviewed, for example diseases, injuries, or operations. It is also important to inquire about the general health status, at which time it is appropriate to ask about medications that the patient might be taking and check for any known allergies. See Chapter 4 for a detailed discussion of History Taking.

VISUAL ACUITY

Visual acuity testing is done to determine if the fovea, which is the portion of the eye used for fine object discrimination and color discrimination, is functioning. The eyes are usually tested for distance vision. Testing for near vision is only performed if the patient is having difficulty reading or distinguishing between objects, or is over the age of 40 (the time at which presbyopia, due to crystalline lens changes, becomes apparent). *A patient's visual acuity should always be recorded on the medical record prior to instillation of any medications into his or her eyes.* This is medically and legally important.

Charts for testing visual acuity are commercially available. The Snellen Eye Chart (Fig. 5–1) is the most commonly used chart to test distance vision, and the

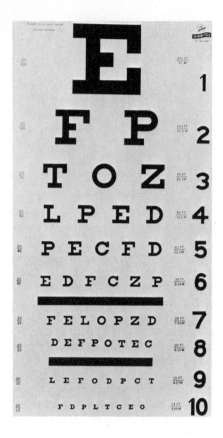

Figure 5-1 Snellen Eye Chart.

Lebensohn Chart (Fig. 5–2) is used to test near vision. The Snellen Eye Chart is available in four types: 1) printed with numbers; 2) printed with letters; 3) printed with pictures; and 4) printed with E's in various positions. The latter type of chart is useful for testing children and illiterates. To facilitate this, the E's are positioned in different directions. The patient being tested is then asked to position their fingers in the same direction as the E's in a particular line of the chart, i.e., right, left, up, or down.

The well-illuminated chart is set up to measure a visual acuity at a distance of 20 feet or 6 meters. The retinal image depends upon the size of the object and its distance from the eye, so it is also possible for the chart to be scaled down for use in a confined space.[2] For example, if a projector is used, the patient may be sitting at a distance of 10 feet from the mirror but the distance is doubled (to 20 feet) by the chart being reflected off a second mirror.

This test will give the examiner a baseline for the patient's central visual acuity. The 20 feet (or 6 meters) will be written as the numerator. The lines of the chart are numbered and are always expressed over the distance of 20 feet (or 6 meters). This is not a fraction (Table 5–1). The patient being tested is asked to read the line that can be seen most clearly. This line will be written as the denominator.[3] Normal visual acuity is considered to have been achieved when a person is able to

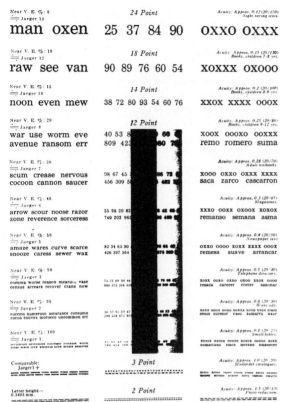

Figure 5–2. Near vision test chart.

read the line marked 20 while standing or sitting at a distance of 20 feet from the chart. Should the patient being tested achieve a visual acuity of 20/30 this means that this person can see at 20 (feet) what someone with normal vision can see at 30 feet. The denominator, therefore varies. It also increases as the vision gets poorer.

If letters (or numbers) are missed or misread when the line is being read, the

TABLE 5–1. RECORDING VISUAL ACUITY

Metric System	Snellen System
6/5	20/15
6/6	20/20
6/9	20/30
6/12	20/40
6/15	20/50
6/21	20/70
6/30	20/100
6/60	20/200
3/60	20/400

reader is debited with the number missed, e.g., 20/30−2. By the same token, if the person reads the line accurately but is only able to read one or two letters in the next line down, then a credit will be given, e.g., 20/30+2.

To take the patient's visual acuity, the following steps should be taken:

1. The chart should be well-illuminated with no shadows.
2. The patient should be seated or standing at a distance of 20 feet (or 6 meters) from the chart and given an occluder (Fig. 5–3).
3. The examiner faces the patient in order to observe any squinting, head tilting, or misplacement of the occluder.
4. Test one eye at a time; cover the other with an occluder. By convention the *right eye (OD)* is tested first and the *left eye (OS)* is occluded.
5. Take the vision without glasses; mark this as s̄c (*without correction*).
6. Remember that corrective lenses include both contact lenses and glasses, and if the patient's vision is being checked with these lenses, then the visual acuity should be recorded as c̄c (*with correction*). Before checking the vision, it is useful to ask the patient wearing glasses if they were prescribed for reading things at a distance or only close up.
7. If vision is found to be less than 20/30, recheck the vision but use a *pinhole*. Record any improvement in the visual acuity as c̄ PH and state whether the patient was tested (with) c̄ or (without) s̄ correction. (An improvement in the visual acuity of either the right or the left eye with a pinhole reading indicates the need for a refraction.) *No improvement* in the line of vision is recorded as N.I.c̄ PH.
8. If the patient cannot see the 20/400 line (usually the large E), then walk him or her toward the chart until the top figures *are* seen. Now estimate the distance you have between the chart and where the patient is standing, and record the first line which is seen as __#__ feet/meters from the chart; e.g., 3/200. This means that at 3 feet this patient can see what a person with normal visual acuity would be able to see at 200 feet.
9. Return the patient who cannot see either the 200 or 400 letter to the chair

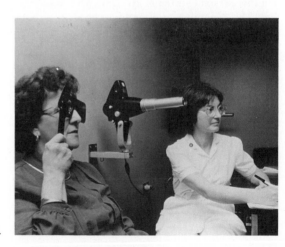

Figure 5–3. Use of an occluder.

(or original position of testing) and record the distance at which this person can count the number of fingers you are holding up. This will be recorded as C.F. (*Count Fingers*). Record the distance you are holding your hand from the patient's eye, 1 foot, 1 meter, etc.

10. If the patient is unable to count fingers, determine the ability to discern hand movements. Record this as H/M (*Hand Movements*) at 1 foot, 1 meter, etc.

11. A patient might only have the ability to perceive light. A penlight should be shone in the eye and then switched off. The patient is asked to tell whether the light is on or off. Record this as L.P. (*Light Perception*). However, the patient might be able to tell where the light is being directed from as it is projected into the eye from different quadrants. This will be recorded as L.P.c̄ P. (*Light Perception with Projection*).

12. If no light is perceived, record this as N.L.P. (*No Light Perception*). This is the term that should be used for an eye with no recordable vision.[3] However, *legal blindness* is officially considered to be evident when a person sees 20/200 or less with correction in the better eye, or a visual field of no more than 20 degrees in the better eye.[1]

By assessing the visual acuity, the health care professional ascertains how much help the patient in a hospital setting will need. This assessment will be referred to as the *functional vision*.

Near Vision Testing

When in a state of rest, the eye is adapted for parallel rays coming from a distant object. In order for divergent rays from a near object to be focused on the retina, there must be an increase in the refractive power of the eye. This change is known as *accommodation*.

Accommodation is an increase in refractive power of the lens as a result of the contraction of the ciliary muscle. This makes the lens more spherical, increases the curvature of the anterior surface, and causes increased refractive power. Accommodation is primarily designed to provide clear vision at a near distance. Accommodation is invariably associated with both convergence of the eyes and pupillary constriction. The association of these three activities is known as the *near reflex*.

Testing for near vision is done for refractive error and presbyopia. Measurement usually does not become a part of the ocular examination unless a person is over the age of 40 or appears to have difficulty seeing objects at close. The nurse should remember that a person may have 20/30 or 20/40 distance vision and will not complain about it, but will complain about reading. This can indicate that there is a need for reading glasses or that there is a macular problem.

The Jaeger Type Chart (which is seen as part of the Lebensohn Near Vision Test charts; Fig. 5–2) has differerent sizes of print which are used for testing and recording near visual acuity. The chart is held at a distance of about 14 inches and the person being tested is asked to read the line that is seen most clearly. The type which can be tested is equal to printed material such as want ads, the telephone directory, newspaper text, magazine type, or music. Vision is recorded according to the corresponding type as J.2, J.3, J.5, J.6, etc. This test is used by the ophthalmologist as a guide to refracting the patient for near vision correction.

Assessing the Child's Vision

Newborn. The premature and term neonate should demonstrate primitive visual responses, such as turning toward subdued daylight through a window. However, if the infant makes a reflex eye movement toward lights or brightly colored objects (fixation reflex), it may be considered that vision is grossly intact.[4]

Six Weeks. The baby tracks lights; however, eye movements may be irregular.[5]

Three Months. By this age, accurate and steady fixation and smooth following movement are anticipated.[4]

Four to Six Months. The child exhibits binocular coordination, following slowly moving objects with ease. The child also demonstrates hand-eye coordination by grabbing at objects.[5]

One Year. The child is interested in tiny objects but should also be able to discriminate simple geometric forms.[6]

Three Years. Visual acuity may be tested with a picture or the illiterate "E" chart and should be at least 20/30.

Four to Five Years. Visual acuity may be tested with the illiterate "E" chart and should be 20/25 or 20/20. Many times, it might be appropriate for a mother to "play" the "E" game with the child prior to having the visual acuity checked, so that the child will respond correctly when being tested.

Visual Fields

Normal visual fields are shown in Figure 5–6 on page 62. Retina, optic nerve, and optic pathway function is tested by performing central and peripheral visual field tests. Central field examination is useful in detecting disorders associated with macular diseases, glaucoma, optic neuritis, malingering, or hysteria. Peripheral visual field examination is most useful in detecting disorders that cause constriction of peripheral vision in one or both eyes such as retinal detachment, retinitis pigmentosa, glaucoma, and intracranial lesions which affect the optic pathway.[1] The following entries describe the many methods used to examine a patient's visual fields.

Amsler Grid. The Amsler grid is designed as a series of horizontal and vertical lines which form 5 mm squares, in the center of which is a black dot (Fig. 5–4). It is used for testing the central 20 degrees of field at reading distance, when analysis of maculopathies is required. The manner in which the patient describes patterns to be altered (curvilinear metamorphopsia in a serous retinal separation, scotoma in optic nerve disease)[4] may provide clues to the patient's complaint of "not seeing too well."

1. Have the patient wear his or her corrective glasses, if appropriate.
2. Test each eye separately. Occlude one eye, (a patch or tissue tucked behind the glasses works well) and have the patient look at the Amsler grid at reading distance (about 13 or 14 inches ($\frac{1}{3}$ meter) away).

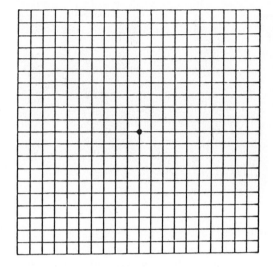

Figure 5–4. Amsler grid (*printed in black on white for convenience of recording*).

3. Ask the patient:
   a) if the black dot can be seen and;
   b) if when looking at the dot, all four slides of the grid can also be identified as straight lines.
4. If there is any blurred or distorted area described, the patient can be asked to reproduce what he or she actually sees using a pencil and paper.

This technique is especially helpful when elucidating all central and paracentral scotomas.[4] The ophthalmologist will use the information in conjunction with ophthalmoscopic evaluation.

Confrontation Methods. The confrontation method of testing visual fields depends upon the patient's subjective response to a visual stimulus.[4] With confrontation, the examiner compares the patient's field with his or her own while in a face-to-face position and without using a tangent screen or perimeter.

The examiner sits approximately 1 meter in front of the patient. One eye is tested at a time, while the other one is occluded. The standard against which the patient's field is compared is the examiner's, which is assumed to be normal. To test the patient's right eye, the left eye is occluded and he or she is asked to fix his or her gaze on the examiner's left eye. The examiner's right eye is occluded.

Finger Counting. The target used in this instance is either the examiner's fist or fingers, which are kept equidistant between patient and examiner. The most widely used clinical technique involves moving a target from outside the field toward the fixation point, and the patient is asked to indicate immediately when he or she notices the examiner's fingers coming into his or her line of vision.

Next, the examiner presents either fist or fingers in each quadrant of the patient's visual field (Fig. 5–5). If the patient successfully identifies the test object,

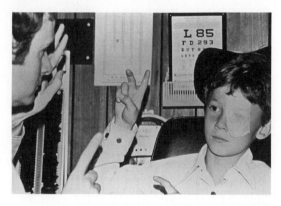

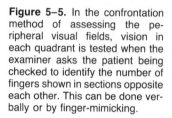

Figure 5–5. In the confrontation method of assessing the peripheral visual fields, vision in each quadrant is tested when the examiner asks the patient being checked to identify the number of fingers shown in sections opposite each other. This can be done verbally or by finger-mimicking.

the examiner can present fingers on both sides of fixation to test horizontal, vertical, and oblique meridians. This is repeated with "wiggling" fingers. The patient is also asked if there is any difference in the clarity of the fingers or if they appear the same. If a difference is noted, the questionable area will need to be pinpointed. A similar area should also be looked for in the other eye. The questionable area will need further testing with tangent screen or perimeter.

The examiner will need black-tipped straight pins, and test objects ranging from 1 to 10 mm (white on one side and black on the other) which can be interchanged on a hand-held black wand.

Tangent Screen Examination. The tangent screen is usually made of black felt, with concentric circles and lines radiating from a central fixation point (rather like a spider web). The screen is hung on the wall in such a way that when the patient is seated 1 meter (3¼ feet) away from it, he or she is at eye level with the central fixation point. (The circle in the center of the screen.)

The examiner will need black-tipped straight pins to test objects ranging from 1 to 10 mm (white on one side and black on the other) which can be interchanged on a hand-held black wand.

The patient's best corrected visual acuity is tested, so that if glasses are worn for distance, they are left on. One eye is tested at a time; a hand-held occluder (or a tissue tucked behind the glasses) covers the untested eye.

The examiner stands by the side of the screen, facing the patient, ensuring that the patient's gaze does not wander from the central point of fixation as the test object is brought in from the peripheral concentric circle, to where it can be identified. If the visual acuity is good (say 20/20) in the eye being tested, then the smallest test object of 1 mm should be used.

The patient is directed not to look for the test object, but merely to acknowledge it when it comes into his or her field of vision. The test object is moved from the periphery of the screen at 30-degree intervals.

As each acknowledgment of observation is made by the patient, the examiner places the black-tipped pin in the tangent screen to "plot" out boundaries of the patient's *central visual field,* an area which is the 25 degrees surrounding the fixation point.

Next, the examiner will identify the patient's physiological blind spot (the point that correlates with the optic nerve head or disc, in which there are no photoreceptors). This can be found 12 to 15 degrees temporal to the central fixation point, approximately 1.5 degrees below the horizontal meridian, extending approximately 7.5 degrees in height and 5.5 degrees in width.[7]

The examiner now tests how well the patient can see within his or her visual field. In order to accomplish this, the black-sided test object is placed within each 30-degree interval, then it is turned over and the patient is requested to identify it when he or she sees it. Suspicious areas are those in which there is failure to identify the test object. These areas should be retested for size, shape, and also with different colored test objects. These areas should be carefully recorded, for they will need further investigation.

Color Comparison. The optic nerve and chiasm functionally may be considered macular structures, i.e., predominantly subserving the *central field.* In optic nerve disease, central depression (scotoma) may be easily elicited by asking the patient to describe changes in his or her perception of the color of the largest test object moved away from or toward the central point of fixation.[4] Alternatively, two similar targets may be used, one placed centrally and the other eccentrically, and the patient asked to describe differences in color intensity.[4]

It is important to record the patient's name, age, visual acuity, and pupil size. The size, shape, and color of the test object, and the distance between patient and screen must also be noted. Other information such as contrast, brightness of the room, alertness, and cooperation of the patient should be recorded, as well as the date on which the test was performed.

The tangent screen is useful in assessing the progression and regression of central scotomas most commonly found in optic neuritis, and the centrocecal field defects associated with tobacco–alcohol nutritional amblyopia. Glaucoma field defects can also be assessed, as can those caused by lesions in the optic tract. However, more sophisticated equipment is available for more accurate identification of peripheral field defects.

Perimetry. While visual acuity gives a clue to the condition of the foveal area of the retina, the only way of determining the sensitivity or "visual acuity" of the rest of the retina is by *perimetry.* Therefore, it is useful in detecting retinal detachment, retinitis pigmentosa, choroiditis, and cerebral tumors. Central and peripheral fields are indicated in intracranial pathology and destruction of sensitivity caused by glaucoma.

The tangent screen is a useful method by which to measure central fields, but it only tests the central 25 degrees of vision, while the normal peripheral field extends to 60 degrees nasally and out to 85 degrees temporally. This leaves a large important area referred to as the *peripheral field* unstudied. The instrument to measure the entire field is called a *perimeter.*

Perimeters come in many types, which vary from the simple office universal perimeter arc, to static perimetry, and finally the large, complex hemispheric and even computerized projection instruments.

The simple office perimeter has a radius of 33 cm. The test target sizes range from $\frac{1}{4}$ mm, 1 mm, 2 mm, 3 mm, and 5 mm, and can be either flat or spherical.

They are placed on a short wand for the peripheral field, while those used in central fields are on a long wand. Test targets are then brought in from the periphery to the fixation point, and the patient is asked to state when he or she first sees the target. The result is then noted and plotted. The arc is rotated and another meridian is tested. It is possible to cover the entire peripheral field with eight meridians being tested. It is more accurate than the confrontation test, and the isopter can be plotted with different-sized test targets. Methods of measuring visual fields are changing very rapidly, and soon all visual fields will be accomplished by automated perimetry.

The *Goldman perimeter* was the first hemispheric perimeter and its uses a projection system similar to the later projection models of the universal perimeter. However, the Goldman is more complex in that it is connected with a pantograph which traces the fields onto a chart as they are being done (Fig. 5–6).

When fields are plotted on tangent screen or with simple office perimeters, the isopters are designated with the numerator being the size of the test target in millimeters and the denominator being the distance to fixation point, also in millimeters. A 1 mm test object isopter in a central field would be 1/1000; the same test target used on an office perimeter would be 1/330. With the more advanced instruments, recording is done in logarithmic units or decibels.

Automated Perimetry. Patients with uncontrolled glaucoma lose their vision so gradually that loss is often hard to detect. All methods of testing visual fields rely on the cooperation of the patient and the skill of the technician. One of the most recently developed computerized perimeters is called the *OCTOPUS.* With this particular instrument the variables have been greatly decreased, allowing a much more standardized test. Also, a greater field of vision can be tested in a shorter length of time. The instrument is also useful in testing patients with neurological problems where loss of vision is suspected.[8]

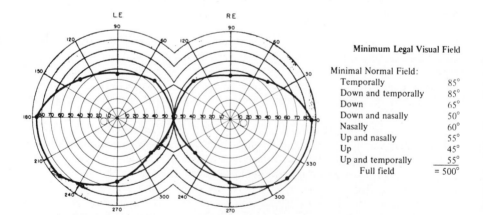

Minimum Legal Visual Field

Minimal Normal Field:	
Temporally	85°
Down and temporally	85°
Down	65°
Down and nasally	50°
Nasally	60°
Up and nasally	55°
Up	45°
Up and temporally	55°
Full field	= 500°

Figure 5–6. Normal peripheral visual fields. *(Reproduced from Vaughan D, Asbury T: General Ophthalmology, 10th ed. Los Altos, Calif: Lange, 1983, p. 380, with permission.)*

The OCTOPUS runs on the principle known as static perimetry. A microcomputer controls measurements, and examination results are stored on floppy diskettes. This collected data can be printed out in various modes, and it can also be used as a baseline for future measurement. The instrument itself really consists of two parts, connected by cables (Fig. 5–7).[8]

The Perimetric Unit is made up of the perimeter cupola, which is actually a hemispheric projection screen (inner radius of 500 mm) with a pure white, flat interior coating for the presentation of the stimulus (test object). A fixation light is located in the center of the visual field of the projection surface. Luminance is standardized and is automatically adjusted by the computer before and after each examination so that background illumination is uniform. The stimulus projector which generates the stimulus light beam is behind the cupola. The sizes of the circular-shaped stimuli are determined by the supervisory controlled aperture which, when selected by the terminal, is automatically turned into the light beam by the computer. The exposure time is also computer controlled.

Projector rings or centering points of four different diameters can be projected into the cupola to the center of the visual field as well as at an angle of 18 degrees to its right side. In the first position, these rings serve as a fixation light, due to a central scotoma. The second position serves as a fixation aid for the examination of the center of the visual field.

The proper head position is achieved by an adjustable chin rest, while two adjustable, lateral supports hold the head sideways and to the front. These supporting structures can be moved to facilitate the examination, since the eye under examination must always be positioned in the center axis of the cupola. The head fixation can accommodate corrective lenses. (The technician will need to check the patient's glasses on the lensometer to ascertain the refractive correction.) The eye not being tested is covered by a cup attached to the instrument. For examinations of the center of the visual field, the head fixation is turned to the right, up to the stop, around its own axis.

The patient response button is to be pressed each time stimuli are noticed, and this way the computer is advised of an aknowledged stimulus. However, by

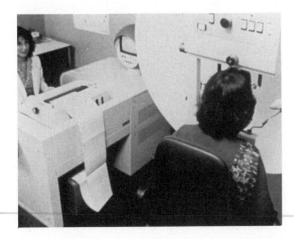

Figure 5–7. Automated perimetry: The OCTOPUS.

pressing the button constantly, the patient can inconsistently interrupt the program.

The patient's seat is rather like a seat in a spaceship, with its powerglide mechanism for forward, backward, and vertical motion. A patient needs to be warned about this, as it can be a rather frightening experience being propelled toward the cupola.

The Control Unit is a desk that contains the computer. This is a microprocessor which has a combined internal RAM memory. It serves to control and supervise the functions of the perimetric unit according to the examination programs selected, the evaluation of the patient's replies, the calculation of the values of the visual field for the output of the data in the desired mode of display and for further tasks such as supervision of functions, etc.

The disk drive and memory units are housed in two separate places; the right-hand unit contains the diskette with all the programs for examination, evaluation, and modes of display. The diskettes inserted into the left-hand unit serve for storing the measured values of each patient either for subsequent examinations or immediate printout.

The input and output terminal receives the patient's data and examination data, and after the examination the typewriter prints out the results in the desired mode of display. There are three alternative ways of printout: the display can be in density steps ''gray scale'' (Fig. 5–8), profile display, or numerical table.

On the desk is the Eye Fixation Control. This consists of a closed television system (in the Perimetric Unit) and a monitor mounted on top of the control desk, so the operator can observe the magnified eye during the whole period of examination. Blinking of the eye is tolerated, but a lasting closure of the eye cancels the stimulus automatically, and can temporarily interrupt the examination. There is a small blinking IR-spot (which can be seen in the center of the pupil as corneal reflex) which enables the operator to ascertain minor deviations of fixation, and allows him or her to cancel the stimuli shown during this period.

The diskettes are used as a means of storage. Each instillation needs one program diskette and a varying number of patient diskettes.[8]

The operator, usually a specially-trained technician, will need to learn how to operate the OCTOPUS, set the paper, insert the diskettes, select the programs and type of program required for the particular patient, select the operating mode, and start the examination.

As with all tests, the name of the patient, date of birth, selected eye, state of correction, patient number, examination time and date, size of stimulus, and the program number should be recorded.

Color Vision

Color is dependent upon hue, saturation, and brightness. Objects appear to have a particular hue primarily because they reflect, irradiate, or transmit light of certain wavelengths. The addition of black to a given hue produces the various shades. Saturation of a color is therefore an indication of its purity, while brightness is the aspect of perception most closely related to light intensity.[1]

Defects of color vision are classified according to the trichromatic or Young-Helmholts theory, which implies the presence of three types of cone receptors which have three primary colors: red, green, and blue. Individuals who have the

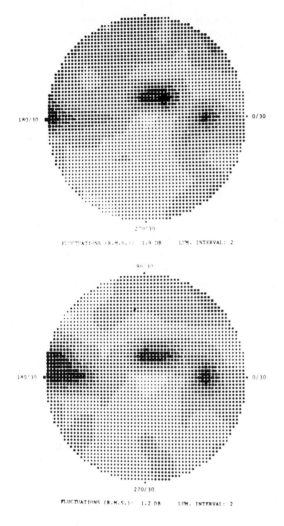

Figure 5–8. Computerized visual field "gray scale" readout. *(From Spaeth GL: Glaucoma surgery, in Spaeth GL, (Ed.), Ophthalmic Surgery: Principles and Practice. Philadelphia: Saunders, 1982, p. 238, with permission.)*

proper complement of cone pigments are called normal trichromats. However, approximately 8 percent of all males and 0.5 percent of all females have insensitivity to one or more of these pigments and are considered "color defective." Color blind (since visual acuity is excellent in most cases) is not an accurate term.

Pseudoisochromatic plates such as *Ishihara* and *Hardy-Rand-Rittler* (HRR) can be useful in detecting such defects. The Ishihara color plates test for color vision is based on the patient's ability to trace patterns in a series of multicolored charts.[1] The value of the Hardy-Rand-Rittler Pseudoisochromatic Plates (printed by American Optical Company) is that they are excellent for use in clinics, schools, and office practice. They give a comprehensive, inexpensive, and rapid test of color vision. They can rapidly separate normal color vision from abnormal; then with further quick testing can determine mild, medium, or strong red/green or blue/yellow defects and can even further help diagnose them as caused by Protan (lacking input from the R cone—erythrolabe), Deutan (lacking input from the G cone—chlorolabe), Tritan (lacking input from the B cone—cyanolabe), or Tetartan (all three pigment cones) anomalies.

Farnsworth-Munsell tests use Munsell color chips mounted in caps. The colors have the same saturation and brightness and differ only in hue. There are two tests: the D-15 and the FM-100. The hues of the D-15 test were chosen so that mild color defectives (anomalous trichromats) can pass. It does not distinguish between mild and moderate color deficiency. It is felt that those who pass the test can perform almost all functions in our society that depend upon hue discrimination.[9] Recording for the D-15 test is done on the score sheet provided (Fig. 5–9). The FM-100, a much more complex test, was designed for two purposes: the first, to separate persons with normal color vision into classes of superior, average, and low color discrimination; and the second to measure the zones of color confusion of persons with either congenital or acquired color vision.[9] This test also has its own score sheet on which the cap scores are plotted.

Color defects that are congenital will be found to be the same in both eyes. Acquired color defects will quite often differ from one eye to the other.[10]

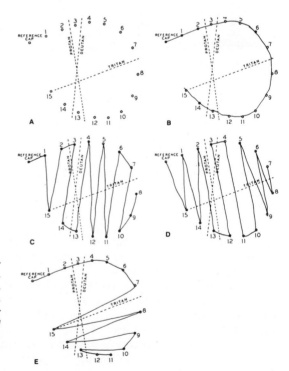

Figure 5–9. A. Score sheet for the D-15 color test. **B.** Normal trichromat. **C.** Deuteranope. **D.** Protanope. **E.** Tritanope. *(From Benson WE: Introduction to color vision, in Duane TD, (Ed.), Clinical Ophthalmology. Philadelphia: Lippincott/Harper and Row, 1985, 3(6) p. 14, with permission.)*

REFERENCES

1. Vaughan D, Asbury T: General Ophthalmology, 10th ed. Los Altos, Calif.: Lange, 1983, pp. 34–42
2. Scheie HG, Albert DM: Textbook of Ophthalmology, 9th ed. Philadelphia: Saunders, 1977, p. 408
3. Boyd-Monk H: Examining the external eye, Part I. Nursing 80, 10(5): 58–63, 1980
4. Glaser JS: Neuro-ophthalmologic examination: General considerations and special techniques, in Duane TD, (Ed.), Clinical Ophthalmology. Hagerstown, Md.: Harper & Row, 1979, 2(2): pp. 1–38
5. Wassenberg C: Common visual disorders in children, in Boyd-Monk H, (Ed.), Nursing Clinics of North America. Philadelphia: Saunders, 1981, 16(3): p. 479
6. Gwinup K, (Ed.): Assessing the function of the eye, in Physical Assessment: Eye and Ear Instructors Manual. Costa Mesa, Calif.: Concept Media, 1977, pp. 7–17
7. Dowen PA: Subjective tests, in Diagnostics. Springhouse, Penn.: Intermed Communications, 1981
8. Interzeag AG: Automatic Perimeter System. Octopus Operating Instructions and Description Manual. Schlieren, Switzerland: Interzeag, c. 1978
9. Benson WE: An introduction to color vision, in Duane TD, (Ed.), Clinical Ophthalmology. Hagerstown, Md.: Harper & Row, 1982, 3(6): pp. 1–19
10. Schaffer DB: Congenital abnormalities of the retina, in Duane TD, (Ed.), Clinical Ophthalmology. Hagerstown, Md.: Harper & Row, 1978, 3(8): pp. 1–8

BIBLIOGRAPHY

Smith JF, Nachazel J: Ophthalmologic Nursing. Boston: Little, Brown, 1980

6

Techniques of Refraction and Examination

NEW TERMS

Aphakia: without a crystalline lens.
Diopter: measurement of refractive power of lenses (D = abbreviation).
Minus lenses: concave lenses that diverge parallel light rays.
Plus lenses: convex lenses that converge parallel light rays to a focus.
Refraction: measurement of the bending of light rays.

OPTICS

The optics of the eyeball can best be described as being similar to a camera (Fig. 6–1). The sclera is the covering that supports inner structures of the eye including the lens system and film carrier. The lens system is composed of the cornea and crystalline lens (a doublet system) with the cornea being the stronger refractive element. Between this doublet lens system is the iris, which in the normal eye adjusts the light entering the system. The retina acts as the "film" upon which the light rays are focused. The lids act as a sunshade or "lens cap" for the eye.

Focusing of the light rays upon the retina is determined by the *refractive power of the lens system, and the axial length of the eye.* When the light rays come to focus on the retina's macula area of the resting eye, the condition is called *emmetropia* (Fig. 6–2). Failure of correlation of the length of the globe and the refractive power when the eye is at rest causes the focus to be in front of or behind the retina. When the focus is in front it is called *myopia* or nearsightedness (Fig. 6–3). If the focus is posterior to the retina it is called *hypermetropia* or farsightedness (Fig. 6–4).

Regular *astigmatism* occurs when the curvature of the cornea is greater in one meridian than another, and the focus is not a point but two separate lines at right angle to each other. Irregular astigmatism usually occurs after trauma and cornea scarring, and the lines of focus are not at right angles.

Refractive errors are corrected with lenses. Simple hypermetropic errors are corrected with *spherical convex lenses* that move the focal point forward to the retina. Myopic errors are corrected with *spherical concave lenses* which move the focus back to the retina.

Astigmatic errors are corrected by *cylindrical lenses* instead of spheres. Cylin-

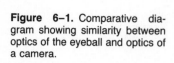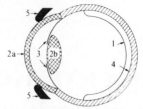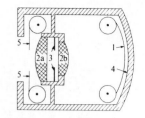

Figure 6–1. Comparative diagram showing similarity between optics of the eyeball and optics of a camera.

drical lenses only have curvature along one side, and since they are formed by cutting a small glass cylinder in half with the curved surface refracting the light rays into a line, they are able to correct the astigmatic error. A *spherocylinder lens* is used to correct both the spherical component and the cylintrical error of *compound myopic astigmatism, compound hypermetropic astigmatism or mixed astigmatism.*

Anisometropia is the term used for an unequal refractive error in the two eyes; for instance, a 1 diopter myopic error in one eye and a 2 or 4 dioptric error in the other eye.

Aniseikonia is a rare condition in which the brain interprets the visual images to be different sizes or shapes. Anisometropia may be a cause or there may be a difference in the retinal layer. Some evidence is also found for interpretation in the brain. Some of the latter causes are difficult to diagnose and require specific instrumentation. Correction of these uncommon cases of aniseikonia once they are diagnosed is achieved by using special lenses known as *iseikonic lenses.*

Presbyopia occurs when the crystalline lens looses its elasticity with age, and focusing the eye for near (accommodation) becomes more difficult. When the ability to read at 14 inches becomes difficult new lenses for near must be used. This loss of reading ability usually begins at about age 42, and is corrected by using

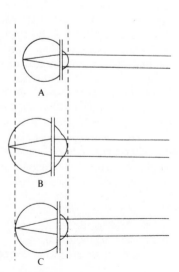

Figure 6–2. Focus of light rays in an *emmetropic* eye. **A.** Smaller than normal; **B.** larger than normal; and **C.** normal size.

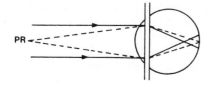

Figure 6–3. Focus of the light rays in the *myopic* eye.

hypermetropic correction "add" onto the distance vision lenses. These lenses are referred to as *bifocals.*

Aphakia occurs when the crystalline lens is removed because of cataract or dislocation, thus weakening the strength of the refractive system and moving the image behind the retinae. In order to correct this, a strong hypermetropic correction is needed to bring the focus forward onto the retina. With the removal of the crystalline lens there is an associated chromatic and spherical aberration, and also a 35 percent increase in the size of objects. It is nearly impossible for a person with unilateral aphakia to wear glasses to correct vision in the aphakic eye if the unoperated eye has good vision. The patient can realize the difference in image size between the two eyes, which is usually unacceptable. A contact lens or intraocular lens implant can reduce these aberrations and facilitate comfortable binocular vision.

Determination of the axial length of the eye is an important step in identifying the power of the intraocular implant which must be used after cataract surgery. These measurements are now easily calculated by a computer attached to an ultrasound measuring instrument.

An automatic *refractometer* can give the lens power necessary to correct the failure of correlation between axial length and the refracting power of the eye. These are computerized instruments.

Hard contact lenses can correct the astigmatism either by covering up (neutralizing) the curvature or by having the astigmatic correction ground or pressed into the plastic lenses. Newer *soft contact lenses* are being made with correcting cylindrical curvature for astigmatism errors. These are difficult to fit and take a great deal of patience on the part of the wearer to become accustomed to them.

Subjective Examination

Refraction is the term used to test and determine the refractive error of an eye. It may be performed without the aid of drugs or drops and is known as a *manifest refraction.* The focusing ability of the eye is intact and must be considered when giving the final determination.

When eyedrops are used to temporarily paralyze the ciliary muscle and the

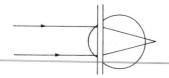

Figure 6–4. Focus of the light rays in the *hypermetropic* eye.

ability of the eye to focus, it is called *cycloplegic examination*. In a cycloplegic examination the eye is at rest and a more definite refractive error determination is reached. The pupil is also dilated by the drops and the peripheral rays of the light are included in the refractive examination and not just the central rays. At this time the interior of the globe can easily be examined using an ophthalmoscope.

Muscle Balance. Normally the eyes move together and the images seen by each eye are fused into one image. If this is interferred with by weakness or paralysis of the extraocular muscle or muscles, double vision (diplopia) is produced. This can be measured by using a wedge of glass or plastic known as a *prism*. This wedge (prism) bends the rays of light entering one of its surfaces away from the apex and toward the base. By placing the prism or prisms of different strengths in front of one eye until the light or object is seen as one with both eyes, a subjective measurement of the deviation can be made. This examination can be made in the sixth cardinal direction (of gaze), as well as straight ahead.

Cross Cylinder. Another subjective test to determine the axis and strength of the cylinder in an astigmatic patient is the use of a combination of plus and minus cylinders in a special holder with a handle. This is known as a *cross cylinder* and the strength of the cylinders can be a +.50 D with a −.50 D lens or a +.25 D with a −.25 D lens. By strandling the axis and flipping the cross cylinder the axis angle can be refined, or by adding the plus or minus axis of the cross cylinder to the axis of the corrective cylinder a stronger or weaker cylinder or sphere or both may be determined.

Objective Examination

The corneal surface regularity can be examined by use of a *keratoscope*. This is a hand-held instrument with illuminated, white concentric rings and a lens or hole in the center of the rings. When held in front of the cornea being examined, the concentric white rings are reflected off the corneal surface and can be observed by looking through the central hole (Fig. 6–5). Distortion of the reflected rings are seen in keratoconus and corneal scarring. Larger, more expensive instruments can also make a polaroid photograph of these reflected rings for inclusion in the patient's record.

   Keratometry is the measurement of the curvature of the anterior surface of the cornea. The older keratometers permitted the examiner to observe reflections of white rings and crosses on the patient's corneal surface. These images could be brought into alignment by rotating calibrated wheels on either side of the observing scope. The axis could be determined by rotating the scope and reading the axis off a protractor surrounding the scope. The numerical measurement ("K" readings) of the curvature can be read off the calibrated wheels, while the axis is read off the protractor. Modern computerized instrumentation gives a printout of the curvature and the axis rapidly and accurately once the person operating the machine has mastered its use.

   Retinoscopy is an objective means of measuring the total refractive power of the eye or even a camera. The hand-held instrument passes a column of reflected light rays into the eye from a slanted mirror in which there is a central hole. The light rays are reflected from the retina of the eye which is being examined and the

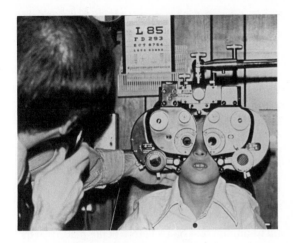

Figure 6–5. Retinoscopy being performed using lenses in the Phoroptor.

light reflex is seen by the examiner when looking through the central hole in the mirror. By moving the instrument from side to side or up and down, a movement of the reflex is also noted. If the movement is *with,* the same direction as the instrument is moved, then plus lenses of varying strength are interposed in front of the examined eye until the movement of the reflex is reversed. Similarly, if the reflex movement is against the movement of the instrument, minus spherical lenses are used to reverse the movement. The end point is reached when the movement is reversed, and the power of the sphere needed to achieve this point is the *refractive error* of the eye. A constant of +1.00 or +1.50 diopters must be subtracted from this number to compensate for the distance the examiner is from the eye being examined (Figure 6-5).

Correction of Refractive Error. Strength or power of lenses are measured in units known as *diopters.* In a convex or plus lens, the strength is the reciprocal of the focal length in meters. If the parallel rays of light are brought to a focus at 1 meter or 1/1 meter = 1 diopter. If the rays are brought to a focus at 2 meters then the power of the lens is $\frac{1}{2}$ meter or 0.5 diopters. On the other hand, if the focal length is $\frac{1}{2}$ meter then $1/\frac{1}{2}$ = 2 diopters. With negative or concave lenses that diverge the rays there is no focus. It is necessary to project the diverged rays back through the lens to an imaginary point in front of the lens and measure this point from the lens. Thus if a minus lens has a focal length of 1 meter the power would be $1/-1$ meter = -1.00 diopter.

The power of prisms are measured in *prism diopters* ($\triangle$). If the prism will displace a ray of light 1 cm at 1 meter then the power of the prism is 1 prism diopter (1 $\triangle$). If it displaces 2 cm then it is 2 $\triangle$.

The Trial Case. A trial case is a case of assorted lenses of both plus and minus lenses in spheres and cylinders. The spheres are in pairs in $\frac{1}{4}$ diopter increments from 0.25 to 4.00 diopters, then in $\frac{1}{2}$ diopters to 8.00, and from then to 20.00 diopters in 1 diopter steps. The cylinders are + and −, and go only to 8.00 diopters in similar steps. Prisms vary in steps and after 4$\triangle$ they only occur singly and in increasing larger steps to 20Δ. These trial case lenses are used in a trial frame and are slipped into the spaces on the frame. There is usually one space or well on the posterior surface of the frame, and space for two or three lenses on the front surface of the frame depending upon the thickness of the lenses.

In place of the trial frame a phoropter, an instrument with many lenses on a wheel which can be rotated in front of the patient's eye, is quicker and less tiring to the patient. This instrument comes with both + *and* − spheres, but has only + *or* − cylinders. Prisms can also be measured.

Measurement of glasses power is done by using a *lensometer*. Computerized lens analyzers are taking the place of hand-operated lensometers, and anyone can determine the strength of glasses without prolonged training.

Care of Contact Lenses. The care of hard lenses is relatively easy. They can be cleaned with lens cleaner by gently rubbing between fingers and subsequently soaked in disinfecting solution for a minimum of 4 hours before being placed on the eye. Soft lenses must be handled with care as they are fragile and can be torn. Although chemical disinfection seems to be more popular now, heat disinfection is also a way of sterilizing the lenses. Soft lenses are cleaned then disinfected and should be stored in the case in fresh sterile saline until they are put in the eye. Extended wear soft lenses can be cleaned by surfactant, which breaks up and emulsifies the debris, or by enzymes. These contact lenses vary in water content and fragility. Wearing schedules will be determined by the contact lens fitter and the physician.

It should be stressed that only sterile solutions should be used for cleaning and storing contact lenses (Fig. 6–6). The hands should be thoroughly washed before removing or inserting the contact lenses. The hard rigid lenses should never be wetted by saliva or placed in the mouth. If any irritation from the contact lenses occurs, an ophthalmologist should be consulted immediately.

Nursing intervention for inserting and removing hard and soft contact lenses are as follows (Fig. 6–6):

Hard contact lenses—to insert the hard contact lens:

1. Moisten the lens with wetting solution and place the cleaned, wetted lens on the index finger.
2. With the other hand, gently part the upper and lower lids and place the contact lens directly on the cornea.

To remove a hard contact lens:

1. (a) Pull the eyelids to the outer canthus to narrow the palpebral fissure, and the lens should squeeze out into a cupped hand.
   (b) Alternately, use a little DMV plunger or suction cup which is placed directly on the lens (on the cornea) and lift it off.

Soft contact lenses—to insert the soft contact lens:

1. Remove the lens from the solution in which it has been stored and place it on the index finger for a couple of seconds to allow it to dehydrate a little. This procedure will make it easier to place on the eye.
2. Using the other hand, part the upper and lower eyelids.

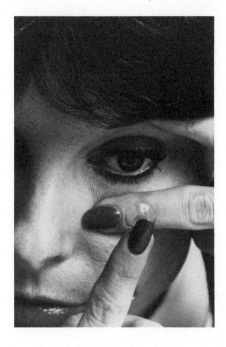

Figure 6–6. Inserting a soft contact lens. *(From Barnes-Hind, Inc., San Diego, Calif., with permission.)*

3. Ask the patient to look down and place the soft contact lens on the superior portion of the sclera. As the patient closes the eye it will slide on to the cornea.

(a) An alternative method is to place the lens directly on the cornea.

To remove the soft contact lens:

1. It must be well-hydrated; otherwise it appears to be sticking to the cornea and is not freely moving.
2. Ask the patient to look up, and pull down the lower eyelid as the contact lens is pinched off the cornea with the finger and thumb; or alternately slide the lens off inferiorly.

Care of Contact Lenses in Fitting and in Practice. Recent information from the Center for Disease Control in Atlanta included the following recommendations for preventing possible transmission of Human T-Lymphotropic Virus Type III/Lymphadenopathy-Associated Virus from Tears:[1]

> The following precautions are judged suitable to prevent spread of HTLV-III/LAV and other microbial pathogens that might be present in tears. They do not apply to the procedures used by individuals in caring for their own lenses, since the concern is the possible virus transmission between individuals.
>
> 1. Health care professionals performing eye examinations or other procedures involving contact with tears should wash their hands immediately after a

procedure and between patients. Handwashing alone should be sufficient, but when practical and convenient, disposable gloves may be worn. The use of gloves is advisable when there are cuts, scratches, or dermatologic lesions on the hands. Use of other protective measures, such as masks, goggles, or gowns, is *not* indicated.

2. Instruments that come into direct contact with external surfaces of the eye should be wiped clean and then disinfected by:
   (a) a 5 to 10-minute exposure to a fresh solution of 3 percent hydrogen peroxide; or
   (b) a fresh solution containing 5,000 parts per million (mg/L) free available chlorine—a 1:10 dilution of common household bleach (sodium hypochlorite); or
   (c) 70 percent ethanol; or
   (d) 70 percent isopropanol.
   The device should be thoroughly rinsed in tap water and dried before reuse.

3. Contact lenses used in trial fittings should be disinfected between each fitting by one of the following regimens:
   (a) Disinfection of trial hard lenses with a commercially available hydrogen peroxide contact lens disinfecting system currently approved for soft contact lenses. (Other hydrogen peroxide preparations may contain preservatives that could discolor the lenses.) Alternatively, most trial hard lenses can be treated with the standard heat disinfection regimen used for soft lenses (78–80°C [172–176°F] for 10 minutes). Practitioners should check with hard lens suppliers to ascertain which lenses can be safely heat-treated.
   (b) Rigid gas permeable (RGP) trial fitting lenses can be disinfected using the above hydrogen peroxide disinfection system. RGP lenses may warp if they are heat-disinfected.
   (c) Soft trial fitting lenses can be disinfected using the same hydrogen peroxide system. Some soft lenses have also been approved for heat disinfection.

Other than hydrogen peroxide, the chemical disinfectants used in standard contact lens solutions have not yet been tested for their activity against HTLV-III LAV. Until other disinfectants are shown to be suitable for disinfecting HTLV-III LAV, contact lenses used in the eyes of patients suspected or known to be infected with HTLV-III LAV are most safely handled by hydrogen peroxide disinfection.

REFERENCES

1. CDC Recommendations for Preventing Possible Transmission of Human T-Lymphotropic Virus Type III/Lymphadenopathy-Associated Virus from Tears. MMWR, 34(34): 533–534, 1985

BIBLIOGRAPHY

Ledford JK: Saving time: Efficiency in the routine ophthalmic examination. Journal of Ophthalmic Nurs & Tech, 4(1): 33–35, 1985
Suitt B: Keratometry—Theory and practice. Insight, 10(1): 6–7, 1984
Vaughan D, Asbury T: General Ophthalmology, 10th ed. Los Altos, Calif.: Lange, 1983

7

Ophthalmic Drugs

Ophthalmic drugs are used frequently for diagnostic purposes as well as therapeutic measures. Nurses, physicians, technicians, and patients are all required at sometime to instill eye medications. The correct technique should be used. The correct medication should be instilled to the correct eye. The hands should be clean. The tip of the bottle or tube should never be contaminated by the eyelashes or lid margin. To avoid systemic absorption, the puncta should be occluded. If more than one drop is to be instilled, there should be at least a 30-second time lapse between the two medications. The tops of the bottles or tubes should be tightly capped when not in use. Old medications should be discarded.

Each of the drug categories discussed in this chapter will be reviewed in an easy reference table form. Table 7–1 lists topical anesthestics, while Table 7–2 presents a review of mydriatics and cycloplegics.

DRUGS USED IN THE TREATMENT OF GLAUCOMA

The variety of drugs used to control the glaucoma patient's intraocular pressure actually work at many different sites, and therefore are used in combination with one another at the lowest possible dosages. The direct-acting cholinergic (parasympathetic) drugs (Table 7–3) like pilocarpine and carbachol increase the outflow of aqueous humor by their action on the ciliary muscle and the sphincter muscle of the iris. The anticholinesterases, i.e., physostigmine and phospholine iodide, prevent the rapid destruction of the normal chemical neurotransmitter acetylcholine, which increases the parasympathetic activity. The resultant pupillary constriction (miosis) is common to all parasympathomimetic drugs, with the result that these drugs are labeled *miotics*. Miosis is actually a side effect and may be responsible for a complaint of visual blurring. Because of this side effect, poor dark adaptation, caused by failure of the pupil to dilate normally in response to reduced illumination, is evident. Miosis also produces general depression in the visual field. Adrenergic sympathomimetic drug action (epinephrine or dipivefrin, a prodrug) has empirically been shown to reduce aqueous production and increase outflow (Table 7–4).

Timolol is a nonselective beta-blocker that is currently available for treatment of glaucoma. It is a derivative of propranolol (Inderal). It is now a treatment drug of choice for glaucoma and it has the advantage of not affecting the size or action of the pupil. Levobunolol is another nonselective beta-blocker similar to timolol. A newer drug betaxolol is $beta_1$ (cardioselective) and will be used where there is a hidden bronchospasm risk; for example, in glaucoma patients who also have a history of asthma.[1,2]

TABLE 7–1. TOPICAL ANESTHETICS

Topical anesthesia of cornea and conjunctiva can be achieved by administering one or two drops of the following anesthetic eye drops. The medication may need to be instilled again during the procedure.

Drug and Available Strength (%)	Dosage and Indications for Use	Onset of Action
Proparacaine hydrochloride (Alcaine, Ophthetic, Ophthaine) 0.5% solution	1. Topical anesthesia used prior to tonometry, minor surgical procedures, irrigation for chemical burns, gonioscope, subconjunctival injury. Corneal foreign body and suture removal. 2. Enhances penetration and effect of phenylephrine	Within 20 sec
Tetracaine hydrochloride (Pontocaine) 0.5–1% Cocaine 2–10% solution	Topical anesthesia used prior to surgical procedures 1. Minor surgical procedures 2. 2% used in diagnosis of Horner's syndrome	Within 1 min Within 20 sec

TABLE 7–2. MYDRIATICS AND CYCLOPLEGICS (PARASYMPATHOLYLICS)

Both mydriatic and cycloplegic drugs dilate the pupil; cycloplegics also paralyze the power of accommodation (the patient is unable to focus on near objects, e.g., reading material). The drugs may be given alone or in combination, so that one potentiates the other. One or two drops are instilled as a series to achieve maximum dilation prior to examination. The drops may also be prescribed two to four times daily as a treatment for uveitis to prevent synechia. Because of the action of dilating the pupil these drugs should not be given to patients who are known to have narrow angles for they can precipitate an acute attack of glaucoma.[2]

Drug and Available Strength (%)	Dosage and Indications for Use	Onset of Action
MYDRIATICS		
Phenylephrine hydrochloride (Neosynephrine, Mydfrin) 2.5% and 10% (AK Dilate) 2.5%	1 or 2 drops in each eye, which may be repeated in 5–10 minutes is given for pupillary dilitation. Used in conjunction with	30 min

Duration	Side Effects	Precautions	Contraindications
15 min	Transient stinging, burning. Conjunctival redness	Warn patient not to rub eyes while cornea is anesthetized—may cause corneal abrasion. Do not permit patients to acquire for prolonged use—may lead to abuse with resultant visual loss	1. Hypersensitivity 2. Prolonged use not recommended, retards wound healing leading to visual loss or corneal perforation
15–20 min	As above	As above	As above
30 min	As above	As above	As above

Duration	Side Effects	Precautions	Contraindications
Up to 3 hr	Iris cell floaters; can cause increased blood pressure in hypertensives	Use 10% with caution in elderly and children. Do not use solution if discolored	Should not be used in patients with narrow angles or shallow anterior chambers; MAO

(continued)

TABLE 7–2. (*Continued*)

Drug and Available Strength (%)	Dosage and Indications for Use	Onset of Action
	cycloplegics to potentiate their actions	
Hydroxyamphetamine hydrobromide (Paredrine) 1%	May be used if patient is allergic to phenylephrine	
CYCLOPLEGICS *Anticholinergic agents*		
Atropine sulfate (Atroprisol, Isopto Atropine, BufOpto Atropine) 0.5%, 1%, 2%, 3% solution. 1% most frequently used. 0.5 and 1% ointment	1 drop twice daily when mydriasis and cycloplegia are desired for a long period of time e.g., amblyopia. Treatment of iritis postcataract surgery without IOL. Refraction in children	30–40 min. Slower onset of cycloplegic in heavily-pigmented eyes
Homatropine hydrobromide (Homatrocel Ophthalmic, Isopto Homatropine) 2–5% solution	Shorter action than atropine and scopolamine; pre-op	30–90 min. Approx. 45–60 min
Scopolamine hydrobromide (Isopto Hyoscine) 0.25% solution	Similar to atropine when much shorter duration of action is desired. Can be used as a substitute for atropine when allergy is present. Inflammatory conditions of the uveal tract	35–45 min
Cyclopentolate hydrochloride (Cyclogyl) 1–2% solution. Combination drug: (Cyclomydril) **cyclopentolate** HCl 0.2% and **phenylephrine** HCl 1.0% solution	1 or 2 drops to each eye; may be repeated after 10 min. Shorter action than atropine or scopolamine. Often given in conjunction with phenylephrine for diagnostic procedure ie, fundoscopy. 1% given for light irides; 2% given for dark irides	15–45 min
Tropicamide (Mydriacyl) 0.5 and 1% solutions	1 or 2 drops of 1% solution in each eye 2 or 3 times at 5 min intervals prior to ophthalmoscopy for diagnostic purposes	20–25 min

Duration	Side Effects	Precautions	Contraindications
			inhibitors; tricyclic antidepressants.
12–14 days. Longest acting cycloplegic	Blurred vision, systemic toxicity, restlessness, flushing, dryness, rapid pulse, fever, mental confusion	Use with extreme caution in infants and children. Keep bottle away from children. Occlude puncta to prevent systemic absorbtion	1. Hypersensitivity 2. Contraindicated in persons with primary glaucoma or shallow anterior chamber
10–48 hr (about 36 hr)	Similar to Atropine	As above	As above
48–72 hr. Duration is shorter in inflamed eyes	As above occasionally causes dizziness and disorientation in elderly people	As above	As above
Up to 24 hr	Burning sensation upon instillation. Systemic: psychosis in children, ataxia restlessness, incoherent speech, hallucinations, disorientation, tachycardia	Use with caution in patients with cardiovascular disease, hypertension, hyperthyroidism, and in the elderly	As above
4–6 hr	Transient: stinging, blurred vision, photophobia	Use in pregnancy has not been established. Keep container tightly closed. Advise patient to wear dark glasses if photophobic	As above

TABLE 7–3. MIOTICS (PARASYMPATHOMIMETICS)

Drug and Available Strengths (%)	Dosage and Indication for Use	Onset of Action
Direct-acting cholinergic agents		
Pilocarpine hydrochloride (Isopto carpine, Pilocar, Pilomiotin) to name but a few generic names. 0.25–10% solutions. Combination drugs: (E-Carpine) **epinephrin** 0.5%, **pilocarpine HCl** 1%, 2%, 3%, 4%, or 6%	1 drop in the eye 4–6 times daily, starting with the lowest effective dose which controls IOP (intraocular pressure). Until recently was the initial treatment of POAG (primary open angle glaucoma). Acute angle closure glaucoma. Counteracts mydriatics and cycloplegics following ophthalmoscopic exam and surgery	60 min
Pilocarpine HCl 4% (Pilopine HS Gel)	Instill half-inch ribbon on conjunctive cul-de-sac daily at bedtime	
Carbachol (Isoptocarbachol) 0.75%, 1.5%, 2.25%, 3% solutions	Instill 1 drop 3–4 times daily. Used in narrow angle and open angle glaucoma. Used as a substitute for pilocarpine acquired allergy or resistance	Slow
Intraocular carbachol 0.01% (Miostat) Intraocular Acetylcholine (Miochol)	Intraocular pupillary miosis during surgery	Immediately
Indirect-acting reversible anticholinesterase		
Physostigmine sulfate (Eserine) 0.25 and 0.5% solution, 0.25% ointment	Reverse atropine mydriasis instill 1–2 drops t.i.d. Acute narrow angle glaucoma. (Largely supplanted by other drugs)	30 min
0.25% ointment	Instill quarter-inch strip in treatment of lice infestations of eyelid margins	

Duration	Side Effects	Precautions	Contraindications
4–6 hr	Transient: headache, myopia, ciliary spasm, blurred vision, conjunctival irritation. Systemic: nausea, vomiting and diarrhea, abdominal cramps, epigastric distress, hypertension, bronchospasm, tachycardia Greatest amount of induced myopia occurs during sleep	Pupillary variation causes changes in visual field— note that patient is on medication when checking visual fields. Use cautiously in patients with bronchial asthma and hypertension. Occlude puncta	1. Hypersensitivity 2. Never use in acute iritis, or acute inflammatory disease of the anterior of the eye (uveitis, corneal abrasion)
8 hr	Similar to above	Use with caution in patients with acute cardiac failure, bronchial asthma, Parkinson's disease, peptic ulcer, hyperthyroidism, GI spasm, urinary tract obstruction Discard unused portion	As above
12–36 hr	Headache, conjunctival irritation, blurred vision	Additive effect if patient is exposed to organophosphate. Discard discolored (pink or rusty) solution or ointment	Allergy to drug

(*continued*)

TABLE 7–3. (*Continued*)

Drug and Available Strengths (%)	Dosage and Indication for Use	Onset of Action
Indirect-acting irriversible anticholinesterase		
Echothiophate iodide (Phospholine Iodide, Echodide) 0.03–0.25% solution	Instill 1 drop twice daily as adjunctive therapy in POAG. Accommodative esotropia	Slow
Demecarium bromide (Humorsol) 0.125%, 0.25% solution	1 drop twice daily (as above)	2–4 hr
Isoflurophate (DFP, Floropryl) 1% in oil; 0.025% ointment	1 drop twice daily, every 12 hr. Infrequently used	

TABLE 7–4. ADRENERGIC (SYMPATHOMIMETICS) AND BETA-ADRENERGIC BLOCKING AGENTS

Drug and Available Strengths (%)	Dosage and Indications for Use	Onset of Action
Adrenergic (sympathomimetics)		
Epinephryl hydrochloride (Epifrin, Glaucon) 0.5%, 1%, 2% solution	1 drop in the eye b.i.d. Used in treatment of POAG. Decreases rate of aqueous formation and increases outflow. Vasoconstriction of superficial vessels to control bleeding. Give before timolol for best effect	Within 1 hr
Epinephrine borate (Epinal, Eppy/N) 0.25%, 0.5%, 1% solution	1 drop in eye b.i.d.	
Dipivefrin (Propine) 0.1% solution	1 drop b.i.d. in the eye. Used in POAG. Penetrates cornea easily and is converted to free epinephrine	
Beta-adrenergic blocking agent		
Timolol maleate (Timoptic) 0.25%, 0.5% solution	1 drop of 0.25% in the eye twice daily. Increase to	30 min

Duration	Side Effects	Precautions	Contraindications
12–26 hr 10 days	Browache. Transient: blurred vision. Cataract formation—time and dose related, iris cysts—reversible with drug discontinuity, retinal detachment. Systemic: Fatigue, weakness, parasthesia, lid muscle twitching, poisoning	To avoid postanesthesia respiratory distress, because of drug's interaction with muscle relaxant *succynl choline* stop drug at least 10–14 days prior to surgery	1. Acute angle closure glaucoma 2. Hypersensitivity 3. Active uveal inflammation

Duration	Side Effects	Precautions	Contraindications
12–24 hr	Severe stinging on instillation; corneal or conjunctival pigmentation due to allergy of levo epinephrine. Systemic: palpitations, tachycardia, extrasystoles	Causes discoloration of lens if placed in eye with soft contact lens in place. Use with extreme caution in patients with cardiac disease	1. Hypersensitivity 2. Narrow angle glaucoma 3. Shallow anterior chamber
12 hr	Same local and systemic side effects of epinephrine, but does not cause conjunctival pigmentation	As above. Use with caution in patients with aphakia. Does not seem to stain soft contact lenses	As above
12–24 hr	Long-term use results in corneal	Assess patient for history of asthma.	Do not use in patients with a

(continued)

TABLE 7–4. (*Continued*)

Drug and Available Strengths (%)	Dosage and Indications for Use	Onset of Action
	0.5% b.i.d. as needed for POAG. Aphakic glaucoma and some types of secondary glaucoma	
Levobunolol (Betagan) 0.5% solution	1 drop of 0.5% in the eye daily to lower intraocular pressure in POAG and ocular hypertension	1 hr
Betaxolol hydrochloride (Betoptic) 0.5% solution	1 drop of 0.5% in the eye twice daily to reduce intraocular pressure	30 min

TABLE 7–5. CARBONIC ANHYDRASE INHIBITORS

Drug and Available Strengths	Dosage and Indication for Use	Onset of Action
Acetazolamide (Diamox) 125 and 250 mg tablets 500 mg capsules 500 mg vial—injectable	250 mg four times daily 500 mg b.i.d. 500 mg intravenously. Useful in reducing IOP in POAG and angle closure glaucoma; as an adjunctive treatment to drops	2 hr (tablets) 5 min (injection)
Methazolamide (Neptazane) 50 mg tablet	50 mg t.i.d. (oral)	2 hr
Ethoxzolamide (Cardrase, Ethamide) 125 mg	125 mg q.i.d. tablets (oral)	30 min
Dichlorphenamide (Daranide, Oratrol) 50 mg tablet	50 mg t.i.d.	

Duration	Side Effects	Precautions	Contraindications
	anesthesia. CNS—confusion	Monitor patient for bradycardia. Occlude puncta to decrease systemic absorbtion	history of asthma or heart failure
24 hr	Some patients receiving beta-adrenergic blocking agents have been subject to severe hypotension during anesthesia. Use with caution in diabetics—may mask symptoms of hypoglycemia	As above. Use with caution in patients with a history of angle closure glaucoma. Known hypersensitivity to other beta-adrenoceptor blocking agents	As above
12 hr	Has produced only minimal effects in patients with reactive airway disease	Assess patient for history of cardiac failure. Use with caution	Hypersensitivity. Do not use in patients with sinus bradycardia

Duration	Side Effects	Precautions	Contraindications
6–8 hr 4–6 hr	Potassium depletion, gastric distress, diarrhea, exfoliative dermatitis, renal calculi; depression, and tingling of the extremities	Sulfonamide derivative, identify any known history of allergy. Monitor for potassium depletion; encourage K+ supplement, e.g., orange or grapefruit juice	Hypersensitivity
10–12 hr	Less GI distress		
7 hr	As above		
Similar to *acetazolamide*			

TABLE 7–6. HYPEROSMOTIC AGENTS

Drug and Available Strength (%)	Dosage and Indication for Use	Onset of Action
Mannitol (Osmitrol) 20% IV solution (500 cc) 25% (50 cc)	1.5 g/kg body weight. Acute angle closure glaucoma, chronic open angle glaucoma and prior to intraocular surgery to lower intraocular pressure. Give over 45–60 min	30–60 min
Urea (Ureaphil, Urevert) 30% IV solution	1 g/kg body weight infused over 1–2.5 hr	30–45 min
Isosorbide (Isosmotic) 100 g/220 ml oral solution	1.5 g/kg body weight. For short term reduction of intraocular pressure	Within 30 min
Glycerin (Glyrol) 0.75%, (Osmoglyn) 50% oral solution	1–1.5 g/kg body weight. (4–6 oz flavored with orange juice over ice) For short-term intraocular pressure reduction pre- and postsurgery	10–30 min

Duration	Side Effects	Precautions	Contraindications
6 hr	Headache, nausea, transient sensation of chills; mild angina-like pain	Monitor solution, warm if crystals are present. Monitor patient for hypovolemia	1. Hypersensitivity 2. Patients with severe congestive heart failure 3. Metabolic edema associated with capilliary fragility in patients with impairment of renal function
5–6 hr	Headache, sloughing of underlying tissue after extravasation	Monitor electrolytes	1. Patients with impaired renal or hepatic function 2. Congestive heart failure 3. Severe dehydration
5–6 hr	Nausea, vomiting, headache, confusion, and disorientation may occur	With repeated doses maintain adequate fluid and electrolyte balance	1. Well-established anuria due to severe disease 2. Acute pulmonary edema
4–5 hr	Nausea, vomiting, headache, confusion, and disorientation. May produce hyperglycemia and glycosurea	Monitor patient to avoid acute urinary retention	Hypersensitivity

TABLE 7–7. ANTI-INFECTIVE OPHTHALMIC DRUGS
The topical antibiotics bacitracin, neomycin, polymyxin, erythromycin, tetracycline, gentamycin, and tobramycin are most commonly used in combination or separately in the treatment of ocular infections associated with the lids, i.e., blepharitis, lacrimal system; i.e., dacryocystitis; conjunctiva, i.e., bacterial conjunctivitis; cornea i.e., keratitis, and prophylactically. More severe intraocular infections are treated with subconjunctival antibiotic injections and systemic antibiotic preparations.

Drug and Available Strength (%)	Dosage and Indication for Use	Onset of Action
1. Antibiotics		
Bacitracin ointment 500 U/g **Bacitracin (fortified)** solution 10,000 U/ml specially reconstituted by pharmacy. Combination drugs: (Polysporin Ophth. ointment): **Polymyxin 10,000 U, Bacitracin 500 U**	half inch 2–4 times daily in conjunctive cul-de-sac. Broad spectrum antibiotic used for prophylaxis during pressure patching of corneal abrasion, and surface ocular infections	Within minutes
Erythromycin 1% (Ilotycin) ointment	half inch 1–2 times daily in conjunctive cul-de-sac. Should only be used when sensitivity studies reveal it to be effective against infecting organism. Treatment of choice in trachoma chlamydia	Approx. 4 hr
Neomycin sulfate	Most frequently used as combination drug. half-inch ointment applied 3–4 times daily in conjunctive cul-de-sac.	Fast
Combination drugs: (Neosporin) ointment: **Polymyxin B** 5000 U, **Bacitracin** 400 U, **Neomycin** 0.25%. (Neosporin) solution: **Neomycin** 0.25%, **Polymyxin B** 10,000 U, **Gramicidin** 0.25 mg. (Maxitrol): See Table 7–8, Topical Steroids. (Cortisporin) ointment/suspension: **Polymixin B** 500 U, **Bacitracin** 400 U, **Hydrocortisone** 1%, **Neomycin** 5 mg	Effective treatment against gram-negative and gram-positive organisms involving conjunctiva and/or cornea	

Duration	Side Effects	Precautions	Contraindications
Variable	Ointments blur vision, retard corneal healing. Prolonged use may led to overgrowth of nonsusceptible organisms including fungi	Warn patients that ointments blur vision. Keep tube closed to avoid contamination and degradation due to light	1. Hypersensitivity 2. Bacitracin interacts with silver nitrate; do not use together
Variable	Slows corneal wound healing. Overgrowth of nonsusceptible organisms with overuse	As above	Hypersensitivity history to erythromycin
4–6 hr	Ocular irritation following prolonged use	Sensitive individuals may cross react to other aminoglycosides (gentamycin). Prolonged use may lead to superimposed infection	1. Hypersensitivity 2. Incidence of allergy 5–10%

(continued)

TABLE 7–7. *(Continued)*

Drug and Available Strength (%)	Dosage and Indication for Use	Onset of Action
2. Tetracyclines		
Tetracycline Hcl (Achromycin 1%) Ophthalmic suspension (Achromycin 1%) ointment	1–2 drops instilled into the affected eye 2–4 or more times daily for treatment of superficial ocular infections susceptible to tetracycline. Apply half-inch ointment to affected area q2hr depending upon severity of infection. Trachoma—used in conjunction with oral therapy. 2 drops in each eye 2–4 times daily, which may be continued for 2 months or longer	Slow
3. Aminoglycosides		
Gentamycin sulfate 3.0 mg/ml (Genoptic, Garamycin) solution and ointment	Ointment: Apply half-inch to affected eye 2 or 3 times daily. Solution: 1–2 drops in affected eye q4hr may be increased to hourly in severe corneal ulcer and intraocular infections where gram-negative organisms are suspected	Within 1 hr
Tobramycin 0.3% (Tobrex) solution	Instill 1–2 drops in affected eye q4hr. In severe infections, may be instilled hourly until improvement is shown against wide variety of gram-negative and gram-positive ophthalmic pathogens	
4. Sulfonamides		
Sulfacetamide sodium (Sulamyd, Bleph 10, Bleph 30) 10%, 30% solution, 10% ointment **Sulfisoxazole** (Gantrisin)	1–2 drops instilled frequently depending upon severity of bacterial conjunctivitis. Active against gram-negative and gram-	Slow

Duration	Side Effects	Precautions	Contraindications
	Hypersensitivity reactions: dermatitis, itching	Overgrowth of nonsusceptible organisms with prolonged use	1. Hypersensitivity to any tetracyclines 2. Incompatible with tyloxapol, a component of Tobrex and Enuclene
	Stinging effect	Possible nephrotoxicity when used in conjunction with systemic preparation. Monitor gentamycin level (of systemic medication) and serum creatinine Prolonged use of topical antibiotic may give rise to nonsusceptible organisms including fungi	1. Hypersensitivity 2. Sterile ophthalmic solution is not for injection
	Lid itching and swelling and conjunctival erythema	As above	Hypersensitivity to aminoglycosides
		Antagonistic to the inhibition of *pseudomonas* by gentamycin. Do not instill medications at	1. Hypersensitivity to sulfonamide preparations 2. Sulfonamide preparations are

(*continued*)

TABLE 7–7. *(Continued)*

Drug and Available Strength (%)	Dosage and Indication for Use	Onset of Action
4% solution, 4% ointment Combination Drugs: (Metimyd) ointment/suspension: **Sulfacetamide** 10%, **Prednisolone Acetate** 0.5%. (Vasocidin ointment): **Prednisolone Phosphate** 0.5%, **Sulfacetamide** 10%, **Phenylephrine** .125%. (Vasocidin solution): **Prednisolone phosphate** 2.5%, **Sulfacetamide** 10%, **Phenylephrine** .125%	positive organisms; use not complicated by secondary fungal infections. Topically effective against trachoma, and inclusion conjunctivitis when used with systemic tetracyclines	

5. Antiviral Agents

Idoxuridine (Dendrite Herplex, IDU) 0.1% solution	1 drop q1hr day and q2hr night, in the treatment of keratitis caused by the Herpes simplex virus (HSV)	
(Stoxil) 0.1% ointment	half-inch ointment strip—5 instillations daily q4hr and at night	
Adenine arabinoside (Ara-A, Vira-A) 3% ointment	half-inch ointment strip to lower conjunctive cul-de-sac 5 times daily for HSV keratitis. Treatment of acute keratoconjunctivitis and recurrent epithelial keratitis due to HSV Types I and II	
Trifluridine (Viroptic) 1% solution	1–2 drops q2hr for a maximum of 9 doses daily (until corneal reepithelialization takes place) then q4hr for 7 days (minimum of 5 doses). Treatment of HSV Types I and II & some adenoviruses	

6. Antifungal Agents

Natamycin (Natacyn) 5% suspension	1 drop instilled in conjunctive cul-de-sac hourly or 2 hourly, then reduced to 6–	

Duration	Side Effects	Precautions	Contraindications
		the same time	incompatible with silver preparations
Short	Ocular irritation, pain, pruritis, inflammation or edema, photophobia	Administer with caution in pregnancy. Protect from light. Stress patient compliance	Hypersensitivity
	Lacrimation, foreign body sensation, conjunctival injection, burning, irritation, superficial punctitate keratitis, and photophobia		Hypersensitivity
	Mild transient burning or stinging upon instillation; palpebral edema; superficial punctitate keratopathy	Drug should not be prescribed for pregnant women unless the potential benefit outweighs potential risk	1. Hypersensitivity reactions; or 2. Chemical intolerance to trifluridine
	One case of conjunctival chemosis and hyperemia has	Shake well before use. Use in pregnancy has not been evaluated,	Hypersensitivity history

(*continued*)

TABLE 7–7. (Continued)

Drug and Available Strengths (%)	Dosage and Indication for Use	Onset of Action
	8 times daily after the first 3–4 days; therapy generally continued 14–21 days. Treatment of fungal blepharitis, keratitis, conjunctivitis	
Amphotericin B (Fungizone) Solution of 2.5 mg/ml of distilled water in 5% dextrose must be made up in pharmacy from powdered drug	Use when above drug is proving ineffective	

TABLE 7–8. TOPICAL STEROIDS

Topical corticosteroids are frequently used for treatment of inflammatory disorders of the eyelids, conjunctiva, cornea, and anterior segment of the globe. The drugs are also available in combination with antibiotics.

Drug and Available Strengths (%)	Dosage and Indication for Use	Onset of Action
Dexamethasone alcohol (Maxidex) 0.1% suspension, 0.5% ointment. Combination drugs: (Maxitrol) **Dexamethasone alcohol** 0.1%, **neomycin** 3.5 mg, **Polymyxin B 6000 U** suspension/ointment. (NeoDecadron) **Dexamethasone phosphate** 0.1%, **neomycin** 3.5 mg	1 or 2 drops topically 4–6 times daily. In severe disease, drops may be given hourly, tapered to discontinuation. Used in allergic and vernal conjunctivitis, uveitis, episcleritis scleritis, phylctenulosis, superficial punctate keratitis interstitial keratitis	Moderate

Duration	Side Effects	Precautions	Contraindications
	been reported Eyelashes mat together.	therefore, drug should be used with caution in these situations Cleanse eye before drop instillation.	
			Hypersensitivity

Duration	Side Effects	Precautions	Contraindications
3–4 hr	Long-term use may be associated with increased IOP. Possible interference with wound healing increases with long-term use, and susceptibility to corneal infection with fungi and viruses. Posterior subcapsular cataracts	Watch for complaints of decreased vision and pain in the eye. Warn patient of side effects of long-term use. Inform patient of necessity of having frequent tonometric exams if long-term therapy is prescribed	1. Hypersensitivity 2. Herpes Simplex keratitis 3. Fungal diseases and active viral diseases of conjunctiva and cornea 4. Acute untreated purulent infection

(*continued*)

TABLE 7–8. (*Continued*)

Drug and Available Strength (%)	Dosage and Indication for Use	Onset of Action
Fluorometholone 0.1% (FML)	As above, but has lower propensity to increase IOP in long term usage	Moderate; dependent upon corneal status
Medrysone 1% suspension (HMS)	1 drop up to q4hr. Treatment of episcleritis, allergic and vernal conjunctivitis	Variable
Prednisolone acetate 0.125% (Econopred Mild, Pred Mild) (Econopred Plus, Pred Forte) 1% suspension	As above	
Prednisolone sodium phosphate 0.125% (Inflamase) solution (Inflamase Forte) 1% solution	1–2 drops topically in eye; may be used hourly, being tapered to discontinuation as inflammation subsides	As above
Combination drugs: (Blephamide, Liquifilm, Sulfapred suspension): **Sulfacetamide** 10%, **prednisolone acetate** 0.2%, **phenylephrine** 0.12% suspension/ointment. (Cetapred): **Sulfacetamide** 10%, **prednisolone acetate** 0.25% suspension/ointment. (Metamyd): **Sulfacetamide** 10%, **prednisolone acetate** 0.5% suspension/ointment. (Vasocidin) **Sulfacetamide** 10%, **prednisolone phosphate** 0.5%, **phenylephrine** 0.12%		
Hydrocortisone acetate 0.5, 1, **and** 2.5% **suspension**	As above	As above

Duration	Side Effects	Precautions	Contraindications
As above	As above	As above	As above
Variable	As above	As above Shake well before using	As above
	As above		
As above	As above	As above	As above
As above	As above	As above	As above

TABLE 7–9. DIAGNOSTIC DYE SOLUTIONS

Drug and Available Strength (%)	Dosage and Indication for Use	Onset of Action
Sodium fluorescein (Ful-Glo) 0.6 mg sterile paper strips; (Fluoreseptic) sterile ophthalmic solution. **Sodium fluorescein** 2% solution in single use disposable units Combination Drug: (Fluress) **Fluorescein sodium** 0.25%, **Benoxinate Hcl** 0.4% solution	Moisten tip with sterile ophthalmic solution, place 1 drop in the conjunctive cul-de-sac. Used as a diagnostic agent for detection of corneal injury, applanation tonometry, and fitting of hard contact lenses	Immediately
Sodium fluorescein 10% sterile solution for intravenous use	Inject 3–5 cc intravenously for fluorescein angiography	Within seconds
Rose bengal (Rose Bengal) 1.3 mg rose bengal per strip	Moisten tip of strip with sterile solution—touch the conjunctiva or lower fornix as required with moistened strip. Used in diagnosis of keratoconjunctivitis sicca; dye stains dead or degenerated epithelial cells of cornea and conjunctiva. Also stains mucus of precorneal tearfilm	Immediately

Duration	Side Effects	Precautions	Contraindications
	Occasional temporary stinging	Avoid tear stain on patient's cheeks	Known hypersensitivity to fluoresceine sodium
Up to 24 hr	Mild dermatological reaction; nausea, vomiting, vasovagal attack; anaphylactic shock; severe stinging	Warn patient that the urine will be orange for the next 24 hrs. Encourage increased fluid intake	As above
		Stains severely, avoid getting on clothes. Topical anesthetic drop used prior to instillation	Known hypersensitivity to rose bengal

TABLE 7–10. ARTIFICIAL TEAR SOLUTIONS

These solutions are instilled in the eye(s) to provide a tear supplement for irritated "dry eye" syndromes. They may be used specifically by either hard contact lens wearer, or the soft contact lens wearer, but usually are not interchangeable. The remaining products are used exclusively as a tear replacement substitute for dry eyes due to mucin-deficient and aqueous deficient conditions. The bland nonmedicated ophthalmic ointment is used for a variety of conditions which include causes for exposure keratitis.

Drug and Available Strength (%)	Dosage and Indication for Use
(Adapt) **Adsorbobase hydroxyethyl cellulose** 0.55%, **thimerosol** 0.002%, **disodium edetate** 0.05%	Instill 1–2 drops prior to lens insertion. Used as a cushioning solution for *hard contact lenses* to prolong wettability and wearing time
(Lacril) **Hydroxypropyl methylcellulose** 0.5% **polysorbate 80, gelatin A, buffered isotonic solution, chlorobutanol** 0.5%	Instill 2–3 drops to counteract dryness of the eyes in the absence of natural tears or for excessive wearing of *hard contact lenses*
(Liquifilm Tears) **Polyvinyl alcohol** 1.4%, **chlorbutanol** 0.5%	Instill 1 drop in the eye as needed or as directed to counteract dry eyes. Used to provide greater comfort and longer wearing of *hard contact lenses*
(Tears Plus) **Polyvinyl alcohol** 1.4%, **povidone, chlorobutanol** 0.5%	Instill 1–2 drops for relief of irritated eyes caused by *hard contact lens wear*
(Tearisol) **Hydroxypropyl methylcellulose** 0.5%, **boric acid, potassium chloride and sodium carbonate benzalkonium chloride, and edetate disodium**	Instill 1–2 drops 3–4 times daily. Tear replacement for minor ocular irritation. Instilled while *hard contact lenses* are in the eye. Used for irritated external ocular tissues after tonometry, as a lubricant for the prosthesis in the postenucleated socket, to relieve discomfort due to dryness of the eye
(Adapettes) **Adsorbobase thimeros 1** 0.002%, **edetate disodium** 0.05%	Instill 1 drop on each lens 3–4 times daily. Sterile lubricating and wetting solution for use with conventional *hard and soft contact lenses*
(Bausch & Lomb Sterile Lens Lubricant) **Povidone with polyoxyethylene thymeros 1** 0.004% **edetate disodium** 0.1%	Instill 1 drop to rewet the *soft contact lens* in the eye 3–4 times daily for relief of irritation, discomfort and burning
(Clērz)[2] **Sodium chloride, potassium chloride, sodium borate, sorbic acid, hydroxy-ethylcellulose, poloxamer 407, thymeros 1** 0.001%, **disodium** 0.1%	Instill 1–2 drops on the eye and blink. For lubricating and rewetting *hard and soft contact lenses*
(Absorbotear) **Adsorbobase hydroxylethyl cellulose thimeros 1** 0.002%, **edetate disodium** 0.05%	Long-acting tear substitute in treatment of "dry eye" conditions related to aqueous or mucin layers' deficiency of the precorneal tear film. 1–2 drops t.i.d. as needed

Precautions	Contraindications
Do not rub Adapt on the lens	Not for use with soft contact lenses
If irritation persists discontinue use of drops and consult a physician	Not for use with soft contact lenses
	Do not use for soft contact lenses
	Do not use with soft contact lenses
If discomfort persists after using solution, patient should remove lens and see an eye-care practitioner	
Keep bottle tightly closed to prevent contamination	Patients with a history of hypersensitivity to mercury compounds (thimerosal)

(*continued*)

TABLE 7–10. *(Continued)*

Drug and Available Strength (%)	Dosage and Indication for Use
(Hypotears) **Lipiden polymeric system,** **benzalkonium chloride** 0.01% **edetate** **disodium** 0.03%	Instill 1–2 drops q4hr as needed. Use a tear supplement in "dry eye" syndrome. Effective in both mucin-deficient and aqueous-deficient conditions
(Tears Naturale) **Duasab polymeric system with dextran,** **benzalkonium chloride** 0.01%, **edetate** **disodium** 0.05%	Artificial tear and lubricant for relief of "dry eye" syndromes. Instill 1–2 drops as frequently as required to relieve irritation or as directed by physician
(Liquifilm Forte) **Polyvinyl alcohol** 3%, **thimerosol** 0.002%	As above
(Lacri-lube) Ophthalmic ointment containing **white** **petrolatum** 55%, **mineral oil** 42.5%, **nonionic lanolin derivatives** 2%, **chlorobutanol** 0.5%	Instill half-inch of ointment in conjunctive cul-de-sac as needed. Useful adjunctive therapy to lubricate and protect the eye following: exposure keratitis due to Bell's Palsy, ectropion, exophthalmos, traumatic lid damage, recurrent corneal erosions keratitis sicca. To lubricate and protect the uninvolved eye during surgery, or just to lubricate and protect the eyes
(Duolube, Akwa Tears) **White petrolatum and mineral oil.** **Contains no preservative**	As above

Precautions	Contraindications

If irritation persists discontinue use and
consult physician. To avoid
contamination, do not touch dropper tip
to any surface. Keep container tightly
closed. Keep out of reach of children

As above

As above

TABLE 7–11. MISCELLANEOUS OPHTHALMIC PREPARATIONS

Drug and Available Strength (%)	Dosage and Indication for Use
1. Decongestant Eye Drops	
Naphazoline hydrochloride 0.012%, **benzalkonium chloride** 0.01%, (Naphcon) solution	2 drops in each eye 2–3 times daily as needed
Naphazoline hydrochloride 0.1% (Vasocon, Muro's Opcon) solution	As above
2. Hypertonic Solution/Ointment	
Sodium chloride 2% **and** 5% solution, **thimerosal** 0.004%, **edetate disodium** 0.1%, (Adsorbonac 2–5%) **Sodium chloride** 5% (Muro-128) solution/ointment	Instill 1–2 drops in the affected eye q3 or 4hr, or as directed by a physician. For temporary relief of corneal edema due to various causes including bullous keratopathy
3. Other	
Cromolyn sodium (Opticrom) 4%	Instill 1–2 drops in eye(s) 4–6 times daily at regular intervals indicated in the treatment of ocular allergy, vernal keratoconjunctivitis, giant papillary conjunctivitis, vernal keratitis

Side Effects	Precautions	Contraindications
	If irritation persists, discontinue and consult with physician. Keep container tightly closed. Keep out of reach of children	Do not use in the presence of narrow angle or angle closure glaucoma because it dilates the pupil
		Hypersensitivity to solution
Transient stinging and burning	Drug should be used during pregnancy only if needed	Hypersensitivity to solution or any of its ingredients

The carbonic anhydrase inhibitors (Table 7–5) are sulfonamide derivatives and all work in the same manner, through inhibition of the enzyme (carbonic anhydrase) responsible for interconversion of carbonic acid with carbon dioxide and water. Primary organs affected by this enzyme inhibition are the kidneys, where diuresis results, and the eye, where aqueous humor production is inhibited.[3] Acetazolamide (Diamox), dichlorphenamide (Daramide), and methazolamide (Neptazane) are all examples of the carbonic anhydrase inhibitors.

Osmotic agents such as mannitol, isosorbide, glycerine, and urea reduce intraocular pressure by making the plasma hypertonic to the aqueous humor (Table 7–6). These agents are generally used in treatment of acute angle closure glaucoma and may be administered pre- and postoperatively to reduce intraocular pressure. Dosage is calculated in grams per kilogram of the patient's weight.

Anti-infective agents have been listed in Table 7–7. These include antibiotic drugs used in combination with one another as well as other categories of drugs such as tetracyclines, aminoglycosides, and sulfonamides. Also included are opthalmic antiviral and antifungal agents. The most frequently used corticosteroids are reviewed in Table 7–8. Diagnostic dye solutions appear in Table 7–9, and Table 7–10 offers a review of the numerous artificial tear solutions that are on the market.

A miscellany of ophthalmic preparations used for a variety of eye disorders which range from allergy to corneal edema are listed in Table 7–11. Though the lists are far from complete, the preparations which have been presented are among the most commonly prescribed by the ophthalmologist, and they will be frequently encountered by ophthalmic health care personnel.

REFERENCES

1. Nurses Reference Library: Eye, Ear, Nose and Throat Drugs, in DRUGS, Pharmacology, Administration, Toxicity, Nursing Implications, 12, 1982, pp. 956–1009
2. Physician's Desk Reference. Oradell, N.J.: Medical Economic, 1987
3. Jeglum EL: Ocular Therapeutics, in Boyd-Monk H, (Ed.), Nursing Clinics of North America, 16(3), 1981, pp. 453–477
4. Vaughan D, Asbury T: General Ophthalmology, 10th ed. Los Altos, Calif.: Lange, 1983, pp. 371–377

BIBLIOGRAPHY

Adler AG, McElwain GE, Merli GJ, Martin JH: Systemic effects of eye drops. Archives of Internal Medicine, 142, December 2293–2294, 1982

8

Operating Room Procedures

NEW TERMS

Cataract extraction: removal of a cloudy lens.
Keratoplasty: corneal transplant.
Scleral buckling procedure: for repair of retinal detachment.
Vitrectomy: surgical removal of the vitreous.

THE ROLE OF THE OPHTHALMIC OPERATING ROOM NURSE

The ophthalmic operating room (O.R.) nurse's role is twofold. First, as a *patient's advocate,* nurses are responsible for protecting the patient's rights and for maintaining the comfort of the sedated and visually-impaired patient. Surgery is a tremendous intrusion on a person's privacy, and the surgical patient must therefore be treated with great understanding. The second role of the O.R. nurse is that of *surgical assistant* to the ophthalmic surgeon. The correct equipment must be available in working order and the surgeon's needs should be anticipated. One of the nurse's responsibilities is protecting the delicate ophthalmic surgical instruments. This chapter will look at the typical O.R. environment in an ophthalmic institution and outline commonly performed eye operations.

Preoperative Interview
It is of utmost importance that the O.R. nurse interviews the patient before surgery, either in the preoperative area of the O.R. or in the patient's room. In addition to establishing a rapport with the patient, the nurse has the opportunity to: 1) *check that the patient's verbal identity corresponds to the name on the wrist band;* 2) identify which eye is the *operative eye* and note that; 3) *the consent form is signed according to the criteria of the hospital.*

Sterilization Procedures
Before sterilization, ophthalmic instruments must be thoroughly cleaned. The ideal method is by *ultrasonic cleansing.* Ophthalmic instruments often have little hidden crevices and with ultrasonic energy, the cleaning of these instruments is achieved by

cavitation—little bubbles in the water produced by the ultrasonic energy expand and then collapse. This motion cleans all parts of an instrument.

Autoclaving. To avoid infection, all surgical procedures are performed under sterile conditions. There are two main methods by which ophthalmic surgical instruments are sterilized. *Autoclaving* kills all microorganisms by steam under pressure. The pressure in the machine is greater than atmospheric pressure and causes the steam to become superheated. The duration that the instrument has to be in the autoclave varies with the material. It is the safest and fastest method of sterilization, but is harsh on micro instruments.

Gas Sterilization. For instruments that are heat sensitive, *ethylene oxide gas* (EO) is preferable for sterilization. Ethylene oxide gas is highly inflammable so it is combined with an inert gas to make it safe. This gas is particularly suitable for ophthalmic instrumentations because many materials, for example the lenses used in indirect ophthalmoscopy, benefit from a more gentle method of sterilization.

Packaging. All items for sterilization must be wrapped in such a manner to allow the sterilizing agent to penetrate the contents and then escape. They must also be wrapped in a way which maintains sterility. An indicator strip should be placed on the outside of the package. This changes color in the sterilizer, indicating that the correct temperature has been achieved. The date when sterility expires should also be clearly marked on each package.

Sterile Technique
Before the surgical procedure can be accomplished nurses and surgeons must prepare themselves in such a way so that sterile technique may be carried out. Length of scrubbing time and method of donning gown and gloves is dictated by hospital policy. The American Society of Operating Room Nurses has recommended that the initial scrub should be at least 5 minutes, with a 3-minute scrub for subsequent cases. Sterile technique must be followed exactly to avoid intraoperative contamination which can lead to postoperative infection, and the O.R. nurse must constantly be on guard for any breaks in technique. It should be remembered that endophthalmitis is a major emergency following surgery (see Chap. 16).

Microsurgery Equipment
The Microscope. The eyes' many delicate structures undergo many intraocular procedures which are facilitated by an operating microscope. Within the body of the microscope is the *objective lens* and attached to the body are the *eye pieces* (oculars) through which the surgeons will view the surgical field. By using a *foot or hand control,* the surgeon can finely control both magnification and focus. Most surgeons prefer a microscope with a *zoom lens* which allows a continuously variable amount of magnification. Stability is a key factor and microscopes are either securely floor- or ceiling-mounted. *Assistant binoculars* can be attached to the body for the surgical assistant, and by attaching a *beam splitter,* the assistant can view exactly what the surgeon is seeing.

Microsurgical Instruments. Microsurgical instruments (Fig. 8–1) are small and delicate, and each instrument is designed in such a way that it will not obscure the surgeon's field of vision. These instruments must be handled with care. The *scrub nurse* is responsible for the protection, cleaning, and sterilization of these instruments. The tips of these instruments should be protected by small plastic covers, ultrasonic cleaning is preferable and instruments should be dried immediately. Gas sterilization is the method of choice.

Sutures. Very small sutures are used to close incisions—as small as 18 μm in diameter—e.g., 10-0 Nylon. The attached small, curved needle is less damaging to the delicate ocular tissues as it passes through them. Great care must be given to such little needles, lest they contaminate the field by inadvertently puncturing gloves or drapes. Careful attention must be given at the end of the procedure to ensure that they are not left near the surgical site, for these fine needles look like an eyelash.

Ophthalmic Anesthesia

Good anesthesia is essential for the success of any operation. General anesthesia is a vital part of the ophthalmic surgeon's armamentarium. It is useful for extensive

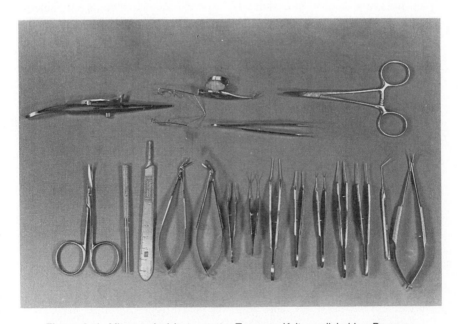

Figure 8–1. Microsurgical instruments. Top row: Kalt needleholder; Barraquer speculum; Barraquer scissors; Lister forceps; Hemostat. Bottom row: Suture scissors; Beaver handle; Bard Parker handle; Castroveijo (left and right) scissors; Bon forceps; Colibri forceps; Castroveijo forceps; McPherson tying forceps—straight and angled; Castroveijo suture tying forceps; spatula; Barraquer needleholder.

operations and open eye injuries where there is a possibility of the patient extruding the ocular contents.[1] It is used for children and uncooperative patients such as those who have arthritis or tremors and cannot lie still. There are certain procedures that require it because the pain cannot be sufficiently blocked with local anesthesia. Local anesthesia is undoubtedly preferable whenever possible. It has a lower incidence of pulmonary and embolic complications, and there is less possibility of postoperative nausea and vomiting. Excellent anesthesia, whether it is local or general, allows for earlier ambulation, which is particularly significant with the growing trend toward same day surgery.

The O.R. *circulating nurse* is responsible for preparing the local injections for the surgeon. Usually, a 10-cc and a 5-cc syringe are used with 1¼-inch 25-gauge needles. The nurse should confirm with the patient which eye is the operative eye and ensure that the correct eye is blocked. Local anesthesia for intraocular procedures consists of the following three parts.

1. Topical anesthesia is administered, e.g., tetracaine hydrochloride 0.5 to 1 percent. It is instilled into the cul-de-sac of both eyes. This lessens the pain from a local injection of anesthetic and also helps lessen the irritation from the iodine used when the patient's eyes are prepped (both eyes are prepped).
2. The surgeon then injects a local anesthetic to paralyze the facial nerve and the obicularis muscle. This prevents the patient from squeezing the lids shut during the surgical procedure. The first injection is given directly anterior to the condyloid in several different directions. This is called the *O'Brien technique*. This block may be reinforced by injecting more anesthetic to the terminal branches of the facial nerve in the direction of the orbital rim. This is called *Van Lint akinesia*. For facial block, carbocaine 2 percent is frequently the drug of choice because of the quick onset. Usually between 8 to 10 cc is injected.
3. A *retrobulbar block* is then administered. Here, the anesthetic is injected into the muscle cone behind the eye. The optic nerve is blocked causing anesthesia of the cornea, conjunctiva, and the uvea. A drug combination of carbocaine 2 percent and marcaine 0.75 percent (the latter because of its long action) is used. Three to five cc is injected.

Local anesthesia in extraocular procedures involves infiltration of the anesthetic agent in and around the region of surgery. Epinephrine is often added to help reduce bleeding.

For both local and general anesthesia cases, the nurse should assess that the patient is adequately sedated. The success of anesthesia is closely related to the patient's emotional status.

Prepping the Patient for Surgery

The *circulating nurse* will prep and drape the patient following these steps:

1. Confirm that the patient is the correct patient for the procedure which is about to be performed, and that the consent form has been signed for the correct eye.
2. Trim the eyelashes at the request of the surgeon (see the discussion on trimming eyelashes in Chapter 3).

3. The nurse dons sterile gloves, and using a sterile prep pack, washes the patient's face with Betadine soap to which water has been added.
   a) If the patient's surgery is under local anesthesia, it is important to tell the patient what is going to be done, because only one side of the face is anesthetized.
   b) If the block is to be done after the prep and drape procedure, as is done in some plastic procedures, then the topical tetracaine hydrochloride anesthetic eyedrops are instilled by the circulating nurse prior to using Betadine to avoid a stinging sensation in the eyes.
4. The soap is rinsed off with sterile water, and the face painted with Betadine solution. The area to be prepped extends from the forehead to under the nose. The nurse must ensure that both eyes are closed to avoid corneal abrasion.
5. The sequence in both washing and painting is for the eyelids to be attended to first, then the forehead, and lastly the nose. The nurse works from inner to outer canthus.
6. To drape the patient, two sterile sheets are used. The first sheet lies under the patient's head. The second is fashioned into a turban and is secured with a towel clip.
7. In a local case, a Mayo stand is placed over the patient and a sterile drape placed over this. The Mayo stand keeps the sheet off the patient's face, thus facilitating breathing.
8. The final stage is performed by the scrub nurse or surgeon, who places a sterile plastic window drape over the eye, and up over the Mayo stand. An opening is cut in the plastic with sterile Stevens scissors.

Corneal Surgery

A clear, transparent cornea is most important if the light rays are to be transmitted onto the retina. Any opacification or disruption of the smoothness of the corneal surface which might occur as a result of abrasion, corneal laceration, ulcer, or endothelial damage will cause decreased vision. Superficial abrasions heal well in a short period of time, but when the cornea is lacerated or opacified, more sophisticated microsurgical techniques become necessary.

Penetrating Keratoplasty. A diseased, cloudy cornea can be successfully replaced with a cornea harvested from a recently deceased human donor. Indications for corneal transplant include a decrease of vision occurring as a result of opacity due to corneal degenerative disease, endothelial damage, or scarring resulting from corneal trauma or ulcer formation.

Penetrating keratoplasty is one of two ways in which a cornea can be transplated, and refers to the procedure in which the whole cornea is replaced with another donor cornea. In a *lamellar keratoplasty* (or partial thickness graft), the deep layers of the host cornea are left intact and only the upper layers are replaced. Penetrating keratoplasty is the much more common procedure (Fig. 8–2).

The quality of the donor eye is of the utmost importance. The age and cause of death of the donor must be known, for the donor material should not be used if the cause of death was a debilitating illness or an acute infection. Prior to being considered for use, and at the beginning of the operation, the donor cornea is

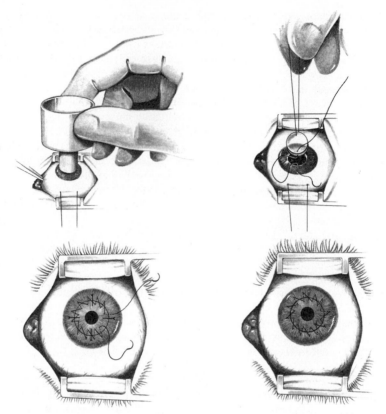

Figure 8–2. Corneal surgery penetrating keratoplasty. *(From Wound Closure in Eye Surgery. Somerville, N.J.: Ethicon, 1977, with permission.)*

carefully examined under the microscope to establish that the endothelium has not been damaged. The donor cornea, which has been dissected from the donor eye also includes a scleral rim and is stored in a special pink tissue medium developed by McCarey and Kaufman (M-K Media). This prolongs corneal viability allowing up to 72 hours for the transplant surgery to be arranged. Most corneal surgeons prefer to use the donor corneas for grafting within 24 to 48 hours.

Before the surgeon begins surgery on the recipient, the donor material is prepared at a separate table. The circulating nurse must carefully pour the cornea onto a petri dish. It is then transferred to a *punching block,* with the *endothelium facing upward.* The "corneal button" is punched out of the donor cornea using a *trephine* of a specific size which is 0.5 mm larger than the trephine used later to remove the host's "corneal button." Attention is then turned to the recipient's eye. A second *trephine* is placed lightly and absolutely vertical on the cornea, and then is turned gently to cut through the epithelium. Left-handed and right-handed *corneal scissors* are handed to the surgeon to cut through the whole cornea.

The new button is placed on the recipient's eye. Four cardinal 8-0 black silk sutures are placed at 12-, 6-, 9-, and 3 o'clock to secure the new cornea. A *Castroveijo needleholder and Colibri forceps* and 10-0 nylon suture will be used by the surgeon to attach the new cornea either with a running suture or with interrupted sutures. Next, the surgeon checks the suture line for wound leaks, using *McPherson forceps,* by pressing on the wound. If no fluid leaks out of the wound it is considered secure. Subconjunctival injections of antibiotic/steroid are given and the anterior chamber reformed with balanced salt solution. A patch and shield are applied after instillation of an antibiotic ointment.

Radial Keratotomy. Radial keratotomy is a surgical procedure which is performed to alleviate myopia. It is an option for those who have difficulty wearing contact lenses.

Eight to 16 radial incisions are made through 90 percent of the thickness of the cornea. These radial incisions have the effect of flattening the cornea, and thus reduce the anterior–posterior length of the eye. This procedure can only reduce myopia by up to 4 diopters and is therefore not suitable for highly myopic patients.

The procedure is performed under topical anesthesia with appropriate sedation. First, the surgeon sets a *diamond knife* at $\frac{9}{10}$ the thickness of the cornea which has been measured very carefully with a *pachometer.* The central optical zone, a circular area of 3 to 4 mm in diameter in the center of the cornea, is marked off with an *optical zone marker;* the surgeon is very careful not to extend any of the radial incisions into this area (Fig. 8–3). The optical zone is kept free so that the cuts do not interfere with the patient's vision. The radial incisions are now made with the diamond knife while *fine-toothed forceps* are used to fixate the globe. Antibiotic ointment is applied and the eye patched overnight.

Repair of a Lacerated Cornea. This procedure is performed as an ophthalmologic emergency. The extent of the damage is established, and the microsurgical repair is accomplished as soon as possible. Often the iris has prolapsed into the wound, and this must be removed or replaced during the course of the surgery. The anterior chamber is then reformed with a #27-gauge irrigation tip. The eye is

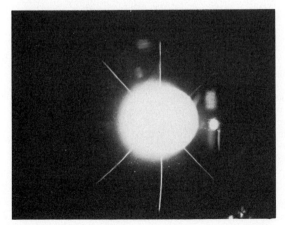

Figure 8–3. Radial keratotomy. By transilluminating the eye, the radial incisions can be seen extending up to the optical zone. *(Photograph courtesy of Juan Arentsen, M.D., Co-director, Cornea Department, Wills Eye Hospital.)*

patched and shielded. If the laceration is in the pupillary region, vision will be decreased by a scar and this patient will be a candidate for a penetrating keratoplasty at a future date.

Lens Surgery

Cataract Extraction. A cataract is an opacity of the lens which causes gradual decreasing vision. It can be removed in one of three ways: 1) extracapsular cataract extraction (ECCE); 2) intracapsular cataract extraction (ICCE) or; 3) phacoemulsification (PE). In each method, the surgeon having inserted the *lid speculum* (obtained from the Cataract Tray [Fig. 8–4]), places a *4-0 silk suture* under the superior rectus muscle using a *Kalt needleholder* and *Lister forceps*. This acts as a traction suture, enabling the surgeon to rotate the globe inferiorly. Next, the conjunctiva is dis-

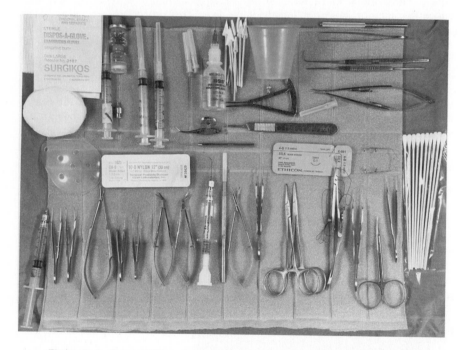

Figure 8–4. Cataract/Glaucoma tray. Top row: Eye patch; Gloves; 3-cc syringe; Miochol and #27G cannula; (2) 3-cc syringes with #18G needles; (2) #25G needles; #21G irrigating cannula on BSS solution; Weck sponges; Medicine cup; Beaver knife handle; Plain forceps (smooth); Muscle hook; Double-ended cyclodialysis spatula; #27G needle; Castroveijo needleholder. Middle row: Eye shield; Suture; Barraquer scissors (De Wecker scissors might be used instead); Iris spatula; Caliper (beneath which is a cautery tip); Bard-Parker knife handle; 4-0 silk suture; Barraquer wire speculum. Bottom row: Syringe with irrigating tip; Straight McPherson forceps; Curved McPherson forceps; Nonlocking Barraquer needleholder; .12 Bonn forceps; Colibri forceps; Left Castroveijo scissors; Right Castroveijo scissors; Healon and #27G cannula; Open-ended Beaver knife handle; Westcott scissors; .12 Castroveijo forceps; (2) Hemostats; Kalt needleholder; .3 Castroveijo forceps; Suture scissors; Lister forceps; Applicator sticks.

sected using *Westcott scissors,* controlling any excess bleeding with *bipolar cautery*. The anterior chamber is then entered via a corneal-limbal incision using a *microblade*.

In an ICCE, the surgeon removes the intact lens, the anterior and posterior capsule as well as the cortex and nucleus. *Alphachymotripsin* can be injected into the anterior chamber to lyse the zonules, making extraction easier. This takes 1 to 2 minutes to perform, and the scrub nurse should monitor the time lapse here. A *cryoprobe* is then placed on the anterior capsule. When this probe reaches −60°F, it freezes on the cataract which can now be extracted. This method has largely been replaced by the other two. With ICCE, the risk of vitreous loss is greater, because the posterior capsule has been removed. Also, the posterior capsule provides excellent support for intraocular lens implantation and most surgeons prefer to leave it intact. The incision at the limbus is closed in a radial fashion using either straight or curved *McPherson forceps* to tie, and a *microneedleholder such as Castroveijo or Barraquer* to hold the 10-0 nylon suture. Westcott scissors are used to cut the suture.

The main goal of ECCE is to maintain an intact posterior capsule. Having opened the anterior chamber, the surgeon proceeds to open up the anterior capsule with a 25-gauge needle (which the scrub nurse bends) or a special hooked needle, called a *cystotome*. This is done in a can-opener fashion and the nucleus is dislocated. The incision is enlarged and the nucleus is delivered using *Allen's hook and loop*. Finally, the cortex is aspirated with a special *irrigation–aspiration machine*. The surgeon may opt to vacuum the posterior capsule using a *Kratz scratcher* on the cystotome handpiece to prevent later opacification. It is at this point that an intraocular lens would be inserted. To prevent the very delicate corneal endothelium from damage as the lens is inserted, *Healon, (sodium hyaluronate)* is first injected into the anterior chamber. This is a viscous preparation which coats the endothelium. The lens is positioned using a *Sinski hook* in either the anterior or posterior chamber depending upon its design and, of course, the status of the posterior capsule. The pupil is constricted with *Miochol (acetylcholine chloride)* injected into the anterior chamber which acts within 30 seconds. Miochol should not be reconstituted until right before use. The Healon is removed lest it causes an increase in intraocular pressure, and the incision is closed using 10-0 nylon sutures. The surgeon may decide to perform a peripheral iridectomy, which is the removal of a small piece of iris at the peripheral aspect as a preventive measure against glaucoma. At the end of surgery the sutures should be evenly placed to avoid postoperative astigmatism.

Phacoemulsification is an alternative method by which the surgeon may decide to remove the cataract. Here, after the anterior capsule, the nucleus and cortex are broken up into minute particles by the ultrasonic waves emitted from a small probe which is placed in the anterior chamber, the emulsification is aspirated through the handpiece which also provides continuous irrigation. The posterior capsule is left intact. The principal advantage of phacoemulsification is the need for only a very small incision of 3 to 4 millimeters. However, this procedure can have a traumatic effect both on the corneal endothelium and the posterior capsule, and Healon is now being used with this ECCE technique to eliminate this potential effect. The procedure of choice today is generally ECCE with the insertion of either a posterior chamber or anterior chamber intraocular lens implant to correct vision. (Patients who are not candidates for the lens implant still have the option of correction by contact lens or spectacles, after surgery.)

A major complication of cataract surgery is rupture of the posterior capsule with vitreous loss. In this event, the surgeon may elect to perform an anterior vitrectomy, and will require vitrectomy equipment, e.g., Ocutome or SITE TXR. Vitreous in the wound both interferes with healing and also carries with it a high incidence of retinal detachment postoperatively. Therefore, it is very important to remove the vitreous from the anterior chamber.

At the end of the surgery, subconjunctival injections of antibiotic and steroid are given, antibiotic ointment is instilled, and a patch and shield is applied.

Glaucoma Surgery
Filtering Procedures. In chronic open angle glaucoma, no longer controllable by maximum medical therapy, the surgeon may opt to perform a filtering operation.

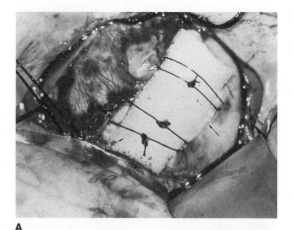

A

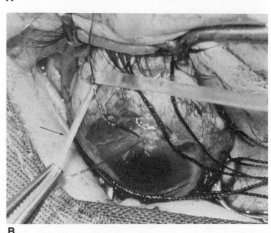

Figure 8–5. Retinal detachment surgery scleral buckling procedure. **A.** "Explant" sewn onto sclera. **B.** Encircling band being positioned. *(Photographs courtesy of William Benson, M.D., Wills Eye Hospital.)*

B

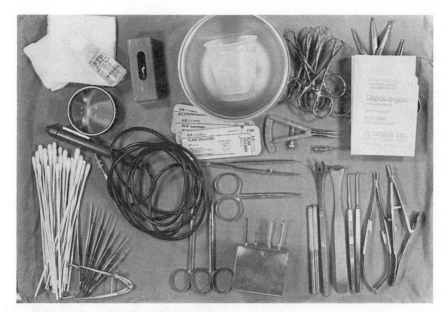

Figure 8–6. Retina tray. Top row: Sterilization indicator under gauze square; BSS; #57 Beaver blade; Metal bowl and plastic medicine cup; 4 Backus towel clips; 4 hemostats; Middle row: Indirect ophthalmoscopy lens; M.I.R.A. cord; Nugent tying forceps; Suture scissors. Bottom row: Applicator sticks; Lister fixation forceps; Bishop-Harmon forceps, Williams speculum; Straight and curved Stevens scissors; M.I.R.A. electrodes; Beaver knife handles; Scheppens retractor; Fisher retractor; Two large muscle hooks; Castroveijo needleholder; Kalt needleholder.

The effect of such surgery is to increase aqueous outflow and thus reduce intraocular pressure. The most common procedure is the *trabeculectomy*. Here, the surgeon exposes the sclera at the limbus using a *#64 Beaver blade* and McPherson forceps and fashions a flap one-half the thickness of the sclera, 4 mm wide and 6 mm long. This flap is hinged at the limbus and is elevated to allow a small piece of trabeculum to be excised, thus creating a new drainage channel. The flap is then sutured, leaving an open cleft at the sides of the scleral flap, which enables aqueous to escape. The conjunctiva is then placed over the flap and a bleb is formed when the aqueous, which is now free to flow from within the eye, "filters" under the conjunctiva. The instrument tray is the same as that used for cataract surgery (Fig. 8–4).

In acute angle closure glaucoma, which is an ophthalmic emergency, the surgery of choice is the *peripheral iridectomy*. Here, a small limbus-based flap is created and a 4-mm incision is made into the anterior chamber using a *#75 Beaver blade*. Counterpressure is applied, using any blunt instrument to the opposite limbus to prolapse the iris. The iris is grasped with McPherson forceps, and a small piece of iris is cut at the periphery using *De Wecker scissors*. Then the iridectomy's patency is checked by *irrigating balanced salt solution* through the hole. The wound is closed in the normal fashion.

It should be noted that many glaucoma conditions that previously required surgery are now treated with laser therapy.

Vitreous–Retinal Surgery

Repair of Retinal Detachment. When the ophthalmologist examines the patient with a retinal detachment preoperatively, he or she makes a detailed diagram of the extent and location of the detachment, through a well-dilated pupil. This diagram is brought to the O.R. where it is displayed, and is a critical aid for it acts as a "map" for the surgery. The procedure for repair of retinal detachment is called a *scleral buckling procedure* (Figs. 8–5A and B). The instruments required for this procedure are shown in (Fig. 8–6). The first part of the operation is indeed localization of the detachment. Having exposed the appropriate extraocular muscles and isolated them with 4-0 silk suture, the surgeon can freely rotate the globe to establish the extent of the area of the retina which is detached. The *circulating nurse* will now place the *indirect ophthalmoscope* on the surgeon's head. This light source will be used to view the fundus during the surgery. Next, *diathermy* will be used to make tiny burns on the sclera to mark where the retinal break has occurred underneath. Throughout the application of diathermy, the surgeon is actively viewing the retina by means of this indirect ophthalmoscope. Next, cryosurgery is used to achieve chorioretinal adhesions to reattach the retina to the choroid. This does not cause the retina to flatten completely, and so the surgeon will request a *plastic implant* which when positioned will cause scleral indentation onto the retina. When this plastic is sutured into position on the sclera it is referred to as an "explant." Often, subretinal fluid has accumulated and at this point this fluid is drained extrasclerially using a needle. A newer method is to drain it intraocularly. This also helps the retina to lie flat. The conjunctiva is closed and atropine sulfate 1 percent eyedrops are instilled to keep the pupil dilated for better visualization postoperatively. Subconjunctival

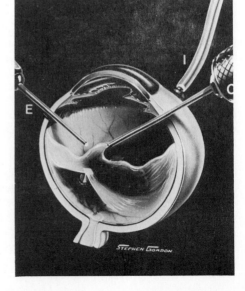

Figure 8–7. Vitrectomy instruments in place. I = infusion, O = cutting/suction instrument, E = endo-illuminator. *(From Boyd BF: Highlights of Ophthalmology, Silver Anniversary ed. Panama, Republic of Panama: Highlights of Ophthalmology, 1(4): 202, 1981, with permission.)*

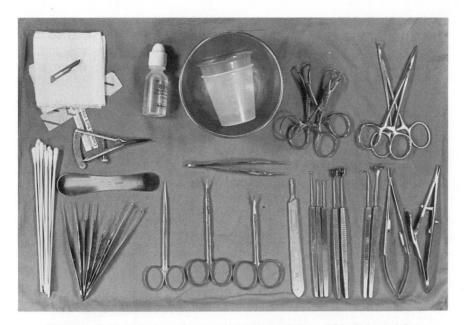

Figure 8–8. Minor lid tray. Top row: #15 Blade; Caliper; BSS (Balanced Salt Solution); Bowl with plastic medicine cups; towel clips; Hemostats. Middle row: Lid plate; Castroveijo forceps. Bottom row: Lister forceps; Bishop Harmon forceps; Suture scissors; Straight Stevens scissors; Curved Stevens scissors; Bard-Parker handle; 4-2-1 Prongs; Rake retractors; Muscle hook; Desmares lid retractor; Castroveijo needleholder; Kalt needleholder.

injections of antibiotic and steroid are given, and a pressure patch applied. Postoperatively, it may be important to position the patient on a certain side to encourage the retina to lie flat.

In cases of severe retinal detachment, such as a "giant tear" (see Chap. 17, Fig 17–13B p. 287) certain other aggressive measures are taken. The patient may be placed on a Stryker frame and turned upside down while the surgeon injects air to push the retina back. On other occasions, Healon in large quantities may be injected into the posterior vitreous cavity—up to 20 cc. Similarly, silicone oil is used to push the retina back into position.

Vitrectomy. A vitrectomy is the removal of the vitreous. Indications include an unresolved hemorrhage, a chronic endophthalmitis, an intraocular foreign body, or vitreoretinal adhesions, membranes, or bands which will lead to retinal detachment. Having performed a peritomy, the conjunctiva is cut 360 degrees, and the extraocular muscles are isolated; then three scleral incisions are made for the irrigation cannula, the fibro-optic light source, and the vitrectomy instrument (Fig. 8–7).

Calipers are used to carefully measure the areas where the incisions are to be made. This region, referred to as the *pars plana,* is about 4 mm from the limbus, and an incision placed in this area will not cause retinal detachment. With the vitrectomy instruments satisfactorily inserted intraocularly, the opaque vitreous is removed and replaced with a basic salt solution into which epinephrine is added to prevent further bleeding. This unwanted material is usually blood; diabetic retinopathy is one of the principle indications for vitrectomy. Sulfhexafluoride (SF^6) or air might be inserted to hold the retina in place. Silicon oil is more frequently used as a vitreous replacement in a patient who has had vitrectomy and who also has a retinal detachment.

Often, during a vitrectomy on a diabetic patient, the surgeon uses the advantage of increased visibility to perform argon laser treatment using an *endolaser* to treat bleeding retinal vessels and seal retinal holes. This treatment may be extensive enough to encompass the whole retina and is referred to as pan-retinal photocoagulation.

When the procedure is complete the incisions are sutured and the eye is patched, after antibiotic subconjunctival injections have been given and antibiotic ointment has been instilled in the cul-de-sac.

Oculoplastic and Oculomotility Surgical Trays

Lid Surgery. Surgical procedures to the eyelids are varied. Figure 8–8 shows the instruments required by the ophthalmologist in order to perform minor lid procedures such as *tarsal resection for entropion* (Fig. 8–9) and *lid-shortening pro-*

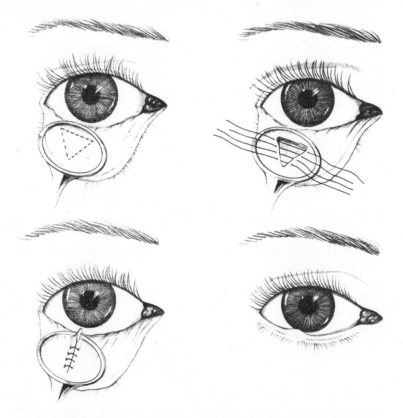

Figure 8–9. Oculoplastic surgery for entropion. *(From Wound Closure in Eye Surgery. Somerville, N.J.: Ethicon, 1977, pp. 18–19, with permission.)*

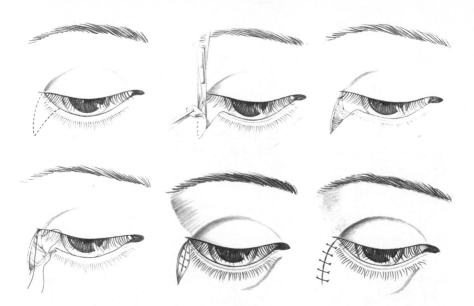

Figure 8–10. Oculoplastic surgery for ectropion. *(From Wound Closure in Eye Surgery. Somerville, N.J.: Ethicon, 1977, p. 7, with permission.)*

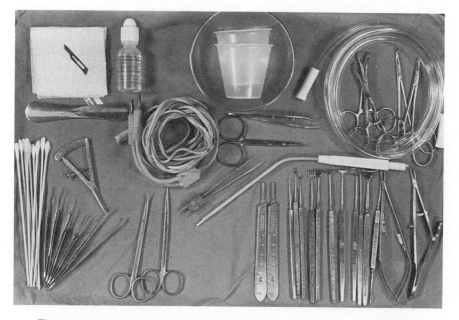

Figure 8–11. Major lid tray. Top row: #15 Blade on top of sterilization indicators (under gauze square); BSS (balanced salt solution); Metal bowl with plastic medicine cups; Suction tubing; Towel clips; Hemostats. Middle row: Lid plate with caliper below it; Bipolar cord; Castroveijo forceps with suture scissors, and bipolar forceps below; Suction tip. Bottom row: Applicator sticks; Lister forceps; Bishop-Harmon forceps; Fixation forceps; Curved Stevens scissors; Straight Stevens scissors; Bard-Parker handles; Skin hooks; 6-4-2 prongs; Rake retractors; Muscle hook; Desmares lid retractor; Castroveijo needleholder; Kalt needleholder.

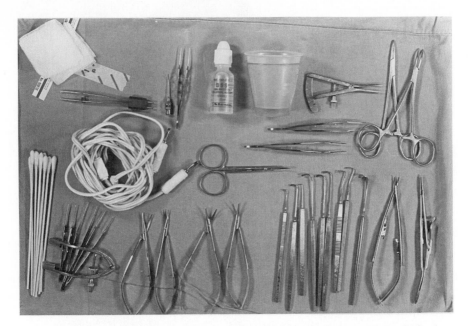

Figure 8–12. Muscle tray. Top row: Sterilization indicators under gauze square; 21G anterior chamber irrigation needle; Bishop-Harmon forceps; BSS; Plastic medicine cup; Jaeger caliper; hemostats. Middle row: Bipolar forceps and cord; Suture scissors; Two Castroveijo forceps. Bottom row: Bishop-Harmon forceps; Two Lister forceps; Westcott right and left scissors; Aebli right and left scissors; Desmares muscle hooks 1–3; Green muscle hooks (2); lid retractor; Barraquer needleholder; Kalt Needleholder.

cedure for ectropion (Fig. 8–10). Major lid procedures such as repair of lid lacerations following trauma and reconstructive surgery require a much more extensive selection of instruments (Fig. 8–11). For other disease entities requiring surgery see Chapter 11.

Muscle Surgery. Extraocular muscle surgery for the correction of strabismus also requires a special set of instruments (Fig. 8–12). For details of muscle surgery for strabismus see Chapter 19.

REFERENCES

1. Libonati MM, Leahy JJ, Elison N: The Use of Succinylcholine in Open Eye Surgery. Anesthesiology, 62: 637–640, 1985

BIBLIOGRAPHY

Gruenoemann BJ, Meeker MH: Ophthalmic surgery in Alexander's Care of the Patient in Surgery, 7th ed. St. Louis: Mosby, 1983, pp. 655–699

III

SPECIFIC EYE PROBLEMS AND THEIR CARE

9

The Orbits and Sinuses

NEW TERMS

Amaurosis: transient recurrent unilateral loss of visual acuity.
Anophthalmia: without an eye.
Enucleation: complete surgical removal of the eyeball.
Exenteration: removal of the contents of the orbit, including the eyeball and lids.
Ophthalmoplegia: paralysis of the extraocular muscles resulting in paralytic strabismus.

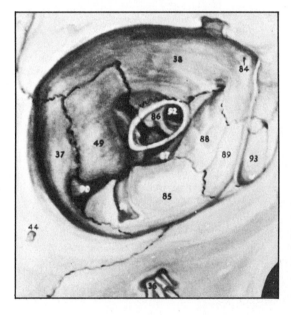

9–1. The orbit: 36. Infraorbital nerve; 37. Zygomatic (Malar) bone; 38. Frontal bone; 44. Zygomatico-facial foramen; 49. Greater wing of sphenoid; 84. Trochlea; 85. Maxilla; 86. Lesser wing of sphenoid; 87. Palatine bone; 88. Lamina papyracea of ethmoid bone; 89. Lacrimal bone; 90. Inferior orbital fissure; 91. Infraorbital groove; 92. Optic foramen; 93. Fossa for lacrimal sac. *(From McHugh G.: Paintings used in The Human Eye in Anatomical Transparencies. Photograph courtesy Bausch & Lomb Optical Co., Rochester, N.Y.: 1957.)*

The bony orbits (or sockets as they are sometimes referred to) form a purely protective function in relation to the eyeball itself. Seven bones make up the orbital cone, the apex of which is directed toward the brain, while the base is formed by the orbital rim. Each orbit looks like a quadrilateral pyramid, with the four walls making up the roof, floor, lateral, and medial walls. The orbital portion of the *frontal bones* form the roof, while paired, paper-thin *maxillae* form the orbital floor.

These bones thicken in the areas that form the inferior orbital rims. Posteriorly the *palatine bones* are part of the orbital floor. The anterior lateral orbital rims are made up by *zygomatic bone,* while the posterior portion is formed by the greater wing of the *sphenoid bone.* On the nasal side the lamina papyracea of the *ethmoid bone* sits behind the *lacrimal bones,* and the lesser wing of the sphenoid bone completes the pyramid. Periosteum, referred to as *periorbita,* lines these orbital bones. The frontal, sphenoid, ethmoid, and maxillary sinuses are paired and surround the orbits. Paired *optic foramen* are the largest of the openings in the orbits. Optic nerves traverse through each foramen, as do the ophthalmic artery and vein which run through the center of the nerve (Fig. 9–1).

Superior and inferior orbital fissures permit passage of blood vessels to the eyeball and motor nerves which innervate the extraocular muscles. The infraorbital artery, vein, and nerve extend through each infraorbital foramen. The supraorbital notch in the frontal bone facilitates the passage of the supraorbital nerves and blood vessels from the orbit. Orbital contents include orbital fat, extraocular muscles, and the eyeball itself.

The four paired sinuses are *frontal, sphenoid, ethmoid* and *maxillary.*

CONGENITAL ABNORMALITIES

Congenital deformities of the orbits are fairly rare and are seldom seen in general ophthalmic nursing practice. The most severe form is seen in anencephaly, where the orbits are shallow with imperfect roofs which point upward rather than forward. The apices are quite deformed with the optic foramina closed or missing. Extraocular muscles are normal but the nerves are degenerated, and the eyes are small or *microphthalmic.* Fortunately, these deformed children do not survive because the central nervous defects are so great that they are lethal.

Craniofacialdystosis
Craniofacialdystosis is a group of congenital malformations which are produced by premature fusion of one or more of the sutures of the cranial bones. Fusion is usually complete at the 24th year, after the need to permit expansion of the growing brain and central nervous system is completed. Limitation of this expansion consequently produce the following: skull deformity with resultant shortening of the orbits; proptosis; compression of the brain; increased intracranial pressure; papillaedema and optic atrophy; blindness; and death. There may also be thinning and digitation of the bones. There are many terms such as oxycephaly (tower skull), scaphocephaly (scaphoid head), playiocephaly (slanting head), etc. which are descriptive terms without etiological significance.

ACQUIRED ANOMALIES

Displacement
Enophthalmos is the retraction inward of the eyeball, giving the patient's eye a sunken appearance. A fractured orbit with displacement of retrobulbar fat into the maxillary or ethmoid sinuses, starvation, and scarring of orbital contents can all cause enophthalmos. History of recent injury can often be elicited. Diplopia may be

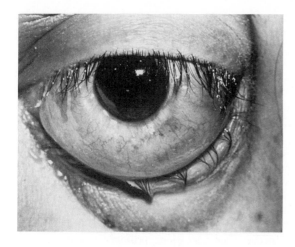

Figure 9–2. Proptosis caused by intracranial lesion.

the patient's chief complaint. Orbital x-rays (Waters' view taken from behind, with the nose and chin resting on the x-ray plate, so that the pyramids are placed down), or CAT scan may be taken to identify the exact cause of the retracted eyeball. Plastic surgical repair might be required in order to correct this problem.

Exophthalmos means abnormal protrusion of the eyeball; a synonym is *proptosis* (Fig. 9–2). These protrusions may be caused by local tumors or by systemic disease, such as disturbance of the thyroid gland.

Orbital edema, the swelling of the orbital contents, is the most striking and severe example and is found in Graves' disease (Fig. 9–3). This disease, caused by an overactive thyroid, has a broad spectrum of activity. There may be moderate involvement of the extraocular muscles which can be demonstrated by CAT scan, with minimal ophthalmological findings.[1,2] The CAT scan has revolutionized and simplified diagnosis of this disease.[3] Treatment, however, remains difficult.

NURSING INTERVENTION
Prednisone 60 mg is given for 3 or 4 weeks, then it is tapered off by about 5 mg/week until a maintenance dose of 20 mg is reached; the dose is cut again by 2.5 mg during the next 2 to 4 weeks until the patient is weaned

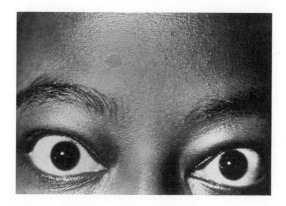

Figure 9–3. Graves' thyroid ophthalmopathy showing bilateral exophthalmus. *(Photograph courtesy Wills Eye Hospital.)*

from the steroid. Treatment results should be seen in the first month after which the patient's condition seems fairly constant.[4,5] Surgical intervention becomes necessary when the degree of swelling is great enough to cause optic nerve compression, and the patient loses vision. Nursing care includes close postoperative monitoring.

Three other conditions that can cause orbital edema are allergic reactions, inflammation, and circulatory disturbance.

Orbital Hemorrhage. *Orbital hemorrhage* is a severe hemorrhage in the closed orbital confines that produces proptosis, forcing the globe forward. Hemorrhage into orbital tissue may be divided into three categories; the (so called) spontaneous hemorrhage seen in hemophilia, scurvy, and anticoagulation therapy. Next, there is a hemorrhage caused by severe straining (as might occur in gymnastics or because of fragile vessels in hypertensives), but by far, the most common cause of orbital hemorrhage is trauma. This can occur after contusion, prolonged labor in the newborn, or penetrating injury. If the hemorrhage is severe enough, the compression can cause closure of the central retinal artery and blindness.

NURSING INTERVENTION
In this type of predicament nursing intervention would be assessment of a visual acuity (if possible)—even if it is only using a flashlight, note the degree of discoloration and/or proptosis; always keep in mind the possibility of a ruptured globe, so handle the ocular area gently. Place ice compresses over the affected eye to halt the hemorrhage and decrease the swelling. Observe for the first sign that compression might be occurring by noting a change in sensorium. Findings should be brought to the attention of an ophthalmologist.

Infection and Inflammation
Periostitis. *Periostitis* is the localization of inflammation or infection in the membrane (periostium) covering the bones of the orbits. The periostium acts as a barrier to inflammation and infection from adjacent structures, i.e., the sinuses. The frontal and maxillary sinuses develop slowly as a child grows; the bones of the medial wall of the orbits (laminae papyracae or paper plate) are thin, and they may even have suture-line dehiscences where mucosa of the sinuses can prolapse into the orbit. In children, the ethmoid sinuses are sites of initial infections, while in adults the paranasal sinuses are implicated.

If the anterior orbital periostium is affected the pain is severe and radiates to the eye and head. There is extreme tenderness on palpation and the tissue is hot. Proptosis is always 180 degrees away from the involved area. When posterior inflammation occurs, the *apex* of the orbit is involved which produces the *orbital apex syndrome*. Conditions such as tumor, trauma, and fracture can produce this syndrome. Altered sensory-motor signs include: globe immobility with internal ophthalmoplegia due to paresis of the III, IV, and VI cranial nerves; anesthesia of the upper lid, side of nose, forehead, temple, conjunctiva, and cornea due to involvement of the first division and part of the second division of the V nerve, and amaurosis due to edema, neuritis, or atrophy of the optic nerve. Treatment of orbital periostitis combines systemic antibiotics with drainage of the infected area.

Osteomyelitis. *Osteomyelitis* can follow orbital periostitis. Fortunately, it is rare; but when it does occur it is very difficult to treat. Antibiotics in massive doses and surgical excision of necrotic bone is necessary.

NURSING INTERVENTION
Nursing intervention includes assessment for early signs and symptoms which may produce the orbital apex syndrome. Encourage compliance with the antibiotic regimen. Monitor vital signs for temperature and sensorium changes. Initiate ocular warm compresses to facilitate drainage of the infected area.

Orbital Cellulitis. *Orbital cellulitis* is inflammatory or infectious involvement of the fatty tissue of the orbit. The clinical picture reveals proptosis, swelling of the lids, chemosis which may be severe enough to cause prolapse of the conjunctiva between the lids, and limitation of movement of the eyeball. The etiology may be from direct trauma such as a penetrating wound or through hematogenous metastatic transmission. Both of these are relatively rare causes. Most commonly, infection is from contiguous areas, sinuses, and the face (by means of venous drainage). Such inflammatory or abscess formation can interfere with the transmission of nerves, resulting in loss of corneal sensitivity, development of keratitis, and even corneal perforation. An acute posterior infection can lead to meningitis or brain abscess with fatal consequences.

NURSING INTERVENTION
Antibiotic therapy is the treatment of choice. Warm compresses are a therapeutic comfort measure and increase the blood supply to the region. If the eye remains exposed it should be protected with a "bubble" shield. Ointment is applied to prevent corneal drying.

Orbital Abscess. An *orbital abscess* is very serious and its seriousness should not be negated. In a recent study of 15 cases, 13 of the patients had radiological evidence of sinus disease with most having more than one sinus involved.[6] Five patients had upper respiratory tract infections; two had chronic sinusitis; and two had dental abscesses which had drained prior to symptoms. Most commonly, *Streptococcus* was the infectious organism. One patient died of osteomyelitis and septicemia and three patients became blind. This condition must be treated vigorously with organism-sensitive antibiotics. Incision and drainage may occasionally be required.

NURSING INTERVENTION
Assess this swollen eye as a serious condition in need of ophthalmological care as soon as possible. Usually the patient is placed on oral systemic antibiotics, and topical antibiotic eyedrops to be instilled following warm compresses. If there is no improvement in the first 24 hours the patient presenting with this condition should return to the ophthalmologist for further evaluation. In severe cases, the patient is admitted into an isolation unit and intravenous antibiotic therapy may be necessary before there is resolution of this acute infection.

Cavernous Sinus Thrombosis. *Cavernous sinus thrombosis* can occur from an orbital thrombophlebitis, with a posterior venous flow from the orbit (central face, throat, and nasal cavities) to the cavernous sinus. Infected areas which drain posteriorly through the orbit into the cavernous sinus can produce this type of disaster. Symptoms include those of the orbital apex syndrome, diminished or absent pupillary reflexes, impaired visual acuity, and papilledema. Lethargy and fever are also evident. Massive doses of systemic antibiotics are given to these patients if they are to survive, and make a good visual recovery.

NURSING INTERVENTION
Assessment of visual acuity and observation of diminished pupillary reflexes should prompt the nurse of the urgency of this condition. Once admitted, nursing care includes monitoring the patient's neurological status and temperature closely for early signs of change in condition. Administer intravenous antibiotics. Ensure that the patient's state of hydration is maintained.

Primary Tumors in the Orbit
Common benign tumors seen early in infant life include:

1. *Choristomas* (dermoid cysts, epidermal cysts, and teratoma), which if they are large, must be excised when they produce cosmetic and functional disfigurement.
2. *Hamartoma* (hemangiomas being the most common tumor in this category), are also seen in early childhood. Treatment of hemangiomas is carried out only if they progress in size or cause deformity. Occasionally, these tumors regress.
3. *Mesenchymal tumors* as a family are varied, interesting, and benign (adipose—lipoma; fibrous—fibroma; myomatous—leiomyoma, rhabdomyoma; cartilaginous—chrondroma; osseous—osteoma.) Osteomas usually do not cause primary problems. They are found on routine roentgenogram and are of little clinical significance, unless they invade from the sinuses. If this happens, they become a problem and require surgical resection.[7]
4. *Neural tumors* (neuroma, neurofibroma, neurilemoma; optic nerve meningioma; optic nerve glioma). Benign neural tumors, because of their close association with the optic nerve and brain, can cause extensive sensory defects, which if overlooked can cause permanent blindness, or even require enucleation.[8]
5. *Epithelial lacrimal gland tumors* may be locally excised in the early stages, but difficulty may arise in making an exact microscopic diagnosis so that the appropriate therapeutic approach can be instituted.[9] If it is malignant, then the tumor should be resected with the part of the orbit which is involved.
6. *Pseudotumors* (lymphoid; chronic sclerosing; plasmacytoid; granulomatous; lipogranulomatosis; fibromatous) can respond to large dose steroid treatment, but may progress with considerable destruction of muscles and nerves before they become arrested.[10,11]
7. *Malignant tumors,* though rare, are serious and in some cases life-threatening. Histological diagnosis should be made so that a block resection is

performed when indicated so as to prevent seeding and recurrence of the tumor in the orbit. Some tumors may be iatrogenic in origin from radiation therapy or radioactive isotopes, e.g., osteosarcoma and rhabdomyosarcoma. However, rhabdomyosarcoma can also be a primary tumor. It is the most common orbital malignancy in children. Combining radiation and chemotherapy in the management of this tumor has been shown to be fairly effective and appears superior to radiation alone. Malignant lesions may first be identified by x-ray, CAT scan, MRI or ultrasound.

Enucleation

NURSING INTERVENTION

There is a need for the nurse to be very supportive to the patient who is about to lose an eye. Many emotions are expressed such as self pity, sadness, denial, and anxiety. Often the patient is devastated at the thought of loss of a body part. In the immediate preoperative period the patient is often uncomfortable, with an eye that may have been causing a lot of trouble for a long time or because of a recent injury. Patients' concerns include anticipated painful surgery; what the site will look like, and how they are going to manage to care for the artificial eye when they receive it. The nurse therefore, will find that she or he has many questions to answer.

At surgery, a plastic *ball implant* covered by the muscles and conjunctiva maintains the contour of the eye's shape, and a plastic *conformer* placed over the conjunctiva maintains the eyelid's integrity while the site is healing over the next 2 to 4 weeks (Fig. 9–4). Postoperatively, the pressure patch over the eye is usually left in place for about 24 hours. Antibiotic or steroid ointment is placed in the cul-de-sac twice a day, until the patient receives the ocular prosthesis. This is made and fitted by an *ocularist,* and the patient may receive the plastic artificial eye, 2 to 6 weeks after enucleation surgery.

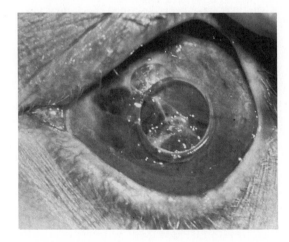

Figure 9–4. Enucleation site with conformer in place.

PATIENT TEACHING

Patient teaching should include the opportunity to inspect the inside of the lower lip, for this is very similar to what the enucleated site will look like. The patient should be taught to instill the ophthalmic drops or ointment correctly. Mucous which collects over the conformer surface may have to be removed by gently irrigating the site. Crying and winking will still be possible, but if the patient had good bilateral vision up to the time of the enucleation he or she will have to learn to judge distances and move the head in a panning fashion to see all around them. The "good" eye should be protected whenever there is any possible hazardous condition.

Inserting a prosthesis is performed as follows:

1. Grasp the prosthesis between the finger and the thumb with the apex pointing toward the nose.
2. Gently insert it under the upper lid and pull down the lower lid.
3. Ask the patient to blink. The artificial eye should then slip into place (Figs. 9–5 A, B, and C).

Removing a prosthesis is performed by gently grasping the prothesis between the finger and thumb of the same hand, slipping the lower lid under the surface of the prosthesis, and pulling. Suction has to be broken before it can be removed. Also available are suction cups which can be placed on the plastic surface, thus facilitating removal (Fig. 9–5D).

Care of a prosthesis: The artificial eye should be washed under running water to be cleaned. Solvents such as alcohol should *never* be used because they destroy the smooth surface.

Exenteration

Care of the exenteration site. This surgical procedure is very extensive, since the orbital contents and the lids are removed. Skin grafting of the orbit may sometimes be done at the time of surgery. The nurse will need to attend to the site from which the skin graft was taken (usually the thigh). The orbit is packed with gauze, which is left undisturbed for 5 to 7 days. The patient may be redressed as an outpatient. It is probably wise to wait until the second dressing before permitting the patient to view the exenteration site. The surgical site may have been described, but actual visualization, and exploration with a glove covered finger may be needed before the patient can come to terms with this disfiguring surgery. Prosthetic devices are not readily available, and therefore the area is usually covered with an eye pad or special dark glasses. Psychological support will be necessary for an extended period of time.

Orbital Injury

Orbital injuries may be divided into soft tissue damage, fracture of the bony orbit, or both.

The orbital contents may be injured by a projectile—bullet, pencils, splinters, knives, or simple contusion. In such conditions hemorrhage, laceration, foreign body retention (Fig. 9–6), and disorganization of the orbital contents can occur followed by infection, abscess formation, hematoma, and necrosis. Treatment should be directed at infection prevention, drainage of abscess and hematoma, and reconstructing the damaged muscles or globe.

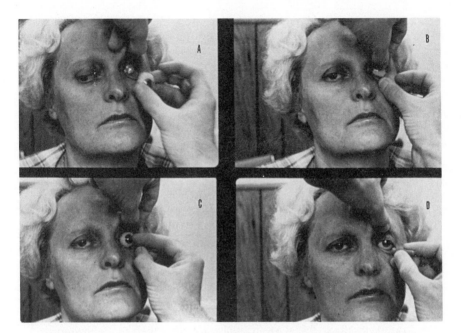

Figure 9–5. Inserting and removing an ocular prosthesis. **A.** Grasp the prosthesis between thumb and finger; **B.** Slide the prosthesis under the upper lid; **C.** When in position have the patient blink and the prosthesis will slip into place. **D.** Removing prosthesis using a suction cup. *(Photographs courtesy Michael Alvin, Philadelphia.)*

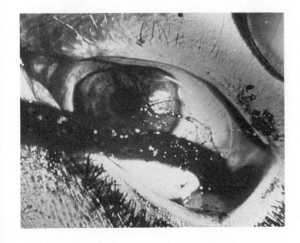

Figure 9–6. Orbital injury due to a rod lodged periorbitally. *(Photograph courtesy Wills Eye Hospital.)*

Fracture of the orbital bones must be diagnosed. If there is leakage of cerebral spinal fluid into the orbit this must be stopped, prophylactic antibiotics must be given, and broken, nonvisible bone must be debrided. Fracture of the paper plate covering the ethmoids must be treated conservatively with antibiotics and nose drops, and the patient should be encouraged not to blow his or her nose or sneeze, otherwise contaminated air from the sinuses will be blown into the orbits, and an orbital abscess formed.

Fracture of the orbital zygoma and temporal as well as facial bones must be repaired surgically.[12]

The most common fracture of the orbit is the blowout fracture of the floor of the orbit caused by a direct blow to the eyeball. Usually the floor gives way and the globe is not smashed. However, if the orbital fat and muscle herniate through the floor into the maxillary sinus they may become trapped, and with muscle entrapment there is restriction in eye movement with resultant double vision[13] (Fig. 9–7).

NURSING INTERVENTION
When assessing the patient the nurse will often elicit a history of trauma. The chief complaint will be pain and diplopia in certain directions of gaze. Orbital swelling and ecchymosis may also be observed. Visual acuity must be obtained. Orbital x-rays will be required. Cold compresses are applied at first, then a switch to warm compresses will facilitate a decrease in swelling. Initial ophthalmologic examination and follow-up at specific intervals should be encouraged. If diplopia persists due to the fracture trapping the inferior rectus muscle, the patient will be scheduled for surgical *repair of orbital floor fracture.*

Postoperatively, the patient will have cold compresses applied to the

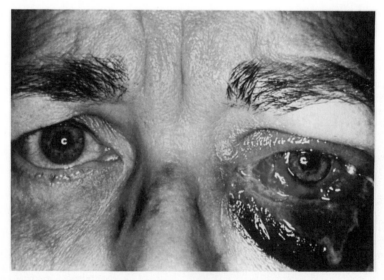

Figure 9–7. Orbital floor fracture as a result of blunt trauma. Double vision was the patient's concern. Note the disparity in the corneal light reflex.

surgical eye at 2- to 4-hour intervals to decrease swelling. A frost suture, taped to the forehead is *in situ* to ensure that the lids are properly closed. The patient's vision is checked prior to leaving the recovery room, and at intervals in the immediate postoperative period. Any complaint of excessive pain should be immediately reported to the physician. Suture removal will be in 5 to 7 days.

Diagnostic Techniques

In 1895, William Konrad Roentgen demonstrated for the first time the imaging of the skeletal system. The next 80 years brought great improvement and sophistication in diagnostic studies, such as *planograms* of the orbits and skull. In 1973, Hounsfield integrated the advanced planogram technique with the computer, and expanded its clinical applications. This has been called *computerized axial tomography* or CAT scanning. With this method of testing, there can be a series of tomograms at different levels and from different angles, which gives different perspectives of the picture. Using this technique, pictures from any angle can be obtained in seconds, and a three-dimensional study is available in minutes.

Another advance in roentgenology is the *Digital Subtraction Angiography*, (DSA). With this method, a skull x-ray is taken, then the circulatory system is injected with an opaque contrast medium after which another x-ray is taken. Then the first x-ray's bright spots are subtracted by computerized DSA technique from corresponding points in the second film, leaving the opaque image clearly seen.

In 1968, *ultrasound* studies were reported. This noninvasive technique uses the reflection of sound waves to record the size and density of tissue structures. This technique has also been computerized, and the body organs can be studied while in motion at the high speed of 30 frames a second.

The most recent experimental instrumentation for diagnostic imaging is *Magnetic Resonance Imaging* (MRI), which is a large powerful magnet which pulses the body or head with a magnetic field. Different types of atoms reemit electromagnetic waves which can be captured on pictures. This is a very new and expensive field which is just beginning to be studied.[14]

Monitoring Exophthalmos. *The Hertel exophthalmometer* is an instrument which is used to monitor degrees of progression or regression of proptosis. The test is performed as follows:

1. Have the patient stand against a wall, directly in front of the examiner.
2. Place the two small concave parts of the exophthalmometer against the lateral orbital margins, and note the bar reading. (This gives the baseline for successive examinations and represents the distance between the lateral orbital walls.)
3. The patient is asked to fix his or her right eye on the examiner's left eye, as the examiner views it in the mirror. The reflection of the cornea is lined up with the reflection on the millimeter scale; the number of millimeters is noted.
4. Repeat the test for the left eye (this time the patient fixes his or her left eye on the examiner's right eye.)
5. Both readings are recorded in millimeters. Typical bar readings are baseline 100 mm—right eye, 16 mm; left eye, 16 mm. Baseline bar readings of

between 12 and 20 are within normal range. Usually the reading is the same for each eye and measures the anterior distance from cornea to lateral margins. When exophthalmos is diagnosed, bar readings may be over 20 mm and/or asymmetric.[15]

REFERENCES

1. van Dyk HJL: A modification of the "NO SPECS" classification. Ophthalmology, 88: 479–483, 1981
2. Lawton NF: Exclusion of dysthyroid eye disease as a cause of unilateral proptosis. Trans Ophthalmol Soc UK: 99(Pt 2): 226, 1979
3. Trokel SL, Hilal SK: Recognition and differential diagnosis of early extraocular muscles in computed tomography. American Journal of Ophthalmology, 87: 503–512, 1979
4. Alpers RC, Oosterhuis JA, Bierloagh JJM: Indications and results of prednisone treatment in thyroid ophthalmopathy. Ophthalmogica, 173: 163–167, 1976
5. Sergott RC, Felberg NT, Savino PS, Blezzard JJ, Schatz NT: Immunological parameters related to corticosteroids therapy. Investigative Ophthalmology, Visual Science, 20: 173–182, 1981
6. Krohel GB, Krauss HR, Winnick J: Orbital abscess, presentation, diagnosis, therapy and sequelae. Ophthalmology 89: 492–498, 1981
7. Blodi FC. Pathologic changes of orbital bone. Trans Am Academy Ophthalmol and Otolaryngol, 81: 26–57, 1976
8. Lloyd GAS: Primary orbital meningiomas. Cl Radiol 33: 181–187, 1982
9. Lloyd GAS: Lacrimal gland tumors: Role of CT and conventional radiology. British Journal of Radiology, 54: 1034–1038, 1981
10. Kleener J: Lymphoma and other lymphoid lesions of the orbit. Acta Ophthalmology 55: 549–560, 1977
11. Young HK, Scian V: Primary orbital lymphomas—Radiotherapeutic experience. Int J Radiol and Oncol Biol Physics, 1: 1099–1105, 1978
12. Serres P: Systematization of primary treatment of orbital fractures—Part 1. General principals, approach, methods of reduction and complications. Ann Oculo, 210: 727–750, 1977
13. Putterman AM: Late management of blowout fractures of the orbital floor. Trans Am Academy Ophthalmol and Otolaryngol, 83: 650–659, 1977
14. Fincher J: New machines may soon replace the doctor's black bag. Smithsonian, 14(10): 64–71, 1984
15. Vaughan D, Asbury T. General Ophthalmology, 10th ed. Los Altos, Calif.: Lange, 1983, p. 25–26

10

The Lacrimal System

NEW TERMS

Dacryoadenitis: inflammation of the lacrimal gland.

Dacryocystitis: infection of the lacrimal sac.

Dacryocystorhinostomy: surgical procedure to correct blockage of the lacrimal sac by making a new opening above the inferior meatus of the turbinate bone.

Epiphora: tearing.

Lacrimal irrigation: probing and irrigation of the lacrimal duct.

Probing: dilation of the lacrimal puncta, canaliculi and duct.

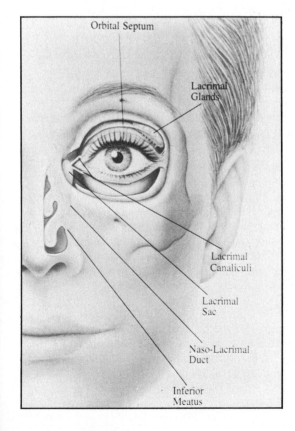

10-1. The lacrimal system. *(From Friedman AL, Desmarest RJ, Westwood WB: Optyl Atlas of the Human Eye. Norwood, N.J.: Optyl, 1979, with permission.)*

139

The lacrimal system is a complete system in itself (Fig. 10–1). The secretory *lacrimal glands* are situated temporally in a fossa located in the frontal bone and behind the superior orbital rim. Tears flow through several *excretory ducts* into the superior temporal fornix of the conjunctiva. Each time a person blinks, tears are washed across the surface of the eye and flow to the *inner canthus* where they pool.

Parasympathetic nerve fibers reach the gland through the facial nerve, and supply the secretory fibers. The sympathetic nerve supply is from the cervical sympathetic, through the carotid plexis.[1]

The drainage portion of the system consists of *lacrimal puncta,* two minute openings through which the tears drain. One punctum is in the upper lid and the other is in the lower lid. The lower lid punctum is angled slightly backwards to the pool of tears. The tears then flow into the *canaliculi,* which join to form the common canaliculus, and then enter the *lacrimal sac,* (or nasolacrimal sac as it is sometimes called). The sac elongates to become the *nasolacrimal duct,* with its openings at the *inferior meatus of the turbinate bone.* Tears drain through this system and then into the nasopharynx.

Tears are secreted by reflex when the lacrimal gland branch of the trigeminal nerve is stimulated by corneal irritation. This reflex action is absent when corneal anesthesia is present.

LACRIMAL GLAND

Congenital Abnormalities

Aberrant lacrimal gland tissue may appear anywhere under the conjunctiva and cornea and may be identified as congenital lacrimal gland cysts, dermoid cysts, or dermolipomas. Biopsy will be necessary to establish histological differentiation from malignancies. Treatment will be surgical excision of the aberrant tissue.

NURSING INTERVENTION
After surgical excision has been accomplished, the eye will be pressure patched for a period of at least 24 hours to control bleeding and decrease swelling. The nurse should observe the site for any signs of bleeding during this period. Cold compresses might be applied to decrease swelling. After removal of the pressure patch, ophthalmic antibiotic ointment, ordered for the suture line, should be applied as requested. Discharge planning should include compliance with outpatient follow-up appointment for suture removal in 5 to 7 days.

Acquired Abnormalities

Acute dacryoadenitis, an inflammation of the lacrimal gland, is a rare unilateral condition which may be seen in children as a complication of mumps, influenza, and other viral infections. It has been known to occur in adults in association with gonorrhea.[2]

NURSING INTERVENTION
Encourage compliance with treatment of underlying cause, which when treated should result in subsidence of this acute inflammatory or infectious process.

LACRIMAL DUCTS

Congenital Abnormalities
During the first few weeks of life, a neonate does not produce tears. When a mother notices that her child is continually tearing, she may become concerned. A chronically tearing eye must be differentiated from the initial stages of congenital glaucoma, and tonometric measurements under anesthesia should be performed if there is any doubt.

Blocked Tear Ducts. Occasionally, a mother notices a mucopurulent discharge in the inner canthus of one or both of her baby's eyes. This is because there is a blockage in the nasolacrimal duct. The discharge may be sufficient to mat the eyelashes, and if a little pressure is applied to the skin over the nasolacrimal sac, a small amount of discharge may exude from the puncta. Persistent tearing may become a problem. Usually the nostril on the affected side is dry. Digital massage of the lacrimal sac area may be prescribed; this is often successful in opening up the ducts. Chemotherapeutic agents or antibiotics might be prescribed for topical administration if there is a secondary conjunctivitis.

If the obstruction persists, as evidenced by continual tearing, *probing and irrigation* of the nasolacrimal duct will be necessary. The procedure should be performed under general anesthesia. However, the age at which a child will be given anesthesia for this procedure depends entirely upon the policies of the anesthesia department, but the procedure is often undertaken when the child reaches about 6 to 8 months of age.[3]

When probing is indicated, the ophthalmologist first attempts to dilate the puncta with a dilator and follows with a lacrimal probe, then irrigates through the lower canaliculus with a fluorescein-stained saline solution using a lacrimal cannula and 2-cc syringe (Fig. 10–2). The hydrostatic pressure may be sufficient to overcome a membranous valve-like obstruction. An applicator or small catheter is placed in the baby's nose to retrieve the solution.[3]

If the solution does not gain entrance to the inferior meatus when the upper punctum is occluded, a single, O Bowman probe is inserted into the upper punctum and is passed vertically for approximately 2 mm along the canaliculus.[3] After removal, irrigation through the lower punctum is repeated. Usually, this is successful in opening the ducts. However, occasionally it is not, and further surgery may be contemplated.

NURSING INTERVENTION
Show the mother how to use her index finger to massage over the baby's lacrimal sac area. In order to encourage compliance, suggest that she do this each time she feeds the baby, and continue doing this for 2 or 3

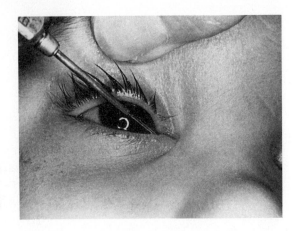

Figure 10–2. Irrigating through the lower canaliculus with a fluorescein-stained saline solution using a lacrimal cannula and 2-cc syringe.

months. The digital massage often is enough to facilitate opening the tear ducts.

The adult patient with blocked tear ducts may have a lacrimal irrigation procedure performed in the office. In this case, the nurse will anesthetize the eye using topical anesthetic drops. The patient is asked to keep the head still as it rests against the headrest, while a lacrimal probe is used to dilate the puncta. Next the lacrimal cannula is inserted into the lower canaliculus. The 2-cc syringe with fluorescein-stained saline solution is attached to the cannula. The lacrimal duct is gently irrigated. If it is patent, the patient will taste the solution in the back of the throat, and will clear it and want to spit. Remember to have tissues or an emesis basin handy for this purpose. Record the procedure, stating which eye was irrigated, and whether the lacrimal duct was patent (irrigation successful) or not patent (irrigation solution did not get into the "back of the throat").

Acquired Abnormalities

Dacryocystitis. *Dacryocystitis,* an infection of the lacrimal sac, is a common acute or chronic disease which usually affects infants or persons over the age of 40. In the intermediate group, it may occur as a result of trauma or fungal infection. Most often it is unilateral, but its occurrence is always secondary to obstruction of the nasolacrimal duct.

Acute Dacryocystitis. In acute dacryocystitis, *Staphylococcus aureus,* or occasionally *Beta-hemolytic streptococcus* are the usual infectious agents identified on smear and culture.[2] The chief symptoms are tearing and discharge from the affected eye, but in an acute episode, inflammation, pain, swelling, and tenderness over the sac area are present. Light pressure applied over the nasolacrimal area will result in mucopurulent material being expressed from the tear sac. If dacryocystitis is left untreated, perforation of the skin and fistula formation may occur. General orbital cellulitis may also result (Fig. 10–3).

Lacrimal probing may be attempted in the adult patient in an effort to help relieve the tremendous pressure which builds up in the lacrimal sac. This is only

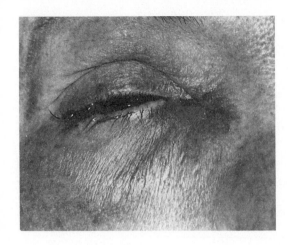

Figure   10–3. Acute   dacryo-cystitis. *(Photograph courtesy of Wills Eye Hospital.)*

occasionally helpful. If the dacryocystitis looks as if it is pointing over the nasolacrimal area, surgical incision and drainage (I & D) may be necessary.[3,4]

NURSING INTERVENTION

Assess the patient who presents with acute pain, swelling, discharge, and inflammation over the nasolacrimal sac area. Inquire as to the duration of the problem. Check, then document, the patient's visual acuity. Before reviewing the antibiotic prescriptions with the patient or parents, ensure that smear, culture, and sensitivity will be done.

If probing of the lacrimal canaliculus is to be done on the adult, assist as necessary by instilling the anesthetic eyedrop and dilating the puncta if protocol permits. It is easier if there is already a sterile tray set up (Fig. 10–4). The incision and drainage which is to be performed on a child with an acute dacryocystitis will be a "dirty case" in the operating room.

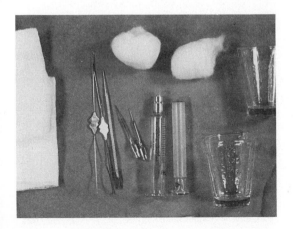

Figure 10–4. Lacrimal irrigation tray. *(Photograph courtesy of Wills Eye Hospital.)*

PATIENT TEACHING

The patient with acute dacryocystitis should be instructed on the correct method of applying warm compresses before instilling the antibiotic eye-drops. Compliance with oral antibiotics (for their full duration) should be encouraged. Patients with dacryocystitis should be cautioned that if the ocular area appears to be getting worse over the next 24 hours they should immediately return to see the ophthalmologist for further evaluation which could include hospitalization for intravenous antibiotic therapy.

Chronic Dacryocystitis. Chronic dacryocystitis is often found to be caused by *Streptococcus pneumoniae.*[4] The patient who has constant tearing as a result of dacryostenosis (narrowing and blockage of the nasolacrimal duct) may elect to have a *surgical dacryocystorhinostomy (DCR)* (Fig. 10–5) to correct this. The nursing assessment should include questions relating to anticoagulant medications, which the patient might be taking. Hematology tests need to be ordered to monitor specific medications as follows:

1. *Heparin* should be stopped 4 to 6 hours preoperatively and a *partial thromboplastin time* (PTT) ordered.
2. *Coumadin* should be stopped 4 days preoperatively and a *prothrombin time* (PT) ordered.
3. Aspirin and aspirin compounds, e.g., Bufferin, Anacin, etc., should be stopped 10 days preoperatively and a *bleeding time* (BT) ordered;
4. *Nonsteroidal, antiinflammatory agents, e.g., Indocin, Motrin, etc.,* should be stopped 4 days preoperatively and a BT ordered.[5]

The DCR procedure is usually performed under general anesthesia. The patient will therefore need appropriate sedation and should have nothing by mouth for a period of at least 6 hours prior to surgery.

NURSING INTERVENTION

The patient should be made aware that in the immediate postoperative period following a DCR procedure, there may be some blood oozing from the nose. This will range from bright red to serosanguineous discharge, even though packing is in place. The "drip" position can be used to

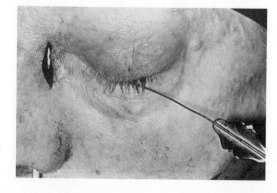

Figure 10–5. Surgical dacryocystorhinostomy, showing incision, lacrimal probe into canaliculus, and lacrimal sac; and probe in nose. *(Photograph courtesy of Wills Eye Hospital.)*

prevent the swallowing of blood. Here the patient lies on the operative side until the bleeding has stopped (maximum of 24 hours, otherwise he or she will develop a crick in the neck). Ice compresses, placed over the pressure patch immediately after surgery, will help to stem the flow of blood.

In about 10 percent of patients the nostril on the surgical side will be packed with ½-inch ribbon gauze. This together with the pressure patch (which covered the eye) will be removed after 24 hours. (A Bandaid may be placed over the small lacrimal incision site if the patient wears glasses). The patient will be assessed at the time the packing is removed, and continuously during the following 24-hour period for any acute bleeding. An acute episode of bleeding—a rare complication of the DCR procedure—will necessitate prompt *medical* intervention. The nose will require repacking with adrenaline saturated gauze. An emergency ENT tray should be kept available, wherever this procedure is performed. Because of this factor, no anticoagulants will be given during the immediate 48-hour postoperative period.

PATIENT TEACHING
The patient is advised not to consume hot beverages for the first 3 postoperative days. The patient should also be advised not to blow the nose for 1 week, to prevent possible bleeding until healing can take place. Afrin Nasal Spray will be prescribed for use twice daily for 1 week. It is suggested that alcohol intake be limited for 2 weeks after discharge from hospital, as alcohol dilates the blood vessels.[5]

Discharge from the hospital will be in 48 to 72 hours postoperatively. A lacrimal sac irrigation may be performed in the ophthalmologist's office. Skin suture removal will be done 5 to 7 days after the surgery as an office procedure.

Trauma
Lacerated Canaliculus. Trauma to the canaliculus may occur in children as a result of a dog bite, a poke in the eye with a stick, or during a fight; or a sporting activity for young adults (Fig. 10–6). When this injury involves the lower canaliculus, it should be repaired as a primary procedure. Failure to do this will result in scarring down of the cut ends (of the canaliculus), and may eventually lead to a much more extensive surgical procedure such as a DCR with glass tube implant.

Surgical repair is accomplished by running a 6-0 black silk or nylon suture through the canaliculi, to keep these ducts patent. The ends of the suture are then taped onto the cheek.[3] Another method used is threading a loop of Silastic through both puncta and bringing it out into the sac or even carrying it down into the nose.[4]

NURSING INTERVENTION
The emergency room triage nurse should be aware that this minute laceration should be treated as an ocular emergency, and will need early surgical intervention, if the patency of the canaliculus is to be maintained. The patient should be treated accordingly, and kept NPO (nothing by mouth) until surgery can be arranged.

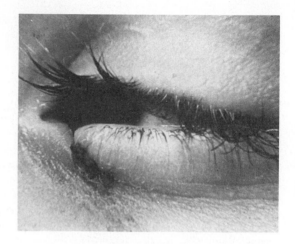

Figure 10–6. Lacerated canaliculus.

PATIENT TEACHING

After the surgical procedure is completed, the patient will be discharged from the hospital, and should understand that the suture or tubing is not to be disturbed for an extended period of time. Compliance with follow-up care by the ophthalmologist should be encouraged, for the suture or tubing will be removed at a later date.

TEARS

The tears essentially form a three-layer meniscus. The outermost *lipid layer* is produced by the Meibomian glands of the lid. The *aqueous layer,* secreted by the main and accessory lacrimal glands, constitutes over 90 percent of the tear film's thickness. The innermost layer of the tear film consists of *mucin,* the product of scattered conjunctival goblet cells.[6]

The tear film covers exposed corneal and conjunctival surfaces of the eye and serves a multitude of purposes. It functions as the anterior refractive surface of the eye, smooths corneal surface irregularities so as to present a suitable anterior surface refraction, and is important for maintaining the corneal and conjunctival epithelium in its normal state.

Tears act as a lubricant for lid movement; they contain antibacterial substances which protect this external surface against infection, i.e., lysozyme and B-lysin, as well as dissolved oxygen, which is necessary for normal corneal epithelium respiration.[6] Tear deficiencies, therefore, can be found to involve any of the three layers.

AQUEOUS DEFICIENCY

Congenital Abnormality

Alacrima, the absence of the secretion of tears, may be present because of the absence of the lacrimal gland. It is usually bilateral, and tears are not shed from birth on. The eyes are irritated and photophobic. Corneal scarring and vasculariza-tion usually result. Treatment ranges from conservative measures such as the fre-quent use of artificial tears to more radical measures, e.g., occlusion of the lacrimal punctum (diathermy and laser are both used for this) to partial tarsorrhaphy, (sutur-ing the eyelids together).

NURSING INTERVENTION
Encourage compliance with frequent instillation of artificial tears (eyedrops).

Acquired Abnormalities
Keratoconjunctivitis Sicca. Keratoconjunctivitis sicca (KCS) constitutes those conditions in which there is either an absolute or partial deficiency in aqueous tear production. Although KCS may occur in males and younger women, aqueous deficiency is more common in females in the 5th and 6th decades of life. (It is predominantly a disorder of menopausal and postmenopausal women.) The disease is bilateral, with insidious onset, and characteristic fluctuations in intensity. Symp-toms include scratchiness, burning, and foreign body sensation. On Slitlamp exam-ination, signs of increased debris in the conjunctival cul-de-sac can be seen. More severe forms of KCS progress to the formation of corneal filaments, and the sharing action created by the lid motion pulls on these filaments causing pain.[7]

There are several systemic diseases associated with KCS, including rheu-matoid arthritis, systemic lupus erythematosus, scleraderma, and Sjögren's syn-drome, as well as dry eyes.

It is also important to remember that in KCS infections occur because the host defense mechanism is compromised. When the classic triad of dry eyes, dry mouth, and arthritis are seen, this is referred to as Sjögren's syndrome.

Decreased tear production can occur after seventh nerve paresis, viral dacryoa-denitis, mechanical trauma, surgical removal of the lacrimal glands, irradiation to the eye, and following chemical burns to the eye.[7]

Two diagnostic tests for dry eyes include the Schirmer test, and staining the eyes with rose bengal, a dye which specifically stains devitalized epithelium and mucin.

MUCIN DEFICIENCY

The bulk of mucin is produced by the goblet cells of the conjunctiva. Mucin is necessary if the tear film is to cover the cornea and conjunctiva adequately, and vitamin A seems to be necessary for its production. In vitamin A-deficiency, the tear film forms with difficulty over these structures. Vitamin A-deficiency may also be due to lack of protein which binds vitamin A. Bitot spots (drying of the cornea) may be seen, and later keratomalacia (noninflammatory melting of the cornea) may occur.

Other conditions which destroy conjunctival architecture, and thereby damage the mucin cells include: phemphigoid (where keratinization of the conjunctival and corneal epithelium occurs), Stevens-Johnson's syndrome (which occurs as a result of drug ingestion), trachoma, and chemical burns.

LIPID ABNORMALITIES

The superficial lipid layer is derived from the secretions of the Meibomian glands and retards evaporation of the aqueous layer. It stands to reason then that pathology such as chronic blepharitis of the lids, exposure keratitis due to seventh nerve paresis, and exophthalmos, as a result of thyroid eye disease can lead to lid-surfacing abnormalities resulting in dry eyes.

Restricted lid movement resultant from symblepharon (which occur in ocular phemphigoid and after chemical burns) and lagophthalmos (occuring at night, in the comatose patient, or as a result of lid trauma) can be contributing factors to lipid abnormalities and consequently dry eyes.

NURSING INTERVENTION
Assess the patient for symptoms of excessive irritation, bulbar conjunctival hyperemia (redness), and pain which might be worse toward the evening.[2] Note any associated alteration in health status such as pregnancy, or systemic disease such as arthritis and inquire if medications are being taken for it. Check, then document the visual acuity of the patient who presents with these "dry eye" symptoms. The ophthalmologist, after Slitlamp examination, will request that a Schirmer Test be performed for anyone suspected of having decreased tear production, for whatever reason.

Schirmer Tear Tests
The Schirmer I tear test is a screening test for the assessment of tear production, and to find out if the cornea is being adequately wetted. The test offers a gross measurement of the quantity of tear film in the conjunctival sac. The Schirmer test (on both eyes), performed without topical anesthesia, measures the function of the lacrimal gland; the irritating nature of the filter paper stimulates the secretory activity of the gland. Schirmer II tear tests performed after instillation of the topical anesthetic measure the function of the accessory glands.

1. Standardized sterile strips are used for the test, and while the plastic packet containing these strips is still sealed, bend the rounded end of the test strip at the indentation. The opposite end of the package is then cut and the two strips removed without contamination.
2. Seat the patient so that the head rests against a head rest or the wall. Warn that the test may be annoying, but will not hurt, and that it is being performed on each eye to measure the amount of tears being produced by the glands which lubricate the eyes.
3. Now ask the patient to look up and draw the lower eyelid gently downward. Hook the rounded bent end of the sterile strip over the eyelid border at the junction of the middle and nasal one-third of the lower eyelid margin (Fig. 10–7). Note the time that the strips are placed in position, and ask the patient to keep the eyes closed during the procedure. Ensure that the patient does not wipe the eyes while the strips are in place.
4. After 5 minutes, remove the strips and measure the length of the moistened

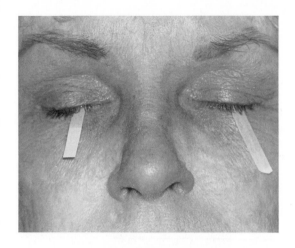

Figure 10–7. Schirmer test strips in place, showing different wetting pattern.

area (against the envelope with the measurement diagram of the strip and millimeter scale printed on it). Measure only from the indentation. Document the results on the patient's chart as follows: The eye; number of millimeters wetted (on the strip) in 5 minutes, e.g., O.D. 10/5 mins.: O.S. 15/5 mins.

5. Evaluation of the results should be assessed in the light of the fact that a measurement of 15 mm (length of the moistened area from the bend) in each eye is regarded as a normal standard for tear production. After 40 years of age, normal values may vary between 10 and 15 mm. If the whole strip is moist, record this as well.

6. Carefully performed Schirmer tests will often reveal a lowered secretion of tears which could be caused by several ocular complaints. Measurement below 10 mm in either eye should be given careful consideration, for in the majority of patients true dysfunction of tear production can be revealed, although false–negative results can occur.[2]

After the tests and examination have confirmed that the patient has dry eyes, the ophthalmologist will prescribe tear supplements. Since the goal of these is to increase the retention time of the tears, this is done by the addition of various cellulose esters which increase the viscosity of the solution, even so, the artificial tears dissipate in 30 to 45 minutes (so the patient must instill eyedrops every 1 to 2 hours during the day and perhaps ointment at night). Patching the eye at night might also be suggested for preservation of existing tears. Preservation of the moist surface of the eye in a patient with exophthalmos might be achieved by using a bubble-eye shield. (Fig. 10–8). Taping the lids of the comatose patient shut will prevent exposure keratitis.

Lacriserts[8], (amethylcellulose pellet) placed in the cul-de-sac might help the condition in some patients, however, topical all-trans retinoic acid (0.01 percent vitamin A ointment), a new orphan drug, is being investigated for use in some patients in which all other treatment modalities have been unsuccessful.[9]

The nutritional status of the patient should also be a nursing concern. It might be appropriate to review a list of foods containing vitamin A.

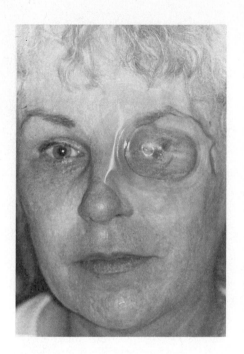

Figure 10–8. Bubble-eye shield.

PATIENT TEACHING
This should include the correct method of instilling eye medications and the correct way to patch the eyes if necessary. Compliance with prescribed treatment should be encouraged. These patients are constantly seeking out the ophthalmologist during the acute episodes and very often management is difficult, and can only be supportive in nature.

LACRIMAL HYPERSECRETION

Excessive lacrimation is normally associated with pain or emotional upset. Neurogenic lacrimation is brought about by reflex stimulation as a result of corneal injury, foreign body, hot air blast, dry wind, or visual irritation.[2]

Epiphora may result from blockage of the tear ducts, or in infants it can be an early symptom of glaucoma.

NURSING INTERVENTION
Assess the patient for possible external causes, and if none can be found refer the patient to an ophthalmologist as appropriate.

REFERENCES

1. Wright WW, (Ed.): The Eye in Childhood. Chicago: Year Book Medical, 1967, p. 129
2. Vaughan D, Asbury T: General Ophthalmology, 10th ed. Los Altos, Calif.: Lange, 1983, p. 43–51
3. Flanagan JC, Mclachlan DL, Shannon CM: Diseases of the Lacrimal Apparatus, in Harley RD, (Ed.): Pediatric Ophthalmology, 2nd ed. Philadelphia: Saunders, 1983, p. 396–411
4. Iliff CE, Iliff WJ, Iliff TN: Oculoplastic Surgery. Philadelphia: Saunders, 1979, p. 171–191
5. Flanagan JC, Boyd-Monk H: The lacrimal excretory system: Treatment of the adult patient. J Ophth Nurs and Techn, 2(4): 163–166, 1983
6. Lemp MA: Diagnosis and treatment of tear deficiencies, in Duane TD, (Ed.): Clinical Ophthalmology, 4(12): 1–9, 1978
7. Alcon Laboratories, Inc., Schirmer Tear Test (package insert). Fortworth, Texas. 1984
8. Jeglum EL: Ocular therapeutics, in Boyd-Monk H, (Ed.): Nursing Clinics of North America, 16(3): 453–477, 1981
9. Scheffer CGT, Maumenee AE, Stark WJ, et al.: Topical retinoid treatment for various dry-eye disorders. Ophthalmology, 92(6): 717–727, 1985

BIBLIOGRAPHY

Boyd-Monk H: Vitamin A deficiency and associated eye disease. J Ophth Nurs and Techn, 2(4): 159–162, 1983

11

The Eyelids

NEW TERMS

Blepharo: Greek root: Blepharon = eyelid.
Lagophthalmos: inadequate closure of the eyelids.
Palpebral: pertaining to the eyelids.
Trichiasis: turning inward of the lashes so that they rub on the cornea.

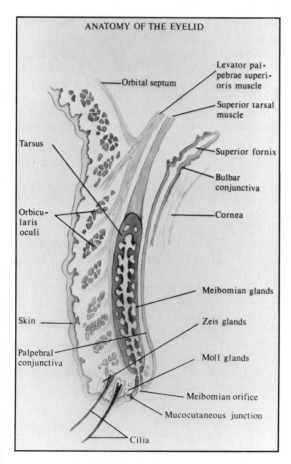

ANATOMY OF THE EYELID

Levator palpebrae superioris muscle

Orbital septum

Superior tarsal muscle

Superior fornix

Bulbar conjunctiva

Tarsus

Cornea

Orbicularis oculi

Meibomian glands

Zeis glands

Skin

Moll glands

Palpebral conjunctiva

Meibomian orifice

Mucocutaneous junction

Cilia

11–1. Anatomy of the eyelid. *(Reproduced from Hospital Medicine, April 1982, with permission of Hospital Publications, Inc., 18(4): 120.)*

The eyelids are movable folds of tissue that cover and protect the orbital structures and are constructed of very loose skin containing much elastic tissue and the fibrous *tarsal plates,* which maintain the lid shape (Fig. 11–1). *Palpebral conjunctiva* lines the lids posteriorly and fuses medially and laterally at the inner and outer canthus to become palpebral tendons. These ligaments attach to the orbital bones. The *palpebral aperture* or *fissure,* is the name given to the space between the upper and lower eyelids.

A barrier, created between lids and orbit by fascia, is called the *orbital septum.* Anterior to this, is the roughly circular *orbicularis oculi muscle* which is responsible for closing the eyes shut and is innervated by the seventh cranial nerve (facial nerve). The *levator palpebrae muscle* inserts into the tarsal plate and is innervated by the third cranial nerve (occulomotor) to elevate the upper lid. An extremely small *Müllers muscle,* originating in the upper lid's levator palpebrae muscle, is also attached to the tarsal plate but is supplied by sympathetic nerves.

Three types of glands are found in the eyelids. The long sebaceous *Meibomian glands,* located in the tarsal plates, secrete an oily layer onto the surface of the tear film. This secretion seals the lid margins together during sleep preventing tear evaporation. There are about 25 of these glands in the upper lid and about 20 in the lower lid. Small, modified sebaceous *glands of Zeis* are connected to the follicles of the eyelashes, while the sweat *glands of Moll,* are unbranched sinuous tubules.

A landmark at both the upper and lower lid margins is referred to as the *gray line.* An incision along this line can split the lid into two portions; the anterior section containing skin, hair follicles, and orbicularis oculi muscle, and the posterior portion containing the tarsal plate and palpebral conjunctiva.

The lids have a well-endowed blood supply derived mainly from the ophthalmic and lacrimal arteries. Lymphatic drainage is by way of preauricular, parotid, and submaxillary lymph glands.

Congenital Abnormalities

Coloboma, a congenital lid defect, can range from a small lid margin indentation, to involvement of the entire lid. The coloboma may be single or multiple, i.e., in one, two, three, or all lids, and the defect may include skin, tarsal plates and conjunctiva, or any combination of tissue. Lesions which may be associated with coloboma are dermoid growths, corneal opacities, coloboma of the iris, lipodermoids of the caruncle, and many other facial abnormalities.[1] Surgical repair is considered when the abnormality may lead to corneal damage through exposure.

NURSING INTERVENTION
Shield the eye with a plastic or metal eyeshield to ensure that the suture line is not disrupted in the immediate postoperative period. Apply ophthalmic ointment which may be prescribed for the suture line. Encourage compliance with any medication regimen, and also with ophthalmologic follow-up care.

Epicanthus. *Epicanthus* (Fig. 11–2) is a semilunar fold of skin seen in the inner canthus, which runs down the side of the nose with the curve directed to the nose. These folds usually occur in both eyes, and vary in height and width. The deformity gives the face a Mongolian appearance. Epicanthus gives the appearance of apparent squint. This can be made to disappear by pinching up the skin over the bridge of the nose into a fold. Simple epicanthus may be transmitted as an inherited dominant characteristic.[2] It is also found frequently in association with Down's syndrome. Plastic surgical correction may be necessary in some severe instances of epicanthus.

NURSING INTERVENTION
Remember, if a squint is suspected in the child with epicanthal folds, perform the corneal light reflex test to assess if a true or pseudostrabismus is present. Refer the child for further evaluation.

PTOSIS

Ptosis is a drooping of and an inability to raise the upper lid; congenital ptosis occurs in various forms. There may be a simple ptosis in which only the lids are affected. This is due to an hereditary dominant failure of the levator muscle to form.[3] In simple congenital ptosis 71 percent are unilateral and 29 percent are bilateral. Complicated cases have other structural involvement, including paralysis of the superior rectus muscle, epicanthal fold, blepharophymosis, external ophthalmoplegia, synkinetic ptosis, and sympathetic palsy. Ptosis is transmitted as a dominant trait and seems to eventually manifest in other associated deformities in succeeding generations.[4]

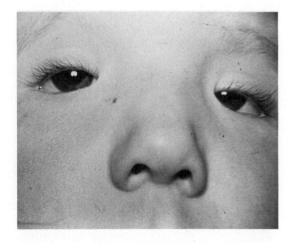

Figure 11–2. Epicanthus is a semilunar fold of skin seen in the inner canthus.

Acquired Abnormalities

Acquired ptosis must be diagnosed and treated. Four groups may be considered:

1. *Neurogenic* (paralytic). Here there is interference with the pathways of a portion of the third cranial nerve supplying the levator muscle of the eyelid (Fig. 11–3).[5]
2. *Myogenic* factors associated with such diseases as muscular dystrophy and myasthenia gravis. Ptosis of one or both lids is often the first sign of myasthenia gravis which is essentially a defect in the humoral transmission at the myoneural junction.[5]
3. *Traumatic* factors.
4. Mechanical factors which include symptoms such as abnormal weight of the lids which prevents the levator muscle from elevating the lids normally; acute or chronic edema or swelling; tumor or extra fatty material.

Some cases of ptosis may be caused by more than one of these four categories occurring at the same time. Even patients having a very slight ptosis may have a visual problem. Because the possibility of ptosis being caused by myasthenia gravis exists even in children, a Tensilon test is usually performed to rule out this disease. Depending upon the cause of the ptosis, plastic surgical intervention may be undertaken to correct the lid abnormality.

NURSING INTERVENTION

When assessing a patient presenting with the symptom of ptosis, the nurse should establish when it occurred. Find out if it is more pronounced at the end of the day. Question if there is a visual problem associated with the drooping eyelid. Further medical investigation is necessary for a newly acquired ptosis.

After surgical correction for ptosis is undertaken, the nurse should ensure that the Frost suture (if one is in place in the lower lid) is not disturbed. No postoperative patch will cover the lid. Ice compresses will be applied to decrease swelling. Ophthalmic antibiotic/steroid combina-

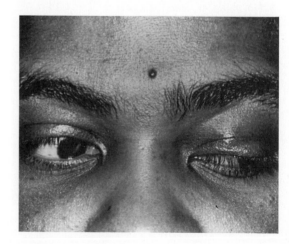

Figure 11–3. Acquired ptosis due to interference with the pathway of the (oculomotor) III cranial nerve. *(Photograph courtesy of Wills Eye Hospital.)*

tion ointment may be prescribed every 3 hours to prevent corneal drying. A plastic or metal shield may be applied to prevent accidental bumping of the site.

PATIENT TEACHING
Patient teaching should include the correct procedure, placement, and frequency of ointment application, shielding the eye as necessary, and compliance with oculoplastic follow-up care by the ophthalmologist who performed the surgery.

Blepharitis. *Blepharitis* is an inflammation of the eyelids and is most commonly of the seborreaic type. Lid margins appear red, irritated, and with waxy scales which cling to the base of the lashes. Ulcers may occur in an infectious blepharitis, and in this case *Staphylococcus aureus* is found to be the causitive agent.[6] Patchy loss of lashes or even trichiasis may also occur. When this condition occurs in children, it can run a chronic course. There can be an associated conjunctivitis and occasionally corneal involvement may occur (keratitis).

NURSING INTERVENTION
The patient should be taught to perform lid hygiene. This should be accomplished morning and evening using a Q-tip and mild baby shampoo, followed by warm compresses. Local antibiotics, prescribed by the ophthalmologist, may be used to circumvent the chronic stage if infection is present. Compliance should be encouraged.

Blepharospasms. *Blepharospasms* are spasmodic tonic contractions of the eyelids. Their etiology may be *functional*—which can be a habit or psychogenic in nature; *organic*—following encephalitis or irritation of the trigeminal nerve and disappearing with the complete destruction of the trigeminal nerve; or *secondary*—blepharospastic reflex occurring after irritation of cornea, conjunctiva, and other structures of the eye and is frequently associated with lacrimation, photophobia, and sneezing.[6]

Treatment of blepharospasm can be medical, psychiatric, or surgical, depending upon the etiology. Severe, incapacitating, chronic blepharospasm may require surgical intervention which is devised to destroy the branches of the facial nerve. One such procedure is the differential sectioning of the seventh nerve.[7] In one study this procedure rehabilitated 75 percent of the patients without significant spasm, however, some patients needed two operations. Complications or side reaction from the differential sectioning include ectropion, severe enough to need surgical correction; epiphoria (tearing) which subsides in a small percentage of patients; moderate lagophthalmos which does not clear spontaneously; exposure keratitis, paresis of the upper lid, and parotid fistula has also been known to occur occasionally. Another surgical procedure is lateral pericutaneous fractional thermolytic destruction of the facial nerve branches which is performed under local anesthesia. Minimal complications such as slight corneal irritation without sequelae may occur.[8] Recently at our institution experimental Botulina toxin has been used to paralyze and weaken the muscle contraction, however, this is only a temporary measure.

NURSING INTERVENTION

Nursing intervention should include an understanding of what might cause the blepharospasm, for example, a patient receiving eyedrops may develop blepharospasm at the thought of something being put into the eye. This can be eliminated by asking the patient to look up with both eyes while putting the drop in the cul-de-sac. If the patient does not see the bottle tip coming toward the eye, reflex blepharospasm can be eliminated. However, the nurse should also be aware of the other causes of blepharospasm, and refer the patient accordingly.

Surgery will be performed under a sterile field, and a sterile dressing will cover the incision site postoperatively. This will be removed after 24 hours, but during this period the patch should be observed to be secure and blood free.

Blepharochalasis. *Blepharochalasis* is atrophy and relaxation of the tissues of the upper lids. It may be a hereditary trait and appear as a congenital or juvenile problem, however, it is transmitted as a dominant autosomal characteristic. It was first reported in the literature in 1836 by Graf with numerous families of five or more generations being identified. The congenital variety can be associated with spasmodic entropion of the lower lid, and also with cleft upper lip and goiter (Ascher's syndrome). The condition manifests itself before puberty with one-third of the patients showing signs before 10 years of age. This type usually starts with lid edema, which leads to looseness of the skin with constant bagginess and wrinkling of the skin. Progressive atrophy of the skin enables the orbital fat to protrude forward and downward into the loose skin. This problem is frequently confused with the aging process called *dermatochalasis* (Fig. 11–4) which occurs much later in life.

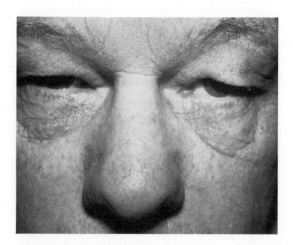

Figure 11–4. Dermatochalasis. *(Photograph courtesy of Wills Eye Hospital.)*

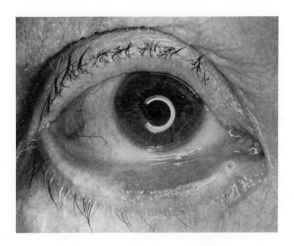

Figure 11–5. Ectropion—eversion or outward turning of the lower eyelid. *(Photograph courtesy of Wills Eye Hospital.)*

Complications of severe advanced cases of blepharochalasis include ptosis and dilated and increased numbers of capillaries. Treatment is surgical.

NURSING INTERVENTION
Nursing intervention includes care of the patient who has undergone lid surgery for this lid structural change.

Ectropion. *Ectropion* is eversion or outward turning of the eyelid and may be classified as congenital, atonic, cicatricial, mechanical, or allergic (Fig. 11–5). Left untreated, tears do not wash over the globe's anterior surface properly, with resultant corneal drying, which can lead to ulcer formation. The tears themselves spill down onto the cheek, and the lysozyme (a lytic agent) causes skin excoriation. Tearing is the chief complaint.

Congenital ectropion may involve both upper and/or lower eyelids and requires plastic surgical correction.

Atonic, involutional (senile) ectropion occurs in older patients. Thermal cautery has been used to correct this, but there is often a recurrence of the problem. Surgical intervention is much more satisfactory. A wedge-shaped segment of the eyelid is removed, and the eyelid sutured (Kuhnt-Szymanowski procedure). Ophthalmic antibiotic ointment is placed on the skin incision b.i.d. Sutures are removed in 7 to 10 days.

Ectropion can also be due to injury or paralysis of the seventh cranial nerve; it may be caused by Bell's palsy (usually subsiding with time), or it occurs as a result of a cerebrovascular accident. Surgical intervention such as medial or lateral canthoplasty is one such procedure performed for eyelid laxity associated with paralytic ectropion. Partial tarsorrhaphy (suturing the eyelids together) is another.

In cicatricial ectropion, scarring results from trauma, burns, or bacterial or viral infections. Surgical intervention such as Z-plasty or free skin grafts (taken from sites such as the other eye, behind the ear, the upper arm near the axilla, or in the male, the foreskin from the penis) may be performed to correct the ectropion. After surgery a mild pressure patch is left *in situ* for 24 hours, and following removal of the patch the graft should be covered with a bland ointment so that it does not dry out.

Mechanical ectropion may be caused by heavy eyelid tumors, or by displacement of tissue as a result of an unrepaired orbital fracture. Tumor excision, or correction of the fracture is necessary to eliminate the ectropion.

Allergic ectropion may be seen secondary to contact dermatitis. The offending irritant should be identified and eliminated.[5]

NURSING INTERVENTION
When the nurse assesses the patient a history of constant, annoying tearing might be all that is complained about. Closer inspection of the lower eyelid may reveal an ectropion. If surgical intervention is undertaken, the patch should be inspected following the procedure and it should be found to be dry and intact. After the patch is removed, apply ointment to the surgical site. In the patient with ectropion secondary to a cerebrovascular accident, corneal damage can occur due to exposure; ointment applied to the eye will prevent drying, until surgical correction can be arranged.

PATIENT TEACHING
Patient teaching should include proper method and placement of the ointment on the surgical site. Outpatient appointment for suture removal will be given to the patient. Compliance with follow-up care should be encouraged.

Entropion. *Entropion* is an inversion of the entire eyelid margin in such a way that eyelashes are in contact with the globe. It may occur congenitally or it may be acquired. Congenital entropion more frequently involves the lower eyelid (although it can involve the upper eyelid). Lower eyelid entropion usually disappears as a child grows older, but surgical correction may be necessary if the lid margin and lashes irritate or abrade the cornea.[9]

Acquired entropion can be of an acute spastic, involutional, mechanical, or cicatricial nature.

1. *Spastic entropion* due to an acute ocular inflammation or injury can temporarily be managed by using tape to evert the eyelid. Eliminating the causative factor will also help. The Quickert suture technique may be performed at the bedside or as outpatient surgery.
2. *Involutional entropion,* the most common form, results from relaxation and lengthening of the retractors of the lower eyelid and orbital septum, and along with redundancy of eyelid skin these processes occur secondary to the aging process. This type of entropion may be treated by intricate plastic surgical procedures.

3. *Mechanical entropion* can result from enophthalmos, where loss of globe support of the eyelids occurs following an orbital fracture. It is seen in the presence of microphthalmic or phthisical globe. Marked proptosis may also be a cause.
4. *Cicatricial entropion* results from tarsal cicatrization secondary to trauma, thermal or chemical burns, or disease such as trachoma. It can also follow other surgical procedures on the eyelids. Both upper and lower eyelids may be involved. Surgical correction is aimed at everting the eyelid margin so that the eyelashes do not rub against the cornea.

NURSING INTERVENTION
The patient seeking help might first describe the symptoms as feeling as if there is "something in the eye." Close inspection will reveal the entropion, which should be referred to a physician for further evaluation. If surgical intervention becomes necessary, depending upon the extent of the procedure, the patient may or may not have a patch on the eye for a 24-hour period. Often for minor procedures the suture line is left exposed, and antibiotic ointment is applied to it. The eye may be shielded. Remind the patient that ointment blurs vision because it smears a thin film over the cornea.

Trichiasis. *Trichiasis* is a misdirection of the lashes which causes them to rub against the cornea instead of bowing outward away from the cornea. This is an ancient condition which was recorded in the Ebers Papyrus in Egypt in the 16th century, B.C.

The many causes of trichiasis include entropion (turning in of the lower lid resulting from spastic and/or senile relaxation of skin and muscle). Most of the causes are due to scarring of the conjunctiva seen in the last stages of trachoma. Trachoma is the most common cause of severe cicatricial scarring. Atrophy of the hair follicles occurs, leading to formation of fine, stubby unpigmented cilia and/or accessory hairs arising from the side buds of the follicles which grow obliquely and inward. Problems created by the cilia rubbing the cornea include tearing, pain, ulceration, vascularization, fibrosis, and eventual, permanent opacification which destroys vision.

Treatment consists of epilation (removal of individual cilia) by forceps. If the cilia returns rapidly, then electrolysis may have to be performed. Surgical intervention is considered when too many lashes are rubbing against the cornea. When entropion is present it should be corrected.

EDEMA

The swelling of the subcutaneous tissues of the lid may be so great that it closes the lids, or just slight enough to cause a feeling of fullness of the lids. The subcutaneous tissue of the lids is quite loose and is the site of extravasation of the edema fluid. This fluid is prevented from spreading to the forehead or cheeks by the fat which is held in the compartment by facial attachments. Because of this extensive swelling, the picture presented is often more frightening than its importance deserves.

1. *Inflammatory edema* may be due to infection, which may have been caused by an infected scratch, or it could arise from an infected hair follical (sty) which is difficult to see. For some infections, i.e., herpes zoster ophthalmicus, the first sign of involvement may be lid edema. Allergic reactions to drugs or animal protein may produce severe, rapidly developing edema.
2. *Traumatic edema* may occur after burns, sunburns, and contusion. Accompanying signs such as erythema, eccymosis, blisters, and lacerations may also be present.
3. *Noninflammatory edema* of the lids can occur with renal disease, blood dyscrasias, as well as local or general conditions which may block the lymphatics (Fig. 11–6). Long standing blepharospasm, in which compression of the veins has occurred, or following a Krönlein operation, may also produce edema of the lids. Another cause would include compression of the veins and lymphatics of the neck. Much more common noninflammatory edema is seen in uticaria, angioneurotic edema, and hereditary edema fugax.

NURSING INTERVENTION
If the edema occurs as a result of an infection, then the nurse would encourage compliance with warm compresses and antibiotic therapy.

Edema occurring as a result of acute trauma may be decreased by the

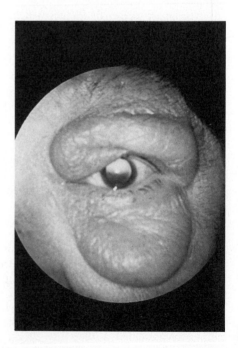

Figure 11–6. Edema of the eyelids. *(Photograph courtesy of Wills Eye Hospital.)*

gentle application of ice compresses. Since compresses also decrease pain, these can be a great nursing comfort measure.

Noninflammatory edema may require that the patient be encouraged to maintain a certain head position. Just raising the head at bedtime might accomplish a decrease in edema of the eyelids, while edema resulting from an allergic reaction would require systemic treatment.

ALLERGY, INFLAMMATIONS, AND INFECTIONS

Contact dermatitis is an eczematous condition of the skin which may result when irritating substances come in contact with the skin either at work, during recreation, or through drug therapy. Evolution of the lesion is from erythema to papule to vesicle. The vesicle then progresses in one of three ways. It can burst and produce what is called ''weeping eczema'' or it can dry and form ''scaly eczema,'' and/or it can become infected and produce pustules which when ruptured form crusts. In old, chronic cases the skin can become thickened and dull.

1. *Primary dermatitis* can be caused by contact with an irritant in sufficient strength, and of duration long enough to injure the cells and produce variable reactions.
2. *Allergic dermatitis* is due to development of hypersensitivity of the skin to repeated contact with the allergen. Some compounds which may excite such lid reactions are ophthalmic drugs, complex chemical compounds, plastics, and bacterial proteins. After these substances are absorbed they continue interaction with protein of the skin provoking antibody formation which enters into the general circulation. When they again reach the skin they form an antigen–antibody reaction which results in eczema. This reaction when associated with direct material is called *contact dermatitis*. When due to drugs in the general circulation it is called *dermatitis medicamentosa,* or if the infection is in proximity to, or distant from, the site it is called *infective dermatitis.*
3. Another type of eczematous dermatitis is seen in *atopic* eczema; it is a genetically inherited dermatitis condition which has an association with hay fever, asthma, and urticuria.

It is important to determine the etiological factor, remove it if possible, and treat the lesion. Antiinflammatory drugs such as steroids are the drugs of choice. Care must be taken, for some preservatives in these drugs can cause dermatological reaction as well as the drugs themselves.

NURSING INTERVENTION
Nursing intervention should include an awareness that an erythematous eyelid may be caused by medications being used by the patient. Patients should be requested to bring all medications into the doctor's office so that the offending medication can be discontinued. If antiinflammatory

drugs have been prescribed, medication compliance should be encouraged. Follow-up care should be stressed.

Hordeolum

Hordeolum, more frequently referred to as a sty (Fig. 11–7), is a commonly encountered infection of one of the glands of the lid. Essentially it is an abscess, with pus formation in the lumen of the infected gland, and is characterized by a localized red, swollen, tender area. If this infection occurs in one of the superficial glands of Zeis (modified sebaceous glands) or Moll (sweat glands), it will be seen pointing on the skin side of the lid margin, and is referred to as an external hordeolum. However, if the infection occurs in the long sebaceous Meibomian glands, it is referred to as an internal hordeolum, and may point on either the conjunctival or skin side of the lid; left untreated this could lead to a cellulitis of the eyelid[5] (see Chap. 9).

NURSING INTERVENTION
Patients suffering from recurrent hordeolum should be referred to an ophthalmologist. Treatment for both internal and external hordeolum consists of warm compresses applied over the affected lid for 10 to 15 minutes, three to four times daily. Antibacterial ophthalmic ointment may also be prescribed by the physician.

PATIENT TEACHING
Patient teaching should include the fact that the ointment should be applied after the compresses have been accomplished. Warn that ointments tend to smear the cornea and thus cause blurred vision.

Chalazion

Chalazion is a sterile, granulomatous inflammation of a Meibomian gland (Fig. 11–8) and can be seen as a bump on the eyelid. Initially it begins with inflammation and tenderness, as that seen in an internal hordeolum, but later, as the bump increases in size, a well-developed chalazion will not have acute inflammatory signs.[5]

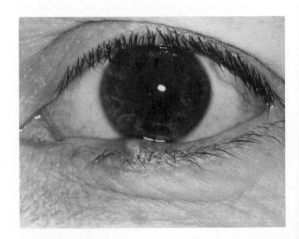

Figure 11–7. Hordeolum of the lower lid.

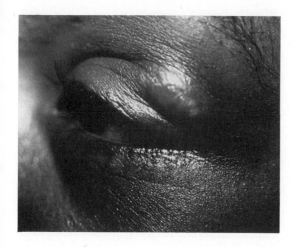

Figure 11–8. Chalazion of the upper lid.

Left untreated, the bump may cause astigmatism as pressure is placed on the cornea. The cause is unknown. Since there are at least 25 Meibomian glands in each upper lid, and about 20 in the lower lid, it is possible that more than one gland can become affected at a time. However, recurrent chalazia in one area should be biopsied to rule out malignancy.

NURSING INTERVENTION

In the early stages, when the patient complains of tenderness, warm compresses applied for 10 to 15 minutes, three to four times daily may help the inflammation to subside. If the patient has an antibiotic or sulfa drug prescribed by a physician, compliance should be encouraged.

However, since most of the enlarged chalazian are treated surgically by the ophthalmologist, the nurse working in an outpatient setting should be aware of the equipment necessary for this "minor surgical procedure," and the sequential care which should be communicated to the patient.

A sterile chalazion tray should contain:

1. A selection of chalazion clamps.
2. Bard-Parker or beaver knife handle and #11 blade.
3. Weaver roter-rooter or curette.
4. Suture and suture scissors.
5. Gauze, applicator sticks, swabs for cleansing the ocular area, and a small medicine glass for the betadine (or other) prepping solution.
6. An eye sheet, for draping the patient prior to the surgical procedure.

The nurse will place a drop of topical anesthetic, i.e., *proparacaine* in the cul-de-sac of the surgical eye; the ophthalmologist will then use a needle and syringe to infiltrate the area with local anesthetic. The ocular area is prepped and draped, and the ophthalmologist accomplishes the surgical procedure (Fig. 11–9).

On completion of the procedure, sterile gauze is held in place under

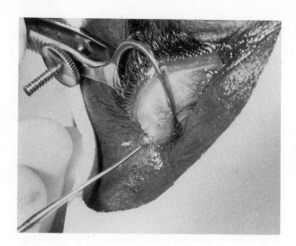

Figure 11–9. Surgical removal of chalazion, showing clamp *in situ* and use of a curette.

pressure, in order to curtail bleeding. Shortly thereafter, antibiotic ointment is instilled in the cul-de-sac, the gauze is changed and a pressure patch is applied over the closed eye.

PATIENT TEACHING

Patient teaching includes a request that the eye remain patched 4 to 6 hours, at which time the patient removes it and starts warm compresses. These compresses and the prescribed antibiotic eye drops should be administered four times a day. Compliance with a follow-up visit should be encouraged. As with any ocular surgical procedure, the patient's visual acuity should be recorded on the chart prior to surgery; it should be repeated at the next visit.

Herpes Zoster

Herpes zoster is a virus infection caused by the varicella-zoster virus which attacks the dorsal root ganglion of the spinal cord or the extramedullary ganglia of the cranial nerves; both sensory and motor nerves can be affected. Usually it occurs in adults, but it can occur in children. It has also been known to occur in the infant born to a mother who was infected during pregnancy.

The word "zoster" comes from the Greek word meaning girdle. Herpes zoster is important in ophthalmology when it involves the gasserian ganglion: the first divison of the trigeminal nerve is usually affected, the second division is rarely affected, but all three have on even rarer occasions been involved. Rarer still is bilateral involvement. Like other virus infections, it may assume grave and even fatal conclusions, especially in persons suffering from nutritional deprivation or with a deficient immune system as found in patients with malignancy.

At first there is tenderness, pain, then erythema over the distribution of the nerve involved; this is followed by edema especially of the lids, and then vesicles filled with clear fluid in which the virus is abundant. These vesicles then burst and scabs form, and after weeks when they finally separate they may leave deep pits.

Pain is of the neurological type, which is burning and severe. It may last for years after the attack. The skin may be left pitted and depigmented with decreased sensitivity, numbness, and pain.

The lesions usually do not cross the midline, and if the nasociliary branch of the trigeminal nerve is involved, ocular complications occur more frequently. This nasociliary involvement is usually demonstrated by lesions on the tip of the nose. Ocular complications may not appear immediately but occur several days after onset, or after the skin reactions have reached their peak. These include conjunctivitis, keratitis, uveitis, retinitis, optic neuritis, optic atrophy, pupillary disturbances, and ocular palsies.[10] The exact mode of action is not clear. It is the feeling that these prolonged, progressive inflammatory and degenerative changes may be due to an occlusive vasculitis.

Treatment is difficult to evaluate since the severity of cases varies widely. It is, however, usually directed at quieting the inflammation with steroids, controlling secondary infections with antibiotics, and the uveitis with atropine and analgesics.

NURSING INTERVENTION
Nursing intervention should include "Ophthalmic Isolation" which really can be considered to be much the same category as wound and skin precautions. Children who have developed herpes zoster ophthalmicus and who have been in contact with other children have been known to contribute to an outbreak of chicken pox amongst these other children, so parents should be cautioned with respect to contact. Medicating these patients as ordered, will contribute to their comfort. Good handwashing technique is important. Soothing solutions such as Burrow's applied to the lesions increase patient comfort. Oral Acyclovir decreases the time the lesions are active.

BENIGN CONGENITAL TUMORS

Primary Tumors of the Lids

1. *Dermoid cysts* occur in about 16.3 percent of lid tumors in children. About 35 percent of these congenital tumors are found at birth or within the first 3 months of life.
2. *Hemangiomas* can occur at birth, may be severe as seen in the port-wine stain of nevus flammeus, and can also be associated with meningeal and cerebral hemangioma.[11]

BENIGN ACQUIRED TUMORS

Many small, benign, easily-identifiable tumors are observed. The following list describes many of these.

1. *Sudoriferous cysts* develop from blocked, specialized sweat glands.
2. The skin and the specialized Meibomian glands can produce *sebaceous*

cysts. Most of these are due to gland orifice blockage with retained secretory substance build-up.

3. The most common benign epithelial neoplasm, *seborrheic keratosis* is referred to by a number of different names, i.e., *basal cell papilloma, seborrheic wart,* or *senile verrucae.* This lesion is seen as a superficial brown or brown-black, slightly elevated, well-circumscribed excrescence.

4. *Senile keratosis,* initially benign, is seen as a well-demarcated, slightly pigmented lesion; however, cutaneous horns will sometimes grow from the base. Occasionally, squamous cell carcinoma develops from this lesion.

5. *Papilloma* is a very common senile eyelid tumor which is composed of cords of fibrovascular tissue surrounded by keratinized epithelium. These cords form finger-like projections which may recur once they are removed.

6. Other uncommon benign tumors of eyelid skin require biopsy and microscopic examination. Included in this group are *calcifying epithelioma* (hair matrixoma), *keratomacanthoma,* and *inverted follicular keratosis.*

7. Some tumors arise from adnexal tissue. These include *trichoepitheliomas* which arise from hair follicles, produce horny cysts, and are located at the lid margins.

8. *Sweat glands adenomas,* seen as small plaques, arise from the sweat gland and are fairly frequent in occurrence.

9. *Nevi* are pigmented tumors, which can occur on lid surfaces as well as lid margins. At puberty or during pregnancy a hormonal reaction causes them to become more pigmented.

10. *Neurofibromas* may be solitary or associated with generalized neurofibromatosis (von Recklinghausen's disease). They are characterized by multiple tumors of the skin, central nervous system, peripheral nerves, and nerve sheaths; unfortunately, this can include the optic nerve.

MALIGNANT TUMORS

1. *Basal cell carcinoma* accounts for over 90 percent of all malignant epithelial eyelid tumors. The most common site is the lower lid, with the inner canthus being affected more frequently than the outer canthus, while the upper lids are least affected. At first these appear as small raised nodules which, as they enlarge begin to ulcerate with a crater that bleeds and scabs over. They gradually enlarge and the edges appear pearly in texture. The tumors vary, some are very invasive and may be scaly, others remain circumscribed and/or go into deeper tissue and bone. In the final stage there may be fungating tumor filling the entire orbit. These tumors usually do not metastasize, but may have multifocal lesions.[12]

2. *Squamous cell carcinoma* is uncommon, comprising only about 5 percent of all malignant lid tumors. Initially the tumor may resemble basal cell carcinoma, with early ulceration, but slower growth. These lesions do, however, metastasize to regional lymph nodes (lower lid tumors to the submaxillary nodes, while tumors of the upper lid extend to the preauricular nodes).

3. *Malignant melanoma* occurs in the lids and may arise from nevi. The lesion may be lightly or heavily pigmented. The degree of pigmentation has nothing to do with the degree of malignancy. These pigmented lid margin nodules enlarge and either become fungating lesions or they may develop pigmented satellite lesions with extension to regional lymph nodes with silent metastasis to internal organs and the brain.
4. *Lymphomas* are rare tumors which can have isolated area infiltration or bilateral lid involvement. Conjunctival and orbital involvement as well as systemic manifestations may occur.

Treatment of benign lesions is simple excision with microscopic examination of all excised tissue. Malignant tissue must be excised, and frozen sections used to determine if the excision has been complete and total.[13,14]

Cryosurgery (using a freezing probe) is being used in some clinics. This technique's drawback is that there is *no* microscopic histopathic diagnosis, so the treatment, final diagnosis, and tumor elimination will not be definite. Recurrence rate varies 1 to 20 percent, in this type of treatment, which leads to doubt. Surgical excision without frozen section monitoring runs about a 4 to 5 percent recurrent risk.[15,16]

NURSING INTERVENTION

Since there is a general trend in nursing today to promote wellness, it behooves the nurse to notice a lesion on or around the eyelid and to inquire the duration of the lesion, and whether any recent changes in appearance have been noticed. A lesion which becomes annoying or unsightly to a person will often prompt that person to seek medical advice, but lesions that tend to scab over are sometimes ignored. These people, though often reluctant, should be persuaded to seek attention for such lesions.

Outpatient surgical clinic nurses must remember how important it is when assisting with surgery to place a biopsy specimen in an appropriate pathology specimen bottle. A specimen smeared onto the glass, which remains untouched by the fixing solution will dry out and will not be able to be identified by the pathologist—to the patient's detriment. If the nurse is responsible for filling out pathology forms, and labelling bottles, the correct information of site and eye should be stated, together with the correct patient's name, age, and date on which the specimen was taken. An amusing way to remember whether the lesion is from an older person or not is that the term "senile" is often used after the age of 40, while juvenile is used before the age of 40.

TRAUMA

Eyelid injuries occur often because the eyelids are an external surface and exist as a defense mechanism to protect the globe. The lids are very vascular, and are capable of a great deal of swelling. Because of the elasticity of the skin they are able to return to their normal shape and size at a later date when the injury has healed. The healing takes place fairly quickly, probably because of the good blood supply.

However, the skin surface is also capable of scar formation. If cicatricial healing occurs it might alter the lids' shape, thus permitting globe exposure, with subsequent visual loss.

Black Eye

A black eye or *ecchymosis* is a frequently seen injury which occurs as a result of blunt trauma, i.e., a fist, ball, bat, etc. The discoloration turns black and blue, then gradually becomes purple, green, and yellow before it finally disappears in 10 days to 2 weeks. The injury itself is not serious, but sometimes the blow might be severe enough to cause damage to intraocular structures, such as the iris, lens, or retina. The injured person might complain the next day about pain in the eye, photophobia, or tearing, all symptoms of *traumatic iritis*. If this injury is accompanied by lid swelling, the complaint might be one of diplopia (double vision).

Ecchymosis may occur following a retrobulbar hemorrhage, seen after a local anesthetic block is given prior to surgery. It also occurs following lid surgery.

NURSING INTERVENTION

Assess the patient who presents with a black eye and discover the cause. Take a visual acuity. If the injury has occurred recently, it might be comforting to place an ice compress over the injured site. Usually ecchymosis takes a little while to make itself evident. The patient should have a Slitlamp examination, and dilating drops should be instilled in the eye to facilitate fundus examination. Usually the black eye is permitted to take its course to resolve, and no further treatment is necessary.

PATIENT TEACHING

Patient teaching should include the information that if any future eye problems develop, the attention of an ophthalmologist should be sought.

Subcutaneous Emphysema

Subcutaneous emphysema or crepitus of the lids may result from a fracture into the ethmoid sinus. When the victim blows his or her nose, air is forced into the loose tissues of the eyelid.[9] Diplopia will then become a symptom. CAT scan or orbital x-rays will establish the fracture's presence.

NURSING INTERVENTION

Caution the injured person not to blow his or her nose when there is a history of blunt trauma to the ocular area. Take a visual acuity. If diplopia is present reassure the person that this disturbing symptom will be followed closely by the ophthalmologist to see if it subsides over a period of time, as the swelling decreases. Ice compresses may be given for vasoconstriction if ecchymosis is also present. Make an appointment for orbital x-rays to be taken and encourage compliance with follow-up care.

Lid Lacerations

Lid lacerations occur from a variety of causes; an injury from a shattered windshield in a car accident, trauma from a stick, scissors, knife, wire, fishhook, glasses that are not shatterproof, dog bite, or human bite, to name but a few. The area will bleed profusely, and often looks much worse than it really is before the lids have been cleaned up. Tissue swelling may be present, but often takes time to reach its full extent. Therefore, the primary repair is usually attempted by the physician as soon as possible. Care has to be taken when repair is undertaken to have the lid margins in apposition to one another, so that lid notching will not occur when the area has healed. Prophylactic antibiotics will be given to the patient both topically and systemically as a measure against infection. The globe must always be thoroughly inspected to ensure that the injury does not also involve it (Fig. 11–10).

NURSING INTERVENTION

Assess the injured area, sometimes this is only possible after the wound has been cleansed, and the blood has been removed from the surrounding tissues. It is important to obtain a visual acuity, sometimes if the degree of swelling is great when the patient presents it might be appropriate to assist the physician in obtaining a visual acuity. Small lid lacerations may be repaired in the emergency room. The area will be cleansed and prepped prior to the procedure being implemented. If the lid laceration is more extensive and warrants surgical repair in the operating room, then the nurse should remember to keep the patient "NPO" (nothing by mouth) until the surgical time is set. Ice compresses to the lid might be ordered to decrease swelling. The area should be cleansed, and it should be covered with a sterile eyepatch or gauze until such time as the patient is taken to the operating room.

A note of interest, if patient comes into an emergency department, and has a piece of the eyelid missing, the nurse should ascertain where the piece of tissue can be located. If it can be found, the surgeon may be able

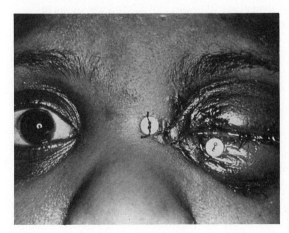

Figure 11–10. Repair of lid laceration. *(Photograph courtesy of Wills Eye Hospital.)*

to replace it. If the missing piece of tissue is brought in with the patient, it should be put in a sterile container, and moistened with sterile saline, and kept in the refrigerator until time of surgery.

Postoperative care will include observing that the pressure patch is dry and intact. Cold compresses may be applied over the patch on return from the operating room. Ointment may be applied to the suture line after the pressure patch has been removed. Very often the eye is only shielded for protection.

PATIENT TEACHING
Patient teaching should include compliance with applying topical ointment, and also follow-up care.

BURNS

Chemical Burns
Chemical burns of the lids occur when chemicals are splashed or thrown into a person's face. Copious irrigation with water from the faucet or saline solution if it is available, should be immediately initiated, and should continue for at least 5 minutes.

Because of the probability that the corneal and conjunctival surfaces are also involved, the patient might be experiencing excruciating pain, irrigation of these structures should be included. Litmus paper will merely establish whether the chemical is acid or alkali. (This will be covered in more detail in the discussion on corneal burns.)

NURSING INTERVENTION
Irrigate the lids copiously for at least 5 minutes. If only one eye is involved, be sure that the head is positioned so that the other eye will not be contaminated. Follow steps for irrigation of the eye. A word of caution to the nurse dealing with chemical contaminants: remember to wash your hands after completing the irrigation, or wear gloves, for nurses have been known to develop contact dermatitis as a result of contact with a patient contaminated with chemicals. Patch the eye for comfort if the patient has to travel a distance for further ophthalmological evaluation.

Thermal Burns
Thermal burns occur when heated material comes in contact with the lid; such things as molten metal and solder can cause structural damage to the tissues. The unfortunate thing is that this type of lid injury could have been prevented if safety glasses or a visor had been worn by the person incurring the injury. Injuries like these occur in both the home and industrial settings. Burns to the lid occurring from fire can be devastating, and may require reconstructive plastic surgery at a future time.

NURSING INTERVENTION

Nursing intervention includes removal of any superficial particulate matter. If metal has become imbedded in the lid, then it would be best to patch or shield the eye until the metal can be surgically removed by an ophthalmologist.

When the burn has been sustained from fire, the area should be covered with sterile, moist gauze pads, and medical care should be obtained as soon as possible. Treatment will include debridement of the area, followed by intensive antibiotic and steroid therapy. Plastic reconstructive surgery may eventually be necessary, and nursing intervention will be the same as for other plastic surgery of the eyelids.

Gunpowder Burns

Gunpowder burns are frequent among children who play with firecrackers and homemade bombs. The wounds have both thermal and intradermal foreign body components which have to be treated, and this is usually undertaken under general anesthesia. X-rays or CT scan may also be ordered to rule out any possible intraocular foreign body. The ophthalmologist will perform an EUA (examination under anesthesia) if the patient is a child; or a fundoscopy if the patient is an adult. The area might need to be scrubbed to remove the intradermal foreign bodies.

NURSING INTERVENTION

In these circumstances, the nurse attempts to get a visual acuity. Carefully ascertain what the patient was doing prior to sustaining such an injury. The eye should be covered until surgery can be arranged. Dilating drops will have to be instilled to facilitate the fundoscopy or EUA. Reassurance of both patient, and in the case of the child, the parents, is a vitally important nursing function. Ascertain the last time food or fluids were ingested. Request the patient to remain NPO prior to surgery.

REFERENCES

1. Crawford JS: Congenital eyelid abnormalities in children. J Pediatr Ophthalmol Strabismus, 21(4): 140–149, 1984
2. Harley RD: Disorders of the lids. Pediatric Clinics of North America, 30(6): 1145–1158, 1983
3. Shannon G, Flannagan JC, Saunders DH: Disorders of the lids, in Harley RD, (Ed.), Pediatric Ophthalmology, 2nd ed. Philadelphia: Saunders, 1983, p. 12–437
4. Spaeth GL, Nelson LB, Beaudoin AR: Ocular teratology, in Duane TD, Jaeger EA, (Eds.), Biomedical Foundations in Ophthalmology. Philadelphia: Harper & Row, 1985, p. 116
5. Vaughan D, Asbury T: General Ophthalmology, 10th ed. Los Altos, Calif.: Lange, 1983, p. 43–51
6. McCulley JP, Dougherty JM, Deveau DG: Classification of chronic blepharitis. Ophthalmology 89: 1173–1180, 1982
7. French B, Callahan A, Dorhbach R, et al.: The effect of differential section of seventh

nerve on patients with intractable blepharospasm. Trans Am Acad Ophthalmol Otolaryngol, 81: 595–602, 1976

8. Battista A: Blepharospasm, a surgical procedure for therapy. Ophthalmic Surgery, 12: 823–829, 1981
9. Sol DB, Winslow R: Surgery of the eyelid, in Duane T, (Ed.), Clinical Ophthalmology. Hagerstown Md.: Harper & Row, 1982, p. 12–22
10. Hedges TR, Albert DM: The progression of ocular abnormalities of herpes zoster. Ophthalmology, 89: 165–177, 1982
11. Stigman G, Crawford JS, Ward CM, et al.: Ophthalmic syndrome of infantile hemangioma of the eyelids. American Journal of Ophthalmology, 85: 806–813, 1978
12. Wesley RE, Collins JW: Basal cell carcinoma of eyelids as indicator of multifocal malignancy. American Journal of Ophthalmology, 99: 591–593, 1982
13. Doxanas M, Green WR, Iliff CE: Factors in successful surgical management of basal cell carcinoma of eyelid. American Journal of Ophthalmology, 91: 726–736, 1982
14. Wiggs EO: Incompletely excised basal cell carcinoma of ocular adnexa. Ophthalmic Surgery, 12: 891–896, 1981
15. Tsunezuki K, Toshihirio T, Mashyoshei M: Cryosurgery for basal cell epithelioma. Japanese Journal of Ophthalmology, 25: 449–456, 1981
16. Fraunfelder FT, Zacarian SA, Limner BL, Wingfield D: Cryosurgery for malignancy of the eyelid. Ophthalmology, 87: 461, 1980

BIBLIOGRAPHY

Bell S: Surgical specimens, treat them right. Journal of Ophthalmologic Nursing and Technology, 4(2): 34–37, 1984

Briggs H: Hereditary congenital ptosis with report of 64 cases conforming to the mendelian rule of dominance. American Journal of Ophthalmology, 2: 408, 1919

Rodin FH, Bakan H: Hereditary congenital ptosis: Report of a pedigree and review of literature. American Journal of Ophthalmology, 18: 213, 1935

12

Conjunctiva

NEW TERMS

Chemosis: excessive edema of the conjunctiva.

Follicles: small, raised parts of the conjunctiva with subepithelial collections of lymphocytes.

Hyperemia: excess of blood in part due to local or general relaxation of the arterioles.

Phlyctenule: an elevated mass of pale inflammatory tissue which occurs at the limbus or on the bulbar conjunctiva.

Symblepharon: an adhesion between the palpebral conjunctiva and the bulbar conjunctiva.

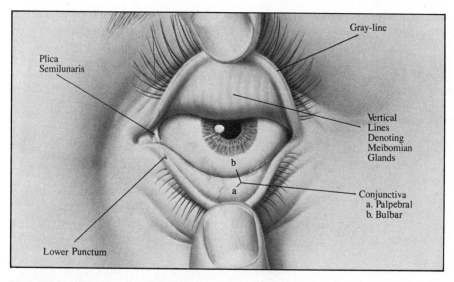

12–1. The conjunctiva, a transparent mucous membrane lines the upper and lower lids (palpebral conjuctiva), folds over on itself at the upper and lower fornix, and also covers the sclera (bulbar conjunctiva) up to the limbus. *(From Friedman AH, Desmarest RJ, Westwood WB: The Optyl Atlas of the Human Eye. Norwood, N.J.: Optyl, 1979, with permission.)*

The conjunctiva (Fig. 12–1) is a transparent mucous membrane which has two portions to it. The area that lines the upper and lower eyelids (up to the lid margins) is called the *palpebral conjunctiva*. It is firmly adherent to the tarsus.

The *bulbar conjunctiva* covers the sclera, up to the limbus (corneal-scleral junction). The folds in the conjuctiva under the lids are referred to as *fornices*. However, the lower fornix is frequently called the *cul-de-sac*.

In the inner canthus two other structures are evident. The *caruncle* is seen as a small, fleshy epidermoid structure, and the *semilunar folds* (Plica Semilunaris) are soft, movable folds of bulbar conjunctiva.

Swelling of the conjunctiva is referred to as chemosis (Fig. 12–2).

CONGENITAL ABNORMALITIES

Fortunately, congenital abnormalities are few in number and rare in occurrence.

Epitarsus consists of an "apron-like" conjunctival fold attached to the inner surface of the lid. Other conjunctival folds have been described, but these are usually of no significance.

Congenital conjunctival cysts and tumors are more common, but often involve other structures as well. Corneal and scleral lesions will be covered in chapters involving those specific structures.

Dermolipoma of the conjunctiva usually occurs in the bulbar conjunctiva, temporally, near the lateral canthus. Clinically, these are subconjunctival, as the conjunctival membranes move freely over them. These congenital lesions are composed of misplaced fatty tissue, and some fibrous tissue, while hair follicles, lacrimal gland tissue, sebaceous glands, and smooth or striped muscle fibers may also be present.

NURSING INTERVENTION
Refer the patient to an ophthalmologist. Treatment may be indicated if the dermolipoma becomes cosmetically disfiguring.

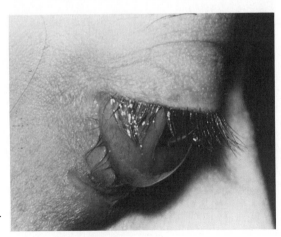

Figure 12–2. Chemosis—excessive conjunctival edema.

Vascular Changes

Congenital vascular changes and tumors of the conjunctiva may be associated with more diffuse pathology. Telangiectasia (a condition characterized by dilation of the capillary vessels and minute arteries, forming a variety of angiomas) and hemangiomata (benign tumors made up of newly-formed blood vessels) are two such changes which can occur.

Hereditary hemorrhagic telangiectasis occurs with dilated, thin-walled capillaries in the skin, conjunctiva, mucosa of mouth, larynx, respiratory tract, and alimentary and genitourinary tracts. The largest number of lesions are found on the head and upper extremities. Because of the thinness of the walls, capillaries bleed very easily.

Hemangiomas of the conjunctiva may occur in Sturge-Weber syndrome or encephalo (ocular) facial angiomatosis. The conjunctival hemangiomas appear on the same side as the port-wine lesions which involve the lids and face.

ACQUIRED ABNORMALITIES

Subconjunctival hemorrhage is a relatively common unilateral disorder which may occur spontaneously, after a vigorous bout of coughing or sneezing, or following trauma. A small blood vessel breaks subconjunctivally, and the hemorrhage appears as a blood-red area under the glistening conjunctiva (Figure 12–3). Frank bleeding is not evident. The hemorrhage itself will absorb and disappear in about 10 days to 2 weeks.

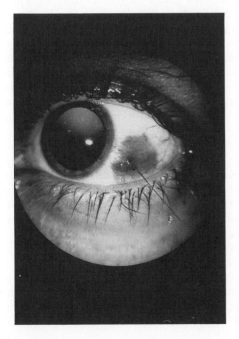

Figure 12–3. Subconjunctival hemorrhage. *(Photograph courtesy of Thomas Farrell, M.D., Director, General Ophthalmology Service, Wills Eye Hospital.)*

NURSING INTERVENTION

Nursing intervention should include eliciting a careful history; children may be reluctant to impart information as to what might have caused such an occurrence because it might have occurred in the conjunctiva following a perforating injury such as that caused by the point of scissors or a pencil. Check the adult's blood pressure, for these hemorrhages occasionally occur in the hypertensive person.

Straining during labor occasionally produces bilateral subconjunctival hemorrhages in the mother at the time of delivery.

Conjunctivitis

Conjunctivitis contributes to a large proportion of eye problems in the western world, and is responsible for an even larger proportion in the rest of the world. Causes of this disease may be classified into three categories: 1) *exogenous;* 2) *endogenous;* and 3) *local spread from contiguous tissues.*

The exogenous mode of conjunctivitis occurs when irritants arrive in the conjunctival cul-de-sac, or on the conjunctiva. These irritants may be air or water borne; transmitted by fingers, flies, or other vectors. They may be mechanical (dust), chemical (ammonia fumes), thermal (flame), radiational (ultraviolet radiation from sun lamps), electrical (wire-carrying current), or due to contamination by microorganisms (bacteria, virus, or fungus); they can also be parasitic (lice or larva).

The endogenous agents causing conjunctivitis may be blood or lymph borne metastatic infection as in virus and other exanthemata (any eruptive disease or eruptive fever). They may be an allergy to some disease or immune disorder. They may result from some general metabolic disorder such as gout.

Finally, there is the local spread of disease from the involved cornea, lacrimal system, lids, nose, sinuses, and orbit to the conjunctiva.

By whatever route the infection arrives, the conjunctiva reacts as mucous membrane usually reacts, by hyperemia (redness—an excess of blood in a part due to local or general relaxation of the arterioles, Fig. 12–4), edema, lymphatic reaction, and pain. The conjunctival insult usually produces tearing to wash the irritant away.

Bacterial Conjunctivitis. *Bacterial conjunctivitis* can be an acute conjunctivitis or a mucopurulent conjunctivitis. There are many etiological bacteria which may cause this condition, but *Staphylococcus aureus* is the prominent organism. The main features of this disease are marked hyperemia and a mucopurulent discharge. At first there is a mild aching or irritated feeling associated with considerable dilatation of the conjunctival blood vessels which is most intense near the fornices (giving the picture of peripheral conjunctival redness or injection). Occasionally, small, subconjunctival hemorrhages may occur. There is mild edema with loss of the translucency of the conjunctiva. The discharge is at first watery due to an increase in tearing, but later becomes thicker with shreds of mucuos, and finally becomes purulent causing the lids to stick together and accumulate in the inner canthus. Some organisms cause punctate staining of the cornea. (These are pinpoint breaks in the corneal epithelium which when stained with fluorescein dye can be

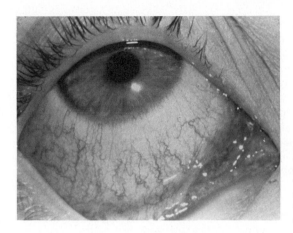

Figure 12-4. Peripheral injection seen in conjunctivitis. Hyperemia due to local relaxation of the arterioles. *(Photograph courtesy of Juan Arentsen, M.D., Co-Director, Cornea Department, Wills Eye Hospital.)*

made visible.) These lesions are found in the lower portion of the cornea and seem to be a reaction to toxins in the tears.

Attempts should be made to identify the offending organisms by smear and culture before antibiotics are started.

NURSING INTERVENTION
Obtain a careful history, keeping in mind the many ways irritants can be introduced into the eyes. Note if the feeling of discomfort is in one or both eyes. Observe the amount and type of discharge from the conjunctiva; inquire if the lids were stuck together in the morning. Note the degree of injection, and its location. Take a visual acuity; the patient's vision usually is not decreased with conjunctivitis. If a smear and culture are ordered, ensure that they are done prior to having the patient initiate his or her antibiotic eyedrops.

Remember that the patient with this conjunctivitis may well have contaminated the nurses' and physicians' working area too, so make sure that equipment which has come in contact with the patient's hands and eyes is cleaned after use.

PATIENT TEACHING
If the conjunctivitis is only in one eye, cross-contamination by the fingers and by fomites is a distinct possibility. Caution the patient to avoid rubbing the irritated eye, and then promptly rubbing the uninvolved eye, for this can contaminate the second eye. Encourage *handwashing prior to instilling eyedrops*. Stress that family members are at risk of developing conjunctivitis if they use the same washcloth and face towel as the person who has the conjunctivitis.

Chronic Conjunctivitis. Chronic conjunctivitis is a disease which reveals slight conjunctival hyperemia and mucous discharge, but includes a great deal of protracted annoyance and discomfort. There is usually an infective element which may have been ineffectively treated; it might be an attenuated infection, reinfection from fingers, or contamination from lids that have not been treated. *Staphylococcus* (*S. aureus* and *S. epidermidies*) is the leading offender. Lid and conjunctival cultures, as well as sensitivity studies, should be performed before vigorous antibiotic therapy and lid hygiene are begun.

There can also be an allergic reaction to these chronic forms of conjunctivitis—either to the organism, the antibiotic used in treatment, or in some cases to cosmetics which have been used. Where an allergic reaction is suspected, conjunctival smear and scraping should be used not only to identify the causative agent, but also to determine if eosinophiles are present. (Eosinophiles are often increased in an allergic reaction.)

NURSING INTERVENTION
Review the method of performing lid hygiene with the patient (see Chap. 3).

Where an allergic conjunctivitis has been identified and the possible culprit may be cosmetics (i.e., a reaction to eye make-up), discuss with the patient the fact that the make-up may have become contaminated, or that it might be necessary to change from that particular brand of make-up. Discourage teenagers from "trading" eye make-up and so cross-contaminating each other.

Purulent Conjunctivitis. Purulent conjunctivitis or blennorrhea (Fig. 12–5) is a very serious disease. It is an acute, violent conjunctival inflammation with copious discharge and pus accompanied by massive lid swelling. Pain may *not* be an important factor because frequently the nerves are so damaged that there is little sensation. Untested, this may lead to loss of an eye. *Neisseria gonorrhoeae* is the usual causative agent, but other organisms may cause similar reactions. Among those other organisms are *Staphylococus aureus, Streptococcus, Diplococcus pneumoniae,* and *Escherichia coli.*

Gonococcal Conjunctivitis. Gonococcal conjunctivitis can occur in the newborn (ophthalmia neonatorium). This is due to direct infection of the newborn from the mother's cervix at the time of birth. It is also seen in children between the ages of 2 and 10, and is found chiefly in girls who have contracted vulvovaginitis and who then transmit the disease to their eyes from their fingers.

NURSING INTERVENTION
Any profuse purulent conjunctivitis should be considered to be a gonococcal infection until proven otherwise by smears and scrapings. Antibiotic sensitivity is very important, because the gonococcal infection must be treated by systemic medications to eradicate any foci of infection in the genitourinary tract, and/or in the gastrointestinal tract.

The Credè procedure is implemented to combat the development of ophthalmia neonatorium. Shortly after a baby's birth, one drop of a 1 percent silver nitrate solution is instilled into the neonate's eyes. Occasionally, this may cause a slight chemical conjunctivitis, which subsides

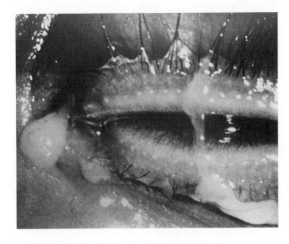

Figure 12–5. Purulent conjunctivitis or blennorrhea may be due to *Neisseria gonorrhoeae, S. Aureus* (or other bacteria), or a TRIC agent. *(Photograph courtesy of Wills Eye Hospital.)*

in a day or so. The Credè procedure is mandatory in all 50 states; however, some states permit use of other ophthalmic antibiotics, such as erythromycin. Penicillin eyedrops are seldom used, because of the later allergy which might be developed.[1]

For the patient who has already acquired gonococcal conjunctivitis—whether it be an infant, child, or adult—treatment of choice is systemic penicillin, administered intramuscularly (or in severe cases intravenously), with a topical antibiotic ointment such as erythromycin or bacitracin instilled in the eyes to prevent a secondary infection.

Patients with a purulent conjunctivitis admitted to a hospital should be isolated. Handwashing to prevent cross-contamination is important for the nurse, patient, and visitors.

Gonococcus infection is a reportable disease in the United States, and therefore the Public Health Department should be notified of its occurrence. Partner contact should also be traced and referred for examination to prevent reinfection.

Acute Membranous Conjunctivitis. Acute membranous conjunctivitis is caused by the diphtheria bacillus. Since mass immunization has been instituted the condition is seldom seen. The bacillus liberates a very destructive exotoxin which causes local necrosis of the mucous membranes. Dissemination of the toxin in the bloodstream produces toxic effects on the myocardium and peripheral nerves.

Treatment is therefore not only isolation to prevent the spread of the disease, but also systemic penicillin and topical erythromycin.

NURSING INTERVENTION
Nurses who have contact with parents of young children should encourage immunization at the appropriate time; this disease has been nearly eliminated through mass immunization.

Other organisms may produce bacterial conjunctivitis. These bacteria are less common and usually are not as dramatic as the previously mentioned types. These organisms include *Streptococci,* which on occasion may have a membrane, *pneumococcus, meningococcus, Koch-Weeks bacillus, bacillus of Pfeiffer (hemophilus influenza group), Shingellae bacillus, Escherichia coli,* and *Proteus.*

It is important for the nurse to realize that the severity of bacterial conjunctivitis has been greatly reduced by the use of specific and potent antibiotics. Improved sanitation and hygiene (which includes good hand-washing technique) have decreased the incidence even further.

Viral Conjunctivitis. *Viral conjunctivitis* seldom occurs without involvement of the cornea. Therefore, virus infections of the external eye are known as keratoconjunctivitis. These viruses may roughly be gathered into four main groups.

1. *Adenovirus,* the largest of the four groups, can be subdivided into three serological groups and types.
2. *Herpes simplex virus.*
3. *Molluscum.*
4. Virus infections which are rare but may be transmitted from animals. Among these are *myxovirus of Newcastle disease* in fowl, and *cat scratch disease.* Systemic viruses can also cause viral conjunctivitis. This is seen early in the course of such viral diseases as mumps, influenza, and infectious mononucleosis.

Adenoviruses. Adenoviruses may be divided into three serological groups:

- Group I is considered nonepidemic and contains Types 3, 7, and 16.
- Group II is the epidemic form and is referred to as *epidemic keratoconjunctivitis* or (EKC). This is usually Type 8; however, Types 9 and 29 are included in this group.
- Group III contains Type 1.

While Type 8 is the main Type responsible for EKC, Type 7 (which is in Group I and is considered nonepidemic), frequently masquerades as EKC, and is more often responsible for respiratory infections than EKC.[2]

Epidemic keratoconjunctivitis is not usually accompanied by respiratory symptoms. Most often its onset is unilateral, with lacrimation and foreign body sensation. There is preauricular lymphadenopathy, and occasionally periorbital pain. Severe conjunctivitis is present and can have a duration of 7 to 14 days. The corneal involvement distinguishes this from other adenovirus infections.

During the first week, superficial epithelial lesions can be observed when stained with fluorescein. Then about 11 to 15 days after onset, subepithelial lesions appear (these lesions can be seen on Slitlamp examination). The subepithelial lesions may intensify for the next 10 to 20 days, and then after about 3 months they begin to fade. In severe cases, subepithelial opacities may last for as long as 2 years. About 50 percent of patients with EKC develop the signs of keratitis (inflammation of the cornea), and half of these will develop the subepithelial infiltrates. In most patients, the second eye also develops signs and symptoms, but the degree of involvement may vary.[3]

Epidemic keratoconjunctivitis was first described in the 19th century in Europe and Asia. During World War II, it broke out in the Marin shipyards in California and gradually worked its way east. In 1955, Jawitz first isolated the infective organism and found it could be recovered from eye and throat up to 14 days after onset of the disease.

Some variants of EKC, in severe infections, may produce swelling of the lids with membranous formation (Fig. 12–6). Follicles may also be present in the palpebral conjunctiva, but the lids must be everted for this to be seen.

In children there is frequently a fever, upper respiratory disease with otitis media, and a rather mild conjunctivitis.

Treatment consists of rest, analgesics, topical antibiotics (to prevent a secondary infection), compresses, and astringents. Steroids, while making the patient feel better initially, will prolong final recovery. Steroid discontinuance may result in an exacerbation of the disease.[4]

NURSING INTERVENTION

On assessment, the most common statement from the patient is that of "feeling as if something is in the eye" (foreign body sensation). Notice that the eye is tearing profusely, and the conjunctive is red (hyperemic). The patient might say that it feels as if the whole eye hurts. If the cornea is involved, then light sensitivity might be a complaint. An enlarged preauricular node can often be palpated on the affected side.

Because EKC is spread by droplet and contact, health care personnel should take precautions since there appears to be a very low level of immunity to this Type 8 virus in the general population of the United States.[3] Infected persons can transfer the agent quite easily. They mop their tearing eyes with a tissue (or their fingers), then touch all the equipment around them. The equipment should be thoroughly cleaned, using a viracidal agent after the patient suspected of having EKC has been attended to. Handwashing is vital if cross-contamination is to be avoided.

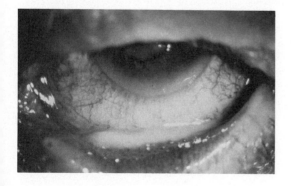

Figure 12–6. Some varieties of epidemic keratoconjunctivitis (EKC) may produce swelling of the lids with membranous formation. *(Photograph courtesy of Juan Arentsen, M.D., Co-Director, Cornea Department, Wills Eye Hospital.)*

PATIENT TEACHING

Patient teaching should include the importance of handwashing, and using only a personal washcloth and towel to prevent cross-contamination of family members; suggestions of comfort measures, such as rest, compresses, and analgesic self-medication; a review of the correct method of eyedrop administration; and encouragement with respect to a commitment to follow-up care by an ophthalmologist.

Herpes Simplex Conjunctivitis. Herpes simplex conjunctivitis is being recognized more frequently. It is characterized by a follicular or pseudomembranous reaction, and may be misdiagnosed as epidemic (adenoviral) keratoconjunctivitis. On first examination only one eye is involved, but later 30 percent of the patients will have bilateral disease. Initial Slitlamp examination will probably not reveal mucosal vesicles or dendritic involvement of the cornea. Later, however, 16 percent will have cutaneous or mucosal involvement, and of these patients, half will develop dendritic keratitis. Definite diagnosis is made with fluorescent–antibody technique.

Correct diagnosis is important because treatment is different from other viral infections. Idoxiuridine, adenine arabinoside, and trifluridine are three antiviral agents (specific for this virus) which may be prescribed for topical use, or the ophthalmologist may choose debridement of corneal epithelial lesions—both of treatments could be beneficial in the herpetic conjunctivitis. Use of steroids could cause serious spread of the herpes simplex virus.

NURSING INTERVENTION

Encourage compliance when antiviral eye medication is prescribed. Stress importance of follow-up care.

PATIENT TEACHING

Patient teaching for the mother who has "cold sores" on her lips should include discouraging her from kissing her baby or children on the eyelids. The same virus is responsible for herpes simplex.

Acute Epidemic Hemorrhagic Conjunctivitis. This viral conjunctivitis was first reported in 1968 in Ghana.[5] It received the name of Apollo II conjunctivitis (because it was identified about the time of the Apollo II space mission). Epidemic outbreaks later occurred in Japan, Taiwan, Hong Kong, India, Morocco, Singapore, Thailand, Indonesia, England, France, and Yugoslavia. In 1981, it was reported in South and Central America, and the Caribbean states. In September and October 1981, 3500 cases were reported in Miami, Florida.[6]

This type of conjunctivitis occurs as a sudden onset of ocular symptoms which peak within several hours. The eyes become red with a foreign body sensation or pain, tearing, discharge, and photophobia. Small hemorrhages also present, are usually seen at the superior temporal part of the bulbar conjunctiva. There is an associated follicular formation and chemosis in all patients. Diffuse superficial corneal epithelial opacities can be viewed with Slitlamp, but they rapidly disappear. Approximately 90 percent of patients have preauricular lymphadenopathy.

It is believed that this disease is produced by a rhinovirus which is a subgroup of the picornavirus. These viruses do not cross-react with other members of the picornavirus such as the enterovirus, poliovirus, and Coxsackie virus. They are extremely small particles, contain ribonucleic acid or genetic material, and there are several types which cause acute epidemic hemorrhagic conjunctivitis.[7,8.]

NURSING INTERVENTION
This disease is spread by droplet infection, and has a short incubation period of 1 to 4 days. The same precautions taken for EKC should be applied if this disease entity is suspected. If it occurs in epidemic proportions then the Public Health Department should be notified.

Molluscum Conjunctivits. Molluscum conjunctivitis is a secondary conjunctivitis resulting from infection of molluscum growing on the lid margin. The virus does not grow in the conjunctiva, but the lesion is a reaction to the virus, debris, and/or the toxin which the virus liberates. Once the lesion is excised from the lid margin, the conjunctiva usually clears.

NURSING INTERVENTION
When a patient has a persistent complaint of having something in the eye which bothers them and what appears to be a chronic conjunctivitis, the nurse should refer the patient to an ophthalmologist for evaluation.

Chlamydia or TRIC Agents
Trachoma is the world's leading cause of preventable blindness, however, it is difficult to develop a clear picture of the specific cause of this condition. The organisms responsible for the disease are known as *Trachoma Inclusion Conjunctivitis* or (TRIC) agents. These organisms have been considered as large viruses under the name of *Bedsonia,* or *Psitticosis-Lymphogranuloma venereum-Trachoma* (PTL), but today they are referred to as *Chlamydia.* They are susceptible to some antibiotics, even though they live intracellularly, and microscopically can be seen as inclusion bodies.[9]

In the early acute stage, there may be marked conjunctival reaction such as redness and the formation of follicles. This conjunctival involvement is found in the superior tarsus. Follicles may also be found at the corneal limbus. After the acute inflammation subsides, there is scarring of the lids, with distortion causing the lid margins to turn in (entropion), and the lashes to abrade the cornea (trichiasis). This irritation causes new vessels to grow in from the limbus, especially from above. This invasion of neovascular tissue is called *pannus* and is a characteristic of trachoma. The follicles at the limbus atrophy and leave depressions called Herbert's pits which are diagnostic of trachoma. They remain visible usually throughout life.

In endemic areas of the world, i.e., North Africa, sub-Sahara Africa, the Middle East, and the dryer regions of the Indian subcontinent, Southeast Asia, and pockets of the southwest United States, the transmission of the organism is through direct contact—mother to child, sibling to sibling, etc.—the contamination occurs via fingers, flies, gnats, and other vectors. Most of the cases of blinding trachoma occur in children, where the disease progresses, eventually leading to deformity and disability in later life.

Treatment consists of a 3-week course of either tetracycline or erythromycin given orally, in doses recommended for systemic infection. Tetracyclines, however, cannot be given to young children, pregnant women, or nursing mothers because of the mottling effect it may have on the child's teeth. Erythromycin also can have side effects which can cause serious physical incapacities. Topical treatment, therefore, is safer and can be as effective if used over a longer period of time.[10,11]

Recent studies demonstrated that the disease could be suppressed if 1 percent tetracycline ointment is given twice daily, 6 days a week for 10 weeks.

NURSING INTERVENTION
Since personal hygiene is often poor in areas where trachoma is rampant, the need for patient teaching is monumental. Methods should be found to improve handwashing techniques; however, where water is a precious commodity, this becomes a difficult task. Maintaining a basin, especially for handwashing, could be encouraged. Religious restrictions may well rebel against this practice, for many feel that only running water should be used for washing. The eyes should be kept free from the dried mucous, which when moist probably encourages the flies to settle in that region. Compliance with medication regimens should also be encouraged.

Inclusion Blennorrhea. Recently there has been a demonstration that the organism that causes inclusion blennorrhea is a TRIC agent. Immunologically, there is a distinction from trachoma, but the organisms are closely related. Inclusion blennorrhea or inclusion conjunctivitis is a common form of ophthalmia neonatorium which is caused by the chlamydia agent. It is transmitted to the newborn from the cervix at birth. Transmission by adults is through sexual contact. Parents should be treated with systemic tetracycline.[9] Diagnosis can be made with the assistance of giemsa stain of the conjunctival epithelial cells, as well as immunofluorescent staining and complement fixation testing of these cells.[10]

Allergic Conjunctivitis. *Allergic conjunctivitis* is one of the most common diseases of the external eye. Even with sophisticated immulogical assessment techniques it is still not always possible to establish a specific diagnosis and treatment for allergic conjunctivitis. Allergic eye problems can be categorized into three major groups.[12]

I. Atopic Conditions
   A. Acute or chronic atopic keratoconjunctivitis can be associated with:
      1. Hay fever; there is a history of allergy to pollens;

2. Sensitivities due to animal proteins, i.e., dander, feathers, and dust;
3. Sensitivities due to ingested material and food.

B. Vernal catarrh: This seasonal disease appears more commonly in warm weather, and although an uncommon entitity, it is bilateral when it occurs. Young boys seem more predisposed to it than girls. Often there is also an associated history of asthma, eczema, etc. In so-called "palpebral vernal keratoconjunctivitis," the upper tarsal conjunctiva has giant papillae that give the conjunctiva a cobblestone appearance (Fig. 12–7).

C. Urticaria of lids may result from insect bites, systemic drugs, and serum sickness. Erythema multiform major (Stevens-Johnson syndrome) is a disease of the mucous membranes and skin, and can fall into this category.

II. Drug Sensitivities

A. Contact dermatoconjunctivitis can occasionally be seen from such frequently used drugs as atropine, scopolamine, or antibiotic drugs such as the mycins. The conjunctiva appears red, the lids (and skin) become indurated in areas with which the drug has come in contact, and the patient complains of itching, burning, and tearing.

B. Chronic follicular keratoconjunctivitis can develop from conditions such as idoxuridine (IDU) after long-term use; D.F.P. (a seldom used miotic); the cleaning and disinfecting solutions for soft contact lenses which have not been properly rinsed from the lenses.

C. Medicamentosa is a conjunctivitis due to ingested compounds such as arsenic and gold.

III. Microbial Allergies

A. Phlyctenular keratoconjunctivitis

1. Delayed tuberculous hypersensitivity due to the products of mycobacteria are seen more frequently in countries where tuberculosis is still a rampant disease.

2. Coccidioidomycoses may, on rare occasions, cause a granulomatous conjunctivitis, which is metastatic from the primary pulmonary infection.

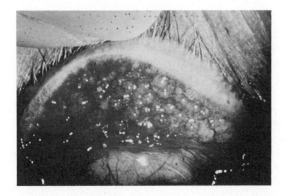

Figure 12–7. Conjunctival cobblestone appearance of vernal conjunctivitis.

3. Bacterial conjunctivitis.
4. *Staphylococci phlyctenular* disease and *phlyctenular pannus* is more frequently associated with delayed hypersensitivity to *S. aureus* in the United States.
   B. Marginal corneal ulcers due to sensitivity to *Staphylococcus*.
   C. Reactions to parasites (onchocerciasis—one of the four leading causes of blindness in tropical underdeveloped countries; and trichinosis).
   D. Possible reactions to chlamydial and viral agents.

The allergic reaction may vary from a pale edema which is very minimal, to a great deal of edema which can close the eye or force a sac of boggy conjunctiva out from under, or between the lids. The most common associated complaints are ocular itching and burning. There can also be classic signs of conjunctival inflammation.

NURSING INTERVENTION

Since treatment consists of instillation of vasoconstrictors in very mild cases, the patient should be encouraged to comply with self-medication. Topical antihistamines can be used too, but these are not very active locally.

Steroids are prescribed, but if used over a long period of time may produce severe glaucoma in the steroid-responder patient. Some patients may even form cataracts from overuse or misuse of ocular steroids. The nurse should therefore attempt to ensure that the patient understands any time constraints which have been placed with regard to administration of steroids.

Elimination of exposure to pollen, dander, bacteria, mold, and dust reduces the severity and frequency of the attacks. The nurse may wish to suggest methods of decreasing patient contact with allergy producing agents. This, of course, would include drugs.

Cromoglycote is a new drug which is useful in the treatment of asthmatics, and has been shown in England to have a beneficial effect on vernal conjunctivitis.

Conjunctival Tumors

All the conjunctival tissues, which include surface epithelium, pigment cells, connective tissue, vascular tissue, lymphatic tissue, and nerves can develop tumors. Congenital tumors which contain cells and tissue normally found in the conjunctiva are called *hamartoma*. Those tumors which contain cells *not* usually found in the conjunctiva, i.e., bone, teeth, and hair, are called *choristomas*.

Benign Congenital Tumors

Dermoid Choristomas. *Dermoid choristomas* are tumors which when cystic are called *dermoid cysts*. These cysts usually contain keratin and sebaceous material. Treatment consists of total excision.

Another dermoid choristoma is the solid *dermoid lipoma* which contains fat cells. These dermoids, usually located in the horizontal plane (at 9 and 3 o'clock), may extend into the orbit, and surround or replace some of the extraocular muscles.

If this is the case, excision is for cosmetic purposes only, and therefore, minimal surgical intervention may be carried out.

Limbal dermoids occur at the junction of the conjunctiva and cornea (Fig. 12–8). These are found on the lateral limbus, and may contain lacrimal glands. About 33 percent are associated with other congenital anomalies, i.e., ear-tags and facial bony structural abnormalities (Goldenhar syndrome).

Vascular Tumors. Vascular tumors have been mentioned under hereditary hemorrhagic telangiectasis. See page 177.

Hemangiomas may be divided into two types: the *capillary (strawberry marks)* usually regress and need no treatment, and *cavernous hemangiomas* which have larger irregular anastomosing channels, lie deeper, and may extend into the orbit. There is less regression in these than in the capillary type.

NURSING INTERVENTION
The nurse may be the first person to notice any one of the above abnormalities in the child's eye. The child should be referred to an ophthalmologist. If surgical intervention is undertaken, the operating room nurse should handle the specimen carefully and correctly prior to sending it the pathology department. Postoperative nursing care would include observation of the postoperative pressure patch, which should remain dry and intact for a prescribed period, usually 24 hours. There should be limited bleeding, with only a little serosanguinous staining on the eyepatch when it is removed. Ointments for lubrication and to increase the contact time of the steroid–antibiotic medication will need to be instilled.

PATIENT TEACHING
Instruct the child's parents with respect to the proper method of instilling eye medications. Compliance with follow-up care is important and should be reinforced.

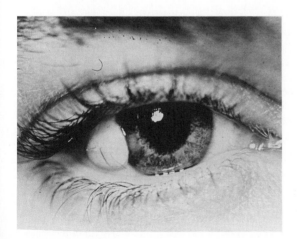

Figure 12–8. Limbal dermoid of the conjunctiva.

Acquired Benign Tumors

Lymphangiomas. *Lymphangiomas* occur rarely. They are benign lesions that progress slowly. Occasionally, the lymphatic channels may be filled with blood because a blood vessel ruptures into the tumor. Treatment is careful excision for cosmetic and, at times, functional reasons.

Lymphatic dilatation or lymphangiectasia occurs frequently and usually regresses soon after appearing. If the crystal clear chain of dilated lymph vessels do not disappear, and they cause the patient psychological and/or cosmetic distress, they can be excised.

Nevi. *Nevi* are conjunctival tumors usually present at birth, but under hormonal stimulation about one-third develop pigmentation. Some of these undergo cystic changes, but unless the lesions are irritated melanogenesis usually remains constant. These lesions can be seen as brown spots on the conjunctiva, and if they become cosmetically and emotionally annoying, surgical excision by an ophthalmologist can be undertaken.

NURSING INTERVENTION

The nurse should be astutely aware of the lesions which suddenly appear or which change in size and shape, and should refer the patient for immediate evaluation.

Acquired Malignant Tumors

Malignant Melanomas. *Malignant melanomas* may arise from nevi or areas of acquired melanosis without any other preexisting lesion. There may also be metastatic lesions from the skin and elsewhere, or extension through the sclera.

Those tumors arising locally from the conjunctiva should be locally excised; those arising from acquired melanosis may be somewhat sensitive to radiation. These should be biopsied prior to initial treatment.

Epithelial Tumors. Familiarity with the following special terms will help the nurse have a better understanding of epithelial tumors.

1. Pseudocancerous lesions—those tumors that clinically and microscopically may resemble cancer, but do not develop into cancer.
2. Precancerous lesions—lesions which may resemble cancer and may, if left untreated, develop into cancer.
3. Cancerous lesions—lesions which have capacity to invade and destroy adjacent tissue and to metastasize.
4. Carcinoma *in situ*—refers to a lesion which has all the histological characteristics of malignancy except that there is no invasion of the underlying stroma.

Bowan's Disease is a specific example of an *in situ* carcinoma of the skin. The name is also applied to *in situ* carcinoma of the conjunctival epithelium. Treatment is by surgical excision.

Multiple Idiopathic Hemorrhagic Sarcoma or Kaposi Sarcoma. This carcinoma is made up of neoplastic vascular endothelial cells, together with other types of cells, such as fibrocytes, phagocytes, and pericytes. These lesions appear as red papules and nodules beneath the conjunctiva. They may also occur in the skin of the lower extremities. Kaposi's sarcoma may be associated with lymphomas. Originally it was known to occur in middle-aged mid-European men, and also young African children where it could be found in association with Burkett's sarcoma.

Recently, it has been reported in very sick homosexual males with acquired immune deficiency syndrome (AIDS). The Epstein-Barr virus is believed to be the cause of African Burkett's sarcoma, and the similar herpes virus may be the exciting agent or occur in these new cases. Researchers have recently isolated a more specific virus responsible for AIDS.

The agent producing AIDS is a retrovirus called "Human T-cell leukemia lymphotropic virus type III" (*HTLV-III*). This virus infects and destroys T-lymphocytes which regulate the human body immunological defenses. With the defenses lowered, the patient can be overwhelmed by other organisms as well as developing neoplasms such as leukemia and Kaposi's sarcoma. The HTLV-III virus has been found in the tears. Whether the virus is infectious or not in such a diluted amount has not yet been determined. However, it is necessary to take extreme precautions when treating or dealing with patients with AIDS.

The ocular manifestation of AIDS in the lids, conjunctiva, and cornea can appear in several forms. Kaposi's sarcoma of the conjunctiva has been seen on many occasions. Subconjunctival hemorrhages do occur and a nonsuppurative conjunctivitis is also seen. Herpes zoster keratitis as well as herpes conjunctivitis can occur, and on some electron microscopic studies of biopsied material cytomegalic virus inclusion bodies as well as the herpes virus has been demonstrated. Severe mulluscum lesions of the lid may also flourish. It seems that the conjunctival signs and symptoms may be mild or minimal, yet there may be serious risk to the examiner unless precautions are taken.[13,14,15]

NURSING INTERVENTION
Gloves should be worn when examining the eye of the AIDS patient. Instruments that come into direct contact with the eye, e.g., tonometers, can be disinfected in a 1:10 dilution of bleach (sodium hypochlorite— Clorox) and clean water for 5 minutes at room temperature. The instruments should then be rinsed in clean water (not necessarily sterile) and wiped dry. Alternatively, the instruments may be soaked in 70 percent ethanol, rinsed and allowed to dry. Note that isopropyl alcohol is not as effective.[16]

Conjunctival Degenerative Diseases
Pinguecula. *Pinguecula* can be seen in adults as a small conjunctival nodule, appearing on both sides of the cornea (but more commonly on the nasal side). The nodule, composed of yellow elastic tissue and hyaline, usually does not increase in size. No treatment is necessary unless it becomes inflamed and irritated.

NURSING INTERVENTION
The patient should be referred for ophthalmological evaluation if the lesion becomes inflamed and irritated.

Pterygium. *Pterygium* may be seen nasally as a triangular, connective tissue overgrowth of bulbar conjunctiva onto the cornea (Fig. 12–9). Pterygia may be bilateral. The people who seem to be susceptible are those who spend most of their lives out of doors in sunny, or dusty or sandy windblown areas. It is thought that this is an irritative phenomenon due to ultraviolet light.

Treatment consists of surgical excision of the pterygium if it encroaches on the cornea, occasionally followed by a postoperative application of Beta-radiation.

NURSING INTERVENTION
Refer the patient to an ophthalmologist if the pterygium is beginning to extend onto the cornea.

After surgical intervention, antibiotic ointment is instilled, and a firm patch is applied to eliminate any bleeding. Later the patch is removed in order that the Beta-radiation application can be given.

PATIENT TEACHING
Encourage compliance with prescribed steroid–antibiotic combination eyedrops. The date of the follow-up visit should be reviewed prior to discharge.

Pemphigoid. Ocular involvement is characterized by progressive shrinkage of the conjunctiva, entropion, trichiasis, xerosis, and finally reduced vision from corneal opacification.

The first symptoms are those of chronic conjunctivitis, with irritation, burning, and tearing. When secondary bacterial infection is superimposed there may also be a mucopurulent discharge. If there is corneal involvement, the patient will complain of foreign body sensation, photophobia, and decreased vision.

Cicatricial pemphigoid is a destructive fibrotic process which occurs beneath the conjunctival epithelium. As the disease progresses, *symblepharons* (Fig. 12–10)

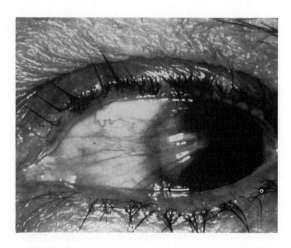

Figure 12–9. Pterygium.

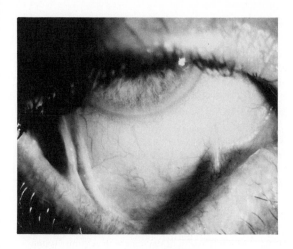

Figure 12–10. Symblepharon. *(Photograph courtesy of Juan Arentsen, M.D., Co-Director, Cornea Department, Wills Eye Hospital.)*

are formed between palpebral and bulbar conjunctiva; the fornices gradually shrink and mobility of the globe is impaired. There is an associated decrease in the tear film.

The disease occurs more frequently in women than in men, and is typically a disease of middle age. It may rapidly progress to blindness. Only the conjunctiva may be affected or all mucous membranes may be involved, i.e., mouth, nose, gastrointestinal tract, vulva, and skin. No treatment is available. On occasions when the disease has progressed to blindness, prosthokeratoplasty has been attempted with variable success.

NURSING INTERVENTION
Encourage the patient to use ocular lubricants and artificial tears for comfort. Give emotional support. Nursing care of the prosthokeratoplasty patient will be discussed in Chapter 13.

REFERENCES

1. Johnson G: Crede's treatment in Nurse's Reference Library Procedures. Springhouse, Penn.: Intermed Communication, 1983, p. 776–777
2. Dawson C, Hanna L, Togni B: Adenovirus Type 8 infection in the United States. Archives of Ophthalmology, 87(3): 258–268, 1972
3. Dawson C, Hanna L, Wood TR, Despain R: Adenovirus Type 8 keratoconjunctivitis in U.S. American Journal of Ophthalmology, 69(3): 473–480, 1970
4. Knopf HLS, Hierholzer J: Clinical and immunologic responses in patients with viral keratoconjunctivitis. American Journal of Ophthalmology, 80(10): 661–662, 1975
5. Kono R, Sasagawa A, Keizo I, et al.: Pandemic of new type of conjunctivitis. Lancet, 1(6): 1191–1194, 1972
6. Sklar VEF, Patriarca PA, Onorato IM, et al.: Clinical findings and results of treatment in

an outbreak of acute hemorrhagic conjunctivitis in southern Florida. American Journal of Ophthalmology, 95: 45–54, 1983

7. Chatergee S, Quarcoopome CO, Apenteng A: Unusual type of epidemic conjunctivitis in Ghana. British Journal of Ophthalmology, 54: 628–630, 1970

8. Yen FY, Portying H, Lon KL, et al.: Epidemic hemorrhagic keratoconjunctivitis. American Journal of Ophthalmology 80(8): 193–197, 1975

9. Dawson CR, Jones BR, Tarizzo ML: Guide to Trachoma Control. Geneva, Switzerland: WHO, 1981, p. 40–43

10. Yondea C, Dawson CR, Daghfous T, et al.: Cytology as a guide to presence of chlamydial inclusion in Giemsa-stained conjunctival smears in severe epidemic trachoma. British Journal of Ophthalmology, 59(3): 116–124, 1975

11. Stenson S: Adult inclusion conjunctivitis. Archives of Ophthalmology, 99: 605–608, 1981

12. Jones BR: Allergic diseases of the outer eye. Transactions Ophthalmological Society, U.K., 91: 441–447, 1971

13. Palestine AG, Rodrigues MM, Macher AM: Ophthalmic involvement in acquired immunodeficiency syndrome. Ophthalmology, 91: 1092–1099, 1984

14. Khademk J, Kalish SB, Goldsmith J, et al.: Ophthalmic findings in the acquired immune deficiency syndrome (AIDS). Archives of Ophthalmology, 102: 201–206, 1984

15. Friedman A: Personal communication. Mt. Sinai Medical Center, Dept. of Ophthalmology, New York

16. Martin JS, McDougal JS, Loskoski SL. Disinfection and inactivation of the human T-Lymphotropic virus, Type III/Lymphadenopathy-associated virus. Journal of Infectious Diseases, 152: 400–403, 1985

BIBLIOGRAPHY

Cugalj N, Moore DS: Current considerations in neonatal conjunctivitis. J Nurse Midwife, 29(3): 197–204, 1984

Kaposi's sarcoma and pneumocystis pneumonia among homosexual males in New York City and California. MMWR, 30: 305–308, 1981

Pavan-Langston D, (Ed.): Ocular viral disease. Int Ophthalmol Clin, 15(4): 19–35; 171–185; 203–210; 187–201, 1975

Recommendations for preventing possible transmission of human lymphotropic virus type III/lymphadenopathy associated virus from tear. MMWR, 39: 533–539, 1985

Vaughan D, Asbury T: General Ophthalmology, 10th ed. Los Altos, Calif.: Lange, 1983

13

The Cornea and Sclera

NEW TERMS

Keratitis: inflammation of the cornea.
Keratoplasty: corneal transplant.
Leukoma: corneal opacity.
Limbus: corneoscleral junction.
Xerosis: dryness of the external surface of the eye.

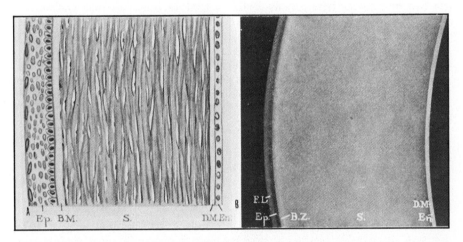

13–1. Five corneal layers. A comparison between histological (A) and optic (B) section of the cornea. F.L., film line; Ep., epithelium; Bm., Bowman's membrane; Bz., Bowman's zone; S., stroma; D.M., Descemet's membrane; En., endothelium. *(From Berliner ML: Biomicroscopy of the Eye. Hoeber Medical Division, New York: Harper & Row, 1949.)*

The clear, avascular *cornea* is the curved structure which forms approximately one-fifth of the outer circumference of the eyeball and is continuous with the *sclera* at the *limbus*. Similar to a watch crystal in nature, its sole purpose is to refract the light rays. The average adult cornea is about 0.65 mm thick and about 11.5 mm in diameter. The five corneal layers are identified as follows (Fig. 13–1).

Epithelium the external, nonkeratinized layer is made up of five or six cell layers in which about 70 sensory nerve endings from the fifth cranial nerve are located. Its very regular and smooth surface is in touch with the precorneal tear film from which it also gets oxygen. The epithelium has its own basement membrane and is able to regenerate and heal without a scar. On Slitlamp examination (SLE) the nonrelucence of the epithelium makes it appear dark.

Bowman's membrane, just beneath the epithelium, is an acellular layer of uniform fibrils. It is nonregenerative and therefore when damaged heals *with* a scar. On SLE, Bowman's membrane appears as a bright interval just posterior to the dark epithelial interval.

Stroma composes 90 percent of the corneal thickness and is made up of parallel layers of loosely adherent lamellae (bundles of collagen fibrils). This parallel arrangement of fibrils accounts for stromal optical clarity. The stroma is dependent upon epithelial and endothelial metabolic actions to maintain its detergency and prevent excessive hydration or swelling. On SLE it can be seen to have uniform thickness and gives a ground glass appearance. Damage to the stroma results in scarring.

Descemet's membrane is an elastic membrane, the product of endothelial cells secretion, which is found on the inner surface of the stroma. In acute ulceration it acts as a barrier to perforation, referred to as a *decemetocele.* It is not usually seen on SLE unless it has been pathologically changed, in which case folds and tears can be identified.

The *endothelium* is a single layer of hexagonal cells which acts as a water pump. It receives its oxygen from the aqueous. These endothelial cells do not regenerate but merely slide over to take the place of damaged cells. Slitlamp examination of the endothelium reveals a mosaic pattern. Since there are no blood vessels in the cornea it receives nutrition from the perilimbal vessels, the aqueous humor, and the tear film.

SLITLAMP EXAMINATION

The Slitlamp (Fig. 13–2) is a necessity in ophthalmic examination. The need for magnification and adequate lighting is fundamental in examining the eye. These principles are best combined in a modern Slitlamp which consists of a binocular microscope, a lamp in a housing, and a patient headrest. The microscope mounted on a sturdy movable arm has a variable power from 5 to 20 times magnification depending upon the instruments' make and model. The light source is a lamp, the beam of which can be focused by lenses on the eye, and the beam size and shape can be regulated by a shutter. A very thin slit of light (which gives the instrument its name—Slitlamp) is made possible by these shutters. This sliver of light when focused enables the observer to localize the depth and size of a lesion in the cornea, anterior chamber, lens, and anterior vitreous. The anterior chamber can be examined for floating cells in the beam. In inflammation of the anterior eye, protein liberated in the aqueous humor reflects the light rays in the beam similar to sun light passing through smoke. The lamp assembly is mounted on another movable arm which can swing from side to side. Both microscope arm and lamp arm pivot on the same post which arises from a platform and which can move sideways, forward, and back. A joystick is used to initiate and control these movements and in some models can also elevate both the lamp and microscope. When the arms are locked

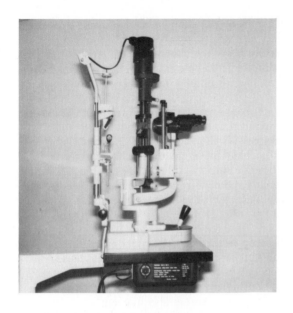

Figure 13–2. The Slitlamp.

together, the observer can sweep the focused beam over the anterior structures as well as deep into the interior of the eye.

The third part of the Slitlamp is an adjustable, comfortable headrest for the patient.

CONGENITAL ABNORMALITIES

Developmental abnormalities include variations in the size, shape, clarity, and structure of the cornea.

Microcornea implies a corneal diameter of less than 10 mm. Usually unilateral, the eye may be normal or microphthalmic (smaller in size). Crowding of the anterior structures may result in glaucoma.[1]

Megalocornea is a nonprogressive, bilateral, symmetric inherited condition in which the cornea is larger than 12 mm in diameter, without evidence of previous or concurrent increase in intraocular pressure which is responsible for the enlargement in size. All modes of inheritance have been described.[2] Subluxation (partial dislocation) of the lens is common.

Cornea plana exists when the corneal curvature is less than normal. Anterior chamber shallowing also occurs. The limbus may not be identified. Refractive and anterior segment abnormalities are associated with this relatively rare inherited (as either dominant or recessive) anomaly.[2]

Dystrophies

Dystrophies are a rare hereditary group of corneal disorders characterized by bilateral abnormal deposition of substances, associated with nonvascular alterations in the normal cornea; usually without manifestation of inflammatory signs and symptoms. Some degree of corneal opacification or clouding is present in these diseases which may result in mild to severe visual acuity loss.[3,4]

Although dystrophies occasionally begin in childhood, most are first seen in the teenage or later years with the disease getting progressively worse in mid-adult life. Dystrophies can be classified as anterior limiting membrane, stromal, or posterior limiting membrane.[4]

Congenital hereditary corneal dystrophy may be seen at birth as full-thickness clouded corneas. These must be examined to rule out congenital glaucoma. Penetrating keratoplasty may be attempted with variable results.

Anterior corneal dystrophies include those involving the epithelium and Bowman's membrane which can become thick and thin, thus resulting in astigmatism, slight decrease in visual acuity, corneal irritation, and decreased corneal sensitivity, e.g., Meesman's dystrophy, Cogan's dystrophy, Fingerprint dystrophy, Reis-Buckler's dystrophy.

Stromal corneal dystrophies are of three types: *granular,* in which fine, whitish "granular" lesions can be seen in the corneal stroma on SLE; *macular dystrophy,* which starts in Bowman's membrane and manifests as a dense, gray central opacity which spreads peripherally—recurrent corneal erosions may occur and vision is severely impaired; and *lattice dystrophy,* in which the stroma becomes involved with linear opacities—recurrent erosions are also frequent.

Posterior limiting membrane or Fuchs's dystrophy begins at about the 4th or 5th decade, is most frequently seen in women, and is a slowly progressive corneal disease in which edema results from the primary metabolic incompetence of the endothelial cells. This leads to stromal opacification and epithelial edema. Bullous keratopathy may eventually occur and when the bullae (vesicles) rupture, the patient experiences the discomfort of pain and foreign body sensation. Vision and comfort may be restored by penetrating keratoplasty.[2]

Keratoconus (conical cornea) is a central noninflammatory ectasia (thinning) of the cornea. It occurs sporadically, is most frequently bilateral, often asymmetric, and is of unknown etiology. There is teenage onset, at about puberty, with progression around the age of 30. The keratoconus hallmarks are irregular progressive astigmatism and distortion of the corneal light reflex. Corneal irregularities can be seen on examination when Placido disc, retinoscope, or corneoscope (fancy Placido disc) are used. When the direct ophthalmoscope is used on +5 the nurse may see an "oil drop" surface. Slitlamp examination reveals early breaks in Bowman's membrane. Descemet's membrane breaks are found as apical thinning which becomes evident later. *Acute hydrops*—actual breaks in Descemet's membrane—may occur and result in corneal scarring. Munson's sign is evident when the conical cornea indents the lower lid as the patient looks down.

Conditions associated with keratoconus include: *atopy,* the history of allergy, eczema, or asthma; patients who have a tendency to rub their eyes; Down's syndrome, retinitis pigmentosa, and Leber's congenital amaurosis.

Identifying the patient who has unstable progressive astigmatism may be difficult at first since the only symptom is progressive poor vision which needs constant change of glasses. Hard contact lenses are used to neutralize the astigmatism, initially. Thermokeratoplasty has also been used to shrink collagen and temporarily make the cornea flatter, thus enabling better contact lens fit. Occasionally, an acute hydrops occurs when Descemet's membrane is stretched to its breaking point; the eye becomes very red and painful, with corneal haze and decreased vision. This condition will be treated medically with cycloplegic eyedrops, oral acetozolamide (Diamox), and an eye patch for comfort. Treatment may continue for 2 months or more and the patient will need much reassurance. Central scarring may result which adversely affects vision. About 4 percent of these keratoconus patients will require corneal transplants.

NURSING INTERVENTION
Nursing intervention includes supporting and reassuring the patient and his or her family during the difficult time of early diagnosis. If hydrops has occurred in the keratoconus patient, encourage medication regimen compliance. Penetrating keratoplasty nursing care will be discussed in detail later in this chapter.

ACQUIRED ANOMALIES

Degenerations
Arcus Senilis. *Arcus senilis* is a commonly seen, bilateral, peripheral gray corneal degeneration which occurs in elderly persons as part of the aging process. When seen in persons under the age of 50, hypercholesteremia should be suspected.

Band Keratopathy. *Band keratopathy* occurs when calcium deposits accumulate in the corneal epithelium, Bowman's layer, and the superficial stroma; this can arise from localized ocular inflammation (e.g., chronic nongranulomatous uveitis) or systemic disease (e.g., hypercalcemia). To correct this, the cornea is anesthetized with 0.5 percent tetracaine hydrochloride eyedrops and an application of a calcium binding chelating agent such as EDTA (ethylenediaminetetraacetic acid) is placed on the cornea.[2] The corneal calcium deposits are now removed by debridement. Visual prognosis depends upon the extent of the diseased cornea.

NURSING INTERVENTION
Seat the patient comfortably at the Slitlamp or lie him or her down (depending upon the physician's preference for performing the procedure). Anesthetize the eye using the prescribed topical anesthetic prior to the surgical procedure being accomplished by an ophthalmologist. At the end of the procedure pressure patch the eye. Assess and medicate for pain as necessary. The eye may be patched and repatched until corneal healing takes place.

Xerophthalmia. *Xerophthalmia* is a major cause of childhood blindness throughout Asia and to a lesser extent in Africa and Latin America. Night blindness occurs early in the disease, while the earliest corneal manifestation is *superficial punctate keratopathy*—microscopic pinpoint holes in the corneal epithelium. Conjunctival xerosis presents with areas that have a "foamy" or "cheesy" appearance known as Bitot's spots.[5] Corneal xerosis seen as mild haziness at first, later develops a dry, pebbly appearance. As the disease progresses, the classic corneal ulcer appears as a punched out lesion which may be plugged by iris tissue. *Keratomalacia,* the full thickness necrotic dissolution of the cornea, may occur in a matter of hours or days.[5] This corneal demise is a result of lack of vitamin A. Protein deficiency appears to be an important contributory factor, for in children with corneal xerophthalmia, serum vitamin A, retinol-binding protein (RBP), and serum prealbumin are very low.[6]

Treatment with vitamin A is essential, but at the same time the protein deficiency should be rectified. Oral administration of 200,000 IU vitamin A on 2 successive days (or in divided doses over 7 to 10 days) or intramuscular injection of 100,000 IU water miscible vitamin A might be given to children with severe systemic disease such as pneumonia and gastroenteritis. Malnourished children should also receive a protein-rich diet as well as prompt treatment of any systemic illness if they are to recover.

Topical antibiotics are prescribed to help prevent secondary bacterial infections in corneal xerosis. Subconjunctival and intravenous antibiotics will be administered in the more advanced corneal ulcers.[6] Use of synthetic vitamin A and carotene to fortify certain foods accounts for about 7 percent of all vitamin A intake in the United States. Vitamin A supplements have been added to staple foods (such as milk), and in this manner, the disease has been eliminated.

NURSING INTERVENTION

To improve the welfare of children suffering from vitamin A deficiency nursing intervention should be directed at their nutritional status. Inclusion in the diet of quantities of beta-carotene rich foods such as dark green leafy vegetables (DGLV), yellow or orange fruits such as papayas and mangoes, and roots, e.g., carrots, will eradicate xerophthalmia. Nutrition education of parents on the use of low-cost locally available DGLV can be done at local child care centers. Where corneal involvement is already present, protection of the globe with a plastic or metal shield is necessary.[6]

Corneal Ulcers

Corneal ulcers may occur as a result of many different causes such as invasion by: a) viruses, e.g., Herpes Simplex Virus (HSV) Type I; b) bacteria, e.g., *Pseudomonas aeruginosa, Streptococcus viridans, Streptococcus pneumoniae, Staphylococcus aureus,* and *Staphylococcus epidermidis* to name just a few; c) fungi, e.g., *Candida albicans, Fusarium, Aspergillus;* d) hypersensitivity reactions to staphylococcus, as may be seen in the marginal ulcer; e) unknown allergens or toxins, as seen in the ring ulcer; f) dietary vitamin A deficiency, e.g., xerophthalmia; g) fifth cranial nerve lesion (neurotropic ulcers); h) unknown cause, e.g., Mooren's ulcer. The ulcer may extend into the stromal layer and even deeper into the corneal layers. Once this occurs the healing process is very slow and leaves permanent scarring.

Viral Ulcers. *Herpes simplex keratitis* is the most commonly occurring corneal ulcer. The patient usually complains of mild irritation, tearing, and photophobia and, if the central cornea is infected, the vision will be blurred. History of a recent

URI (upper respiratory infection) with "cold sores" about the face is often elicited. Inspection of the cornea after it is stained with fluorescein will reveal one or more dendritic ulcers with the characteristic branching appearance (Fig. 13–3). Sometimes this pattern can be seen grossly after staining but it will be more obvious on SLE. Three herpes simplex-specific antiviral drugs are currently available; idoxuridine (IDU), vidarabin (Vira-A) and trifluridine (Viroptic)—the most costly— being the preferred drug of choice for treatment. Steroid use should be avoided. The ulcer has a recurrence rate in about 50 percent of patients, with edema of the cornea leading to scar formation which might ultimately need penetrating keratoplasty if vision is to be restored.

Herpes zoster ophthalmicus (HZV), caused by the same DNA virus that produces varicella (chickenpox), is thought to be due to activation of latent virus remaining within the dorsal root or cranial nerve ganglia of affected patients. It occurs in healthy individuals as well as those who have recently incurred trauma, ultraviolet or irradiation, surgery, immunosuppressive therapy, and malignancy. The full-blown syndrome is characterized by facial cutaneous eruptions over one or more divisions of the trigeminal nerve, kerato-uveitis, and postherpetic neuralgia. Keratitis is one of the most common complications of ocular herpes zoster and the patient experiences photophobia, lacrimation, and pain, and the eye appears red and uncomfortable. Dendritic lesions, identified on Slitlamp biomicroscopy, eventually heal but leave dull gray corneal opacities. Treatment of herpes zoster is nonspecific with symptomatic relief of pain the chief aim. Topical steroids and cycloplegic agents, e.g., 1 percent atropine sulfate or 0.25 percent scopolamine hydrobromide (used for the iridocyclitis) will be instilled in the eye, while soaking will be prescribed for active skin lesions. Acyclovir (ACV) has recently received FDA approval for treatment of HZV and HSV. Its administration can be topical, oral, or intravenous. Two other drugs which may soon be available are bromovinyldeoxyuridine (BVDU), and ethyldeoxyuridine (EDU). Cimetadine (Tagamet), a histamine blocker, has been administered within the first 48 to 72 hours of onset of the disease and has been shown to give rapid relief of pain and itching. A patient hospitalized for this condition will be nursed using an isolation technique.[7,8]

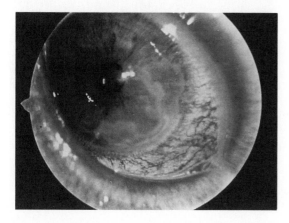

Figure 13–3. Dendritic ulcer caused by the herpes simplex virus shows characteristic branching appearance.

Bacterial Ulcers. When a bacterial corneal ulcer occurs (Fig. 13–4), a predisposing factor can usually be identified, e.g., dry eyes, poor or nonsterilization of contact lenses, corneal exposure, abrasion, a history of surgery, use of steroids or other immunosuppressant drugs. The patient will present with conjunctival injection, mucopurulent discharge, pain, tearing, and decreased vision if the ulcer is central. Hypopion which is usually sterile may be present. When the cornea is stained with fluorescein, a well-demarcated corneal defect will be seen. On SLE, stromal infiltrates (cells on a bed at the bottom of the ulcer) will be evident; ulcer necrosis may also be seen. Bacterial identification is accomplished by scraping the cornea with a sterilized platinium or ring spatula and plating specimens as follows:

1. Smear—three slides are needed for staining, one for Giemsa, one for fungus, and the third for ASB (acid fast bacilli).
2. Cultures plated on blood-agar, chocolate-agar, Thioglycolate (for anaerobic bacteria), and Sauberauds.
3. Antibiotic sensitivities will take about 48 hours to establish a specific diagnosis.

Topical, subconjunctival, and intravenous therapy may be necessary. In mild to moderate cases of corneal ulceration, only topical therapy or combination topical–subconjunctival therapy is used. Intravenous therapy is usually reserved for those cases where perforation occurs.

Fungal Ulcers. *Fungal corneal ulcers* can occur as a result of fungal overgrowth from long-term antibiotics and corticosteroid therapy.[3] Any patient who receives an eye injury which occurs from vegetable matter should also be observed closely for evidence of fungal invasion. Cultures take an extended period of time before results are available. Topical 5 percent natamycin eyedrops instilled hourly, is the treatment of choice for fungal keratitis caused by *Fusarium* and *Cephalosporium* species, while a specially prepared topical solution of miconazole can be used for *Candida* infection.[3]

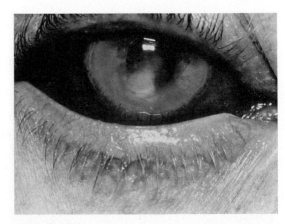

Figure 13–4. Bacterial corneal ulcer is seen as a large opacity on the cornea.

Miscellaneous Ulcers. *Hypersensitivity reactions* such as *marginal ulcers* (which occur as a known sensitivity to staphylococcus, and are found at the limbus) will be treated with frequent steroid drops. Isolation technique is not used if these patients are hospitalized. When the ulcer is due to an allergen or unknown cause such as a Mooren's ulcer, cryotherapy may be used by the physician. This can be done at the patient's bedside or even as an office procedure with close follow-up.

Neurotropic ulcers can occur when corneal exposure results following damage to the trigeminal nerve which supplies the cornea. Plastic surgical intervention of the lid such as a tarsorrhaphy may be necessary to promote healing.

Exposure keratitis can develop when the cornea is not properly covered by the eyelids. This can occur following Bell's palsy, as a result of exophthalmos, or following trauma or lid surgery. Corneal drying occurs and an ulcer may develop in the lower third of the cornea. Treatment will depend upon the underlying cause, however, two other methods of facilitating healing of an ulcer are as follows:

1. Use of a soft contact lens as a bandage lens to prevent the lid rubbing on the slow healing corneal ulcer. The contact lens remains in place even when medications are being instilled into the patient's eye. However, the nurse should be aware that if the patient complains of pain, the physician should be notified, for very often this signifies a need for contact lens removal.
2. A conjunctival flap which is performed as a sterile surgical procedure.

NURSING INTERVENTION
Nursing intervention is to admit the patient with an ocular infection into an isolation or protective care unit. This should be ordered by the physician. Meticulous handwashing should be carried out prior to and after administering treatments to these patients. Nonsterile, disposable gloves should be worn when ocular discharge is excessive. The impending treatment should be explained to the patient. If the patient is to receive eyedrops in both eyes, then the noninfected eye should be cleansed and medicated first.

To clean the infected eye, tilt the patient's head toward the infected side and gently irrigate the closed lid margin, while holding a cotton ball gauze square at the outer canthus (to catch the contaminated irrigation solution). Wipe mucous threads and secretions free. Discard the cotton ball or gauze square. The lashes can be cleansed with a slightly moistened applicator stick. If two antibiotic drops are given at the same frequency of time they should be alternated. For example, gentamycin q.l.h. given on the hour, and fortified bacitracin q.l.h. given on the half hour. Where other eye medications are ordered, a short time lapse should occur between each drop. If warm compresses are ordered they can be demonstrated to the patient and then performed by the patient; these are done prior to instillation of eyedrops. If the eye is tearing and the patient feels the need to mop the tears, he or she should be discouraged from using the same tissue for both eyes as this will be a source of cross-contamination. *An infected eye is never patched.* Bacterial growth increases when the appropriate circumstances are available such as would exist under an eye patch, e.g., warmth, moisture, darkness, and a culture media—the eye! Once the corneal ulcer shows signs of healing and all signs of infection are absent, steroid therapy may be instituted to decrease some of the inflammatory response.

Patients placed in isolation units tend to become very lonely and feel rather cut off from the world and indeed sometimes experience sensory deprivation if left alone too long, so these patients will need a great deal of psychological support during this acute period. Passive leg exercises might be appropriate if the patient is unable to leave the confinement of a room.

Deep Keratitis

Interstitial keratitis results from an allergic corneal reaction to the treponemal antigen in congenital syphilis. The use of antibiotics in the treatment of syphilis has dramatically decreased the incidence of interstitial keratitis, although both tuberculosis and leprosy can be the cause of this corneal insult.[9] In the patient with congenital syphilis, there is acute onset of marked, bilateral, stromal infiltration with severe photophobia, followed by rapid and extensive corneal vascularization. It usually occurs by the end of the first decade. Subsequently these vessels empty of blood and result in the formation of *ghost vessels*. Corticosteroids suppress the immunological inflammation. Instillation of 1 percent atropine sulfate eyedrops may be necessary to prevent posterior synechiae from developing. Dark glasses will relieve the photophbia. Extensive scarring results in decreased visual acuity.[9]

Corneal Pigmentation

Corneal pigmentation may occur with or without ocular or systemic disease. Sometimes the variation may be seen with a penlight, while at other times the subtle changes can only be viewed with the use of a Slitlamp.

Blood Staining. *Blood staining* of the cornea can occur in a small percentage of patients who have sustained a total traumatic hyphema which has rebelled, leading to an increased intraocular pressure. It can be seen as early as 36 hours post-injury on Slitlamp biomicroscopy. Later the cornea appears a golden brown and vision is decreased. This corneal pigmentation gradually clears but takes anywhere from 6 months to 2 years to do so.[3]

NURSING INTERVENTION

In the acute stages of a traumatic hyphema nursing intervention is directed at maintaining the patient's head in an elevated position so that the hyphema can settle by gravity. The injured eye should be shielded to prevent inadvertent, accidental bumping which might precipitate further bleeding. Rebleeding may be seen with penlight as fresh bright red blood in the anterior chamber, but a complaint of an acute, sharp pain in the eye should alert the nurse to its occurrence. An osmotic agent such as I.V. 20 percent Mannitol or oral isosorbide solution may be prescribed to decrease the intraocular pressure and will need to be administered.

Rings. *Kayser-Fleischer ring* is a pigmented ring that has a color ranging from ruby red to bright green, blue, yellow, and brown. It is composed of fine granules immediately in front of the endothelium, about 1 to 3 mm inside the limbus posteriorly. These rings have long been considered pathognomonic of Wilson's disease—a disease in which copper deposits accumulate in the brain, liver, and eye. Specific medical treatment with penicillamine, a copper chelating agent, may dramatically improve a disease that would otherwise be inevitably fatal.[3]

Fleischer's ring can be seen as a brownish or greenish line around the base of the corneal cone that occurs in keratoconus, and is probably due to deposits of iron (hemosiderin).

TRAUMA

Abrasions

Corneal abrasions occur when the superficial corneal epithelium is broken. This structure contains all the sensory nerve endings supplied to the cornea by the fifth cranial nerve and the symptom of acute pain appears to be disproportionate to the size of the injury. The patient seeking attention is often quite unreasonable and difficult to deal with because of the amount of pain being experienced. A red, irritated eye is observed, and the patient experiences photophobia and a decrease in vision if the abrasion is located in the pupillary region. Sometimes the abrasion can be seen with a penlight but examination with a Slitlamp using a cobalt blue filter, after staining the area with fluorescein dye, will give a much more accurate picture of the abraided cornea. Epithelial healing occurs within a 24- to 48-hour period. Cycloplegic eyedrops may be necessary for the iridocyclitis which can also occur, and an antibiotic drop or ointment, to prophylactically prevent infection, followed by a pressure patch will aid in comfort and facilitate healing. Analgesics may be required for pain.

NURSING INTERVENTION

Nursing intervention should include immediate assessment of the patient with acute ocular pain and decrease in visual acuity. A history of "hard contact lens overwear," a "fingernail or paper scratch on the eye" or "something in the eye" may be elicited on questioning. Everting the upper lid may reveal a foreign body under the lid which has caused the corneal abrasion. Instill the prescribed antibiotic and cycloplegic if ordered. Pressure patch the eye ensuring that it is properly closed under the patch.

PATIENT TEACHING

Patient teaching should include an explanation that the patch is to immobilize the eye and facilitate corneal healing and should be maintained for a prescribed period of time. At the time the patch may be removed, the prescribed antibiotic drops should be started. Encourage the patient to return for follow-up care to ensure that the corneal epithelial healing process is occurring appropriately.

Recurrent Corneal Erosion

Recurrent corneal erosion can be identified by classic signs and symptoms of the presenting history. When the patient attempts to open the eyes in the morning the lids pull off loose corneal epithelium and the patient awakes with a seething, continuous pain in the eye which then become red, irritated, and photophobic.

Three types of recurrent corneal erosions can be identified as follows:

1. *Acquired* erosions follow traumatic corneal injury, i.e., abrasion, and then occur several months later at the injury's site.
2. *Familial recurrent erosion* is bilateral and occurs more frequently in women with no history of trauma.
3. *Recurrent erosion associated with corneal dystrophies* is due to a defect in the basement membrane of the corneal epithelium.

Healing is facilitated by pressure patching the affected eye. Keeping the other eye closed also helps. Sometimes the ophthalmologist may consider debridement of the defective epithelium. Healing will occur in 2 to 3 days.[3] Ointment may be prescribed for use at bedtime to prevent recurrence.

NURSING INTERVENTION

Take a visual acuity. Sometimes this will only be possible after an anesthetic 0.5 percent proparacaine hydrochloride eyedrop has been instilled. Apply the pressure patch to the eye for a 24-hour period after the diagnosis has been made.

PATIENT TEACHING

Warn the patient who has sustained a corneal abrasion to inform the physician of this previous injury if there is ever any future eye problem. Request that the eye patch be maintained for the appropriate period, usually until the return visit to the physician's office in 24 hours. Sometimes it must be replaced several times before the erosion heals completely. Suggest keeping both eyes closed for comfort and to facilitate healing. Sometimes a day of bedrest might be encouraged. Analgesic pain medication might be necessary. Encourage compliance with follow-up care and also application of eye ointment at night to prevent recurrence of this problem.

Corneal Foreign Bodies

Corneal foreign bodies can range from an eyelash, a speck of dust, dirt or cinder, to a piece of metal which imbeds on the cornea while a person is in the work area. Therefore, when a patient complains of ocular foreign body sensation, make a note of the time, place, and what the person was doing when the event occurred. Also note what was done before the patient came in for emergency attention. This is important for medical and legal reasons. Visual acuity should be tested prior to attempting removal of the object. Sometimes an irrigation stream might just be enough to remove the eyelash or speck of dust, however, a small corneal abrasion may remain so that the foreign body sensation persists. If nothing can be seen on the cornea, evert and inspect the upper lid to ensure that a foreign body is not imbedded under the eyelid.

A metalic corneal foreign body may leave a rust ring, so this is treated differently. The imbedded foreign body should be removed by an ophthalmologist viewing it through the Slitlamp, using a foreign body spud or even a #21-gauge, sterile disposable needle. A cycloplegic drop may or may not be instilled to decrease the iridocyclitis. Antibiotic ointment or drops are applied and the eye is pressure patched for 24 hours to permit area reepethelialization. The patient must return for rust ring removal the next day. This may be accomplished by the ophthalmologist with Slitlamp magnification, using either a drill, foreign body spud, sterile needle, or cotton-tipped applicator. The eye will again be pressure patched for a period of time, but this time it may be removed sooner, and antibiotic drops started. Follow-up care for this type of industrial injury is imperative for medical and legal reasons.

NURSING INTERVENTION
Assess the patient and take and record a visual acuity. Instill the eye medication. Ensure that the pupil is well-dilated by cycloplegic eyedrop before instilling the antibiotic ointment or eyedrop and applying the pressure patch to the eye. The visual acuity should be rechecked at each subsequent visit. The procedure of medicating and patching the eye may need to be repeated.

PATIENT TEACHING
Patient teaching should include the information that at least two visits will be involved. Follow-up care is important. The foreign body sensation will not disperse until epithelial healing takes place. Analgesics may be used as a comfort measure. Compliance with medication regimen will prevent secondary infection.

Corneal Lacerations and Perforations
Corneal lacerations (Fig. 13–5) and *corneal perforations* result from a variety of accidents and will require surgical repair. Visual acuity should be taken and recorded, even if it is only light perception that is elicited, it is important. Concern is for contamination with vegetable matter, for fungal infection has to be kept in mind. The eye should be patched and shielded, unless the perforating object is protruding, then it might be better only to shield the eye. The patient should be warned not to eat or drink anything, for this injury will need surgical repair under anesthesia.

NURSING INTERVENTION
Assess this patient as an emergency and establish what caused the injury. Try to assess a visual acuity in both eyes but do not attempt to force the lids of the injured eye open. Ask the patient to open his or her eyelid if possible, sometimes the patient *cannot* oblige. A record of light perception assessed with a flashlight might be all that can be obtained at this time. Ascertain the time that the injured patient last ate or drank anything, for the time scheduled for emergency surgery under anesthesia will surely

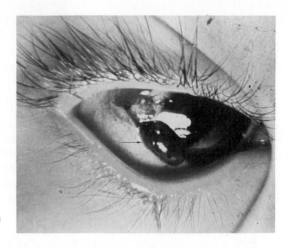

Figure 13–5. Corneal laceration
and iris prolapse (*arrow*).

depend upon whether the patient has a full stomach or not. Gently clean
the periocular area and apply a patch and shield to the eye for protection
from further injury. It might be appropriate only to apply a shield to an
eye with a perforating, protruding corneal foreign body. Administer prescribed antibiotic medications, preoperatively these may include intravenous or intramuscular medications. Postoperatively topical eyedrops
as well as systemic antibiotic coverage will be ordered. A patch and shield
or only a shield may be worn to protect the eye. Assess when the last
tetanus toxoid was given, if not received within the last 10 years it will
need to be given.

Chemical Burns
Chemicals splashed into the eyes should be immediately copiously irrigated with
water or an irrigating solution such as normal saline, for a period of at least 15 to 20
minutes (see Chap. 3). This is a true ocular emergency and should be treated as
such. No attempt should be made to neutralize the chemical substance for this will
just create heat and further irritate the cornea. Litmus paper may be used to assess if
the chemicals were acid or alkali. Topical anesthetic drops such as 0.5 percent
proparacaine hydrochloride, instilled prior to the irrigation to relieve the pain, will
facilitate the irrigation. This may be repeated a second time only. Direct the stream
of irrigating solution, such as normal saline, toward the inner canthus, allow it to
flow over the corneal surface to the outer canthus. To prevent cross-contamination
of the other eye make sure the patient tilts the head to the side being irrigated.
Visual acuity taken after accomplishing the initial irrigation, should be documented
for medical and legal purposes.

Acid burns, depending upon the pH, do relatively well and the corneal hazing
usually clears. Acid coagulates the protein and produces a substance called col-
lagenase. Alkali substances such as calcium hydroxide (lime, found in builders
sand), sodium hydroxide (lye, found in commercial drain cleaners), and ammonium
hydroxide (found in refrigerant gas) do not coagulate the protein and once in the

tissues continue to burn and burn and eventually completely destroy the cornea. Long-term results of corneal damage from alkali burns varies from patient to patient, but the cornea might go on to vascularize and/or perforate, with ultimate treatment being a corneal transplant.

NURSING INTERVENTION
Immediately initiate copious irrigation with water or a normal saline solution for at least 20 minutes. Obtain a physician's order for instillation of a drop of topical anesthetic to improve the patient's comfort level. If both eyes are involved, irrigate them simultaneously if two people are available to perform the task, otherwise irrigate the eyes alternately. The fornices should be cleaned with applicator sticks to remove any particulate matter. Once this is accomplished, assess the visual acuity. Instill a prescribed cycloplegic such as 2 percent homatropine hydrobromide of 0.5 percent scopolamine hydrochloride to prevent the iritis which will otherwise occur. After this, frequent steroids and antibiotic eyedrops, to decrease inflammation and prevent secondary infection, will be prescribed. In the post-injury period, after irrigation, it might be more comfortable for the patient to have both eyes patched. However, the psychological torment of losing sight might be worse than the discomfort sustained by having the lids open. This situation varies from patient to patient.

Administer analgesics for pain as necessary. Sometimes a soft contact lens is used as a ''bandage lens'' to facilitate healing and decrease the abrasive effect of blinking; if this is used then the eye medications are placed in the eye while the contact lens is *in situ*. Nurses should be cognizant of persistent complaints of pain and inform the physician, for in this case it would be appropriate to remove the lens.

TUMORS

Corneal tumors are relatively rare and usually have spread from the conjunctiva, like the squamous cell epithelioma (Fig. 13–6). Diagnosis is established by biopsy and treatment is by excision referred to as *superficial keratectomy*.

CORNEAL TRANSPLANTS

Penetrating Keratoplasty
Penetrating keratoplasty is a very successful surgical procedure for patients with nonvascularized, opaque corneas. Graft success is measured by clarity of the graft and the visual benefit to the patient following surgery.

The most common indications for penetrating keratoplasty are to improve vision in patients with Fuch's endothelial and other corneal dystrophies, keratoconus, herpetic corneal scar, active or chronic corneal inflammations of bacterial or fungal origin, aphakic bullous keratopathy, traumatic corneal scar, interstitial keratitis, chemical burns, dry eye syndromes, congenital corneal opacities, and

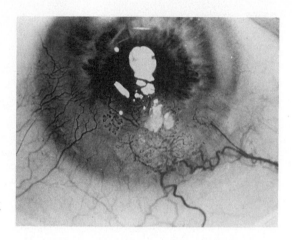

Figure 13–6. Squamous cell epithelioma of the cornea.

corneal degenerations. However, the prognosis is poor for such conditions as chemical burns, vascularized corneas, and dry-eye syndromes.[10]

Any lid abnormalities and tear film dysfunction are assessed and treated preoperatively. Intraocular pressures are measured, and when the corneal opacity is so dense that the posterior structures are not easily visualized, B-scan ultrasonography corneal degenerations. However, the prognosis is poor for such conditions as chemical burns, vascularized corneas, and dry-eye syndromes.[10]

1. If a *penetrating keratoplasty* is planned for an aphakic patient (a patient who has his or her own crystalline lens), then instillation of 2 percent pilocarpine hydrochloride eyedrops 2 hours and 1 hour before surgery, to constrict the pupil and protect the lens, is necessary.
2. The patient who is to have a *combined cataract and keratoplasty procedure,* however, will need to have mydriatics instilled to dilate the pupil to facilitate this surgery. A *triple procedure keratoplasty,* cataract extraction, and intraocular lens implant is also accomplished in some instances.
3. The aphakic or pseudophakic patient may have no drops ordered, or may have pilocarpine instilled to hold the vitreous face back when surgery is being performed.

Antibiotic eyedrops and a face wash may or may not be ordered prior to surgery. An osmotic agent such as intravenous 20 percent Mannitol, given immediately before the surgical procedure reduces intraocular pressure. Surgery may be performed under local or general anesthesia.

Surgery consists of removing the central portion of the recipients' diseased, opaque cornea—referred to as a button—and replacing it with tissue obtained from a donor cornea. The graft is sutured to the recipient with interrupted and/or continuous 10-0 nylon sutures (Fig. 13–7). A single knot tied superiorly is covered by the eyelid. The sutures will be left in place for up to a year while the corneal healing takes place. Occasionally, the interrupted suturing technique is still used.

Postoperatively, a patch and shield is placed on the eye and the patient is

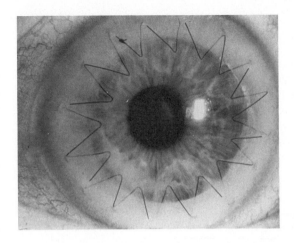

Figure 13–7. Corneal transplant showing sutures in place.

maintained in bed until after the effects of the anesthesia has worn off. A short acting cycloplegic such as 1 percent cyclopentolate hydrochloride of 1 percent tropicamide will be instilled after the first dressing is removed. Combination steroid–antibiotic eyedrops will also be prescribed. Hospitalization is for 2 to 3 days postoperatively and the patient is discharged on the above medications.

Complications include early signs of graft rejection which necessitates the frequency of the steroid eyedrops being increased. A wound leak may be sealed by pressure patching the eye for 24 hours or may even require resuturing. Infection would be a devastating endophthalmitis which would be aggressively treated with topical, subconjunctival, intraocular, and systemic antibiotics. Vitrectomy may even be considered after a diagnostic paracentesis and vitrectomy for bacteriology identification has been obtained.

Other Methods of Grafts. A *lamellar keratoplasty* is a partial thickness corneal graft which is done rarely and selectively. This method of surgery, however, forms the basis for some *refractive surgery* whereby the anterior corneal curvature is modified while the posterior curvature remains unaffected.[10] *Keratomileusis* is a surgical method perfected by José Barraquer in Colombia, in which the anterior portion of the cornea is lathed to a predetermined thickness and curvature to correct refractive errors. In *epikeratophakia,* the addition of a modified piece of donor tissue is placed upon the surface of a deepithelialized cornea correcting for either hyperopia or myopia. While *keratophakia* is the surgical manipulation of the patient's cornea by the implantation of a modified piece of donor tissue placed within a surgically made corneal pocket to correct for hyperoptic errors. The cornea is lathed to steepen the radius of its curvature. The procedure is designed to correct those cases of hyperopia and aphakia in which the traditional methods are not accepted.

A *rotating graft* is really an *autograft.* This method may be used when the patient's cornea is scarred in the pupillary axis but the superior portion of the cornea is clear. A full thickness button is removed from the patient's cornea and then replaced so that the scar is rotated out of the line of vision, thus restoring vision through the patient's own clear portion of the cornea.

NURSING INTERVENTION

Patients who require corneal transplant are placed on a waiting list. When corneas become available, through death of a donor, the patient is given short notice to come in for immediate surgery. Once the corneas are available they are grafted within 24 to 48 hours. Nursing assessment of the patient admitted for keratoplasty needs to take into account that the patient will often be admitted in a rush, for surgery is done when donor corneas become available. Appropriate eyedrops should be instilled for the planned procedure. After checking the chart to see that the surgical consent has been signed and witnessed, the patient is premedicated for surgery and the I.V. osmotic agent, if ordered, is administered. Intraoperative care was discussed in Chapter 8. Postoperatively, the patient's vital signs are monitored until they are stable, as is the intravenous infusion, until it can be discontinued. Medicate the patient for any pain and/or nausea in the immediate postsurgical period. Assist the patient to the bathroom as necessary. Administer steroids for the steroid dependent patient, if prescribed by the physician. After the first eye dressing, instill the cycloplegic and antibiotic–steroid eyedrops. Maintain a patch and shield at night, and protective glasses or shield during the day.

PATIENT TEACHING

Patient teaching should include self-administration of eye medications, an awareness of eye care and protection, and encouragement for compliance with follow-up care. The eye should be shielded at night for at least the next couple of months. Since graft rejection is a possibility, the patient should be advised to seek attention for an eye that has a sudden decrease in vision and is red and/or painful for a period longer than 24 hours. Daily checks should be encouraged.[11] Vision will improve still further when the patient is refracted at a later stage, and given either a contact lens or prescription glasses.

Prosthokeratoplasty

Diseases in which corneal transplant is prone to fail are characterized by a dry eye (no tear secretion) and a hazy vascularized cornea, such as occur in phemphigoid, Stevens-Johnson syndrome, and alkali burns. The idea of replacing the opaque cornea with some other material is two centuries old, but it was not until the development of new plastic and surgical techniques by several ophthalmologists, and the ingenuity of Hernando Cardona that artificial implants became a reality. Of the two types of keratoprosthesis, the "through and through" type is most frequently used. In this procedure, an optical cylinder passes through both the cornea and the upper lid. The prosthesis is fixed to the cornea with multiple sutures and is covered with a piece of periosteum taken from the leg. The eyelid is sutured closed and remains that way permanently. These surgical steps give a better fixation to the prosthesis. The little optical cylinder is seen on the eyelid surface (Fig. 13–8).

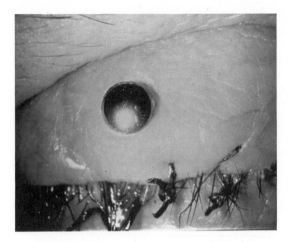

Figure 13–8. Keratoprosthesis.

NURSING INTERVENTION
Postoperatively, care will include gently cleansing any crusted blood from the lid after the patch is removed. Assisting the patient to perform ocular warm compresses for 20 minutes, four times a day, and applying a combination antibiotic/steroid ophthalmic ointment around the prosthokeratoplasty and to the lid margin.

PATIENT TEACHING
Instruct the patient to continue the compresses after discharge from the hospital for the next day or two. The ointment should be applied as prescribed. Since light will enter the eye through the keratoprosthesis, the eye may need to be patched at night to occlude light. Encourage compliance with follow-up care.

Radial Keratotomy
Radial keratotomy is a surgical procedure designed to correct myopia, a refractive error in which the focal point of light rays from a distant point fall in front of the retina. Although still controversial, it offers another option to the patient who is not entirely satisfied with the vision when wearing thick minus lenses or contact lenses. The degree of myopia is measured in diopters (a unit of measurement of strength of refractive power of lenses or of prisms), and candidates for this procedure will have myopia ranging from -2 to -8 diopters.

Preoperative patient evaluation includes visual acuity with and without glasses, SLE, manifest and cycloplegic refraction, specular photomicrographs for endothelial cell count both pre- and postoperatively, measurements of intraocular pressure using applanation tonometry, and axial length of the eye by A-scan ultrasonography. The surgical procedure is accomplished using topical anesthesia eyedrops such as 0.5 percent proparacaine hydrochloride. The surgeon first measures the corneal thickness centrally, and at the 3, 6, 9, and 12 o'clock meridians using an ultrasonic pachymeter. The visual axis is marked with a dull, marking trephine, then a calibrated diamond knife is used to make eight (or more) radial incisions into the corneal surface, which just ride on the trephine mark (Fig. 13–9). A basic salt solution (BSS) is used to irrigate the incisions. Topical 0.3 percent gentamycin and a cycloplegic such as 0.25 percent scopolamine eyedrops are instilled, and the eye is pressure patched for 24 hours.[12,13]

Postoperatively, the patient may experience discomfort for 10 to 18 hours, as well as an aggravating sensitivity to bright lights. Foreign body sensation and photophobia last longer.[12,13] Fluctuation in vision and also anisometropia, until the refractive error in the other eye is also corrected, are patient complaints. This procedure causes the cornea to flatten, thereby placing the light rays appropriately on the retina. Glasses may still have to be worn even after the surgery, but they will probably be less thick.

Long-term follow-up is not yet available for this recently approved outpatient surgical procedure.

THE SCLERA

The *sclera,* composed of collagenous fibers woven together to form an opaque, white, hollow ball, is the skeleton of the eyeball and makes up four-fifths of the globe. It is continuous with the cornea anteriorly at the *limbus* and joins with the dural sheath of the optic nerve posteriorly, where a few strands of scleral tissue pass over the optic disc to form a sieve-like structure called the *lamina cribrosa.* Around the optic nerve, the sclera is penetrated by the *long and short posterior ciliary arteries and nerves.* The horizontal circumference of the eyeball is referred to as the *equator* and in each quadrant, slightly posterior to the equator the *four vortex veins* exit through the sclera. About 4 mm posterior to the limbus, the four *anterior ciliary arteries and veins* penetrate the sclera. The sclera's outer surface is covered by a thin layer of fine elastic tissue, the *episclera,* containing numerous blood vessels which nourish the sclera. The *rectus muscles* insert into the sclera.[6]

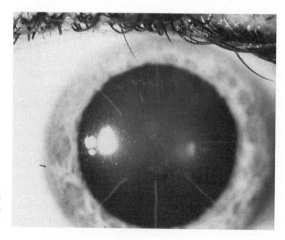

Figure 13–9. Radial keratotomy. *(Photograph courtesy Juan Arentsen, M.D., Co-Director, Cornea Department, Wills Eye Hospital.)*

Congenital Abnormalities

There are certain conditions which cause discoloration of the sclera.

Blue sclera, the most famous anomaly, is a congenital translucency of the sclera which permits the pigmented choroid to be seen and which appears blue. The importance of this condition is in the systemic manifestations of the deficiency. There is fragility of the bones, subluxation of joints, deformities of the cranial bones, and often deafness.

Acquired Abnormalities

Acquired lesions may be divided into those conditions involving the superficial outer coat, the episclera, and the deeper layer, the sclera.

Episcleritis can be either simple or nodular, the latter being found less often than the former. This benign, recurring inflammation usually does not progress to scleritis. Hypersensitivity may be responsible but the cause is not usually known; rheumatoid arthritis, Sjögren's syndrome, syphilis, herpes zoster, and tuberculosis have all been associated with episcleritis.[3] The eyeball develops a localized hyperemia which looks pink or purple on examination. Occasionally, there is an accompanying iritis. Generally, the condition is self-limiting in 1 to 2 weeks. Topical corticosteroids, i.e., dexamethazone 1 percent, shortens the disease's course to days.

Scleritis, on the other hand, is a much more serious and severe disease and is usually accompanied by episcleritis. Although a relatively rare disease, it runs a chronic course when it occurs. The symptoms of scleritis include persistent pain, redness, photophobia, tenderness, and lacrimation. Examination reveals a violaceous, purple-blue, diffusely discolored sclera.[3] Scleritis can occur as a nodular or a necrotizing type. When necrotizing scleritis occurs it may lead to scleral thinning and perforation. There is usually systemic connective tissue disease associated with this severe form. Because the sclera heals very poorly, biopsies are contraindicated. Treatment is directed at supressing the inflammatory reaction.[14]

NURSING INTERVENTION

Assess the patient who complains of a painful red eye in the absence of injury or signs of conjunctivitis for both ocular and systemic disease. Refer the patient to an ophthalmologist for evaluation and encourage compliance with the medication regimen.

Staphyloma. *Staphyloma* is the thinning and stretching of the sclera which is lined by the uvea. If the sclera is just thinned as in blue sclera, it is an ectasia. Staphylomas usually occur in adult life and are caused by increased intraocular pressure, or by pathological processes, i.e., scleritis, syphiloma, tuberculoma, uveitis, and/or trauma to the point where the sclera is weakened by the nerves and blood vessels passing through. When this occurs, a staphyloma appears blue or purple due to the pigmented uvea lining the inside of the bulge. Treatment is difficult since staphylomas are usually progressive. The lowering of intraocular pressure is very important if this is the cause. In severe cases, scleral grafting may be considered.

Trauma. *Scleral rupture* may occur from blunt trauma in which the scleral fibers are torn and as a result the intraocular contents may be expelled or prolapsed.

Following a rupture there is globe softening and perhaps intraocular hemorrhage which leads to decrease in vision. It is essential that systemic antibiotic therapy be instituted immediately. The eye is patched and shielded for protection prior to surgical exploration and rupture repair.

Perforations of the sclera by projectile or foreign substances can also occur. Globe exploration by CAT scan, x-ray, or ultrasound needs to be performed in order to localize any intraocular foreign body prior to surgical removal being attempted by the ophthalmologist. Systemic antibiotic therapy is instituted and surgical repair of the perforation must be made, for there may be prolapse of intraocular contents if not immediately, then after the penetrating object is removed.

In either scleral rupture or perforation, healing does not occur from the scleral fibers themselves but from the episclera or uvea. If the scleral fibers are not closed, then fibrocytic cells may grow down into the eye causing severe damage to the internal structures, and may even produce retinal detachments.

NURSING INTERVENTION
Assess the cause of the injury. A statement by the patient to the effect that "I got something in my eye," should prompt the nurse to inquire what was being done at the time of the injury. Assess and record visual acuity. Shield the eye. Systemic antibiotic therapy will be initiated prior to preparing the patient for exploratory tests and surgical repair. Topical antibiotic and cycloplegic eyedrops may be instilled both pre- and postoperatively. Psychological support is most necessary. Occasionally, the rupture is so extensive that the eye might be lost through this type of injury.

Degeneration. In the aging process there may be deposition of lipids in the deeper layers between the scleral fibers, resulting in the sclera losing its whiteness and becoming discolored with a yellowish hue.

Hyaline changes can also occur. These hyaline deposits appear as grayish, waxy plaques and are usually found to be symmetrical and anterior to the insertions of the lateral recti muscles. Occasionally, the plaques may become calcified, or even deposited diffusely throughout the sclera or at previous scleritis sites. Bone formation has been noted histologically. The main clinical effects brought about by these scleral degenerative changes is the increased scleral rigidity with the alteration it causes in the measuring of intraocular pressure.

NURSING INTERVENTION
If the Schiøtz method of tonometry is used, the increased scleral rigidity may contribute to false readings. The 10-mg weight might have to be used.

REFERENCES

1. Ophthalmologic Staff of the Hospital for Sick Children, Toronto, in Wright WW, (Ed.): The Eye in Childhood. Chicago: Year Book Medical, 1967, p. 165

2. Kenyon KR, Fogle, JA, Grayson M: Dysgeneses, dystrophies and degenerations of the cornea, in Duane TD, (Ed.). Clinical Ophthalmology. Hagerstown, Md.: Harper & Row, 1983, pp. 1–55
3. Vaughan D, Asbury T: General Ophthalmology, 10th ed. Los Altos, Calif.: Lange, 1983, p. 98–101
4. Laibson PR, Waring GO: Diseases of the cornea, in Harley RD, (Ed.). Pediatric Ophthalmology, 2nd ed. Philadelphia: Saunders, 1983, p. 456–514
5. Sommer A: Latest concepts in the diagnosis and treatment of xerophthalmia, in Lim ASM, Jones BR, (Eds.). Vision: World's Major Blinding Conditions. Mt. Elizabeth, Singapore: International Agency for Prevention of Blindness, 1982, p. 47–48
6. Pirie A: Practical aspects of xerophthalmia, in Lim ASM, Jones BR, (Eds.). Vision: World's Major Blinding Conditions. Mt. Elizabeth, Singapore: International Agency for Prevention of Blindness, 1982, p. 49–50
7. Weingeist TA: Herpes zoster and the aging eye. Geriatrics, 36(1): 81–89, 1981
8. Pavan-Langston D: Promising therapy for herpes infections of the eye. Sightsaving, 53(4): 12–13, 1984–1985
9. Bloomfield SE: Clinical allergy and immunology of the external eye, in Duane TD, (Ed.): Clinical Ophthalmology, 1983, p. 16–17
10. Raju VK: Corneal surgery, in Duane TD, (Ed.). Clinical Ophthalmology, 1983, p. 1–28
11. Smith, JF: Nursing care of the patient having penetrating keratoplasty. Journal of Ophthalmic Nursing and Technology, 3(4): 160–164, 1984
12. Fyodorov SN: Radial keratotomy: The Russian experience. Ophthalmic Forum, 1(1), 1982
13. Bores LD, Fyodorov SN, Rowsey JJ, Salz JJ: Round table discussion—Controversies in keratotomy. Ophthalmic Forum, 1(1):38–45, 1982
14. Watson, PG (London), Hayren SS (Iowa City, Ia.): Scleritis and episcleritis. British Journal of Ophthalmology, 60(3): 163–191, 1976

BIBLIOGRAPHY

Boyd-Monk H: A fortunate accident, radial keratotomy. Today's OR Nurse, 6(3): 25–31, 1984
Boyd-Monk H: Vitamin A deficiency and associated eye disease. Journal of Ophthalmic Nursing and Technology, 2(4): 159–162, 1983
Coyne, SA: Advanced Slit Lamp techniques with an understanding of pathology. Journal of Ophthalmic Nursing and Technology, 3(2): 62–75, 1984
Fedukowicz HB: External Infections. Norwalk, Conn.: Appleton-Century-Crofts, 1984.
Introduction to Corneal Dystrophies. Kingswood, Tex.: The Corneal Dystrophy Foundation, 1985.

14

The Uveal Tract

NEW TERMS

Anterior chamber angle: junction formed by the iris and cornea.

Choroiditis: inflammation or infection of the choroid.

Cyclitis: inflammation of the ciliary body.

Heterochromia: difference in color in the two eyes.

Hypotony: soft eyeball—due to low intraocular pressure.

Iritis: inflammation of the iris.

Iridocyclitis: primary inflammation of the iris with secondary inflammation of the ciliary body. Inflammatory cells are seen in the anterior chamber as well as in the anterior vitreous behind the lens.

Phythisis bulbi: shrunken eyeball.

The *uveal tract's* component parts are the *iris, ciliary body,* and *choroid,* and its primary function is to supply nutrition to the eye. Essentially vascular, the uveal tract provides sustenance for the rods and cones (of the retina) through the coriocapilaris (of the choroid) and for the lens through the *aqueous humor.* The muscles of iris and ciliary body respectively control pupillary size, and alter the accommodation of the lens, as well as the refractive action of the eye.[1]

The *iris,* the most anterior portion of the uveal tract, is a musculovascular diaphragm with a central opening, the *pupil.* The iris' function is related to its structure. The degree of iris pigmentation is responsible for the ''color'' of the eye. If the iris stroma is lightly pigmented the eye is said to be blue; when the iris stroma is heavily pigmented, the eye is called brown.[2] Pupillary size is regulated by the *sphincter and dilator muscles,* while the pigmented epithelium acts as a light barrier so that only light passing through the pupil readily reaches the retina. The iris muscles are controlled by the involuntary nervous system; the sphincter, stimulated by the parasympathetic system causes *miosis,* and dilator stimulation by the sympathetic systems causes *mydriasis.* The iris' anterior surface is irregular with furrows and crypts (tiny caverns located between the vascular radiations), which lead into the stroma. The vascular, anterior iris stroma provides for the nutrition of the anterior segment of the eye though diffusion of the aqueous. When inflammation occurs, exudate pours out into the anterior chamber.[1] Arterial blood supply is from the junction of *long posterior ciliary arteries* and the *anterior ciliary arteries* extending from the insertions of the extraocular rectus muscles. The iris forms the posterior boundary of the anterior chamber angle. The thin iris root is continuous with ligaments of the trabecular meshwork. The posterior chamber is limited by the posterior surfaces of the iris anteriorly, and the ciliary body laterally.[1]

The *ciliary body* extends from the root of the iris to the *ora serrata* where the peripheral retina terminates. It is made up of two zones. The *corona ciliaris* or ciliary processes, whose surface consists of many elevations and depressions, which are composed of capillaries and veins that drain through the vortex veins; and the smoother, flatter *pars plana* consisting of a thin layer of longitudinal ciliary muscle covered by ciliary epithelium. The longitudinal, radial, and circular portions of the ciliary muscles form the bulk of the ciliary body. They change the refracting power of the lens by regulating traction on the *zonules*. This results in altered tension on the capsule of the lens, which gives the lens variable focus for both near and more distant objects in the field of vision. The zonular fibers, which hold the lens in place, originate in the valleys between the ciliary processes. There are also two layers of ciliary epithelium, an external pigmented layer and an internal non pigmented layer—the inner cell layer which induces aqueous humor formation by active "secretion."[1] Both of these continue as pigmented layers over the iris' posterior surface. The pigment epithelium represents the forward extension of the pigment epithelium of the retina.[3] The blood vessels to the ciliary body come from the major circle of the iris.

The *choroid* extends from the ora serrata to the optic nerve and is located between the sclera and the retina. It consists mainly of blood vessels, with a profusion of nerve fibers and pigmented cells set in a loose, connective tissue matrix. It is supplied by branches of the posterior and anterior ciliary vessels derived from the opthalmic artery, and drains via the four vortex veins into the ophthalmic veins, and eventually, through the superior orbital fissure into the cavernous sinus.[4]

Microscopically, the choroidal layers may be identified as the *suprachoroid,* the *large-vessel layer,* the *medium-vessel layer,* the *choriocapillaris,* and *Bruch's membrane.* The suprachoroid is the space between the inner pigmented sclera, and the three layers of blood vessels. The *large vessel layer,* is the outermost layer of the choroid. The *medium-vessel layer,* composed of medium-sized blood vessels, is located in the center of the choroid. The innermost small blood vessel layer (composed mainly of capillaries), the *choriocapillaris* is separated by *Bruch's membrane* from the retina pigmented epithelium. The primary functions of the choroid are to supply nutrition to the rod and cone layer of the retina, and also to shield the retina from extraneous light.

CONGENITAL ANOMALIES

Congenital anomalies, which result from primary dysgenesis of mesoderm and neuroectoderm, mean that disruption occurred very early in the developmental stages of these embryological structures. As a result, clinical manifestations of anomalies of lens, pupil, iris, ciliary body, and choroid may occur with one or more structures being affected. Fortunately, these anomalies are relatively rare in the general population, but when they occur they often impede normal visual development.

Aniridia

Aniridia (iridiremia) is the apparent absence of the iris on clinical examination. A primary failure of the optic cup to grow may result in a rudimentary iris (always present) which is actually hidden behind the corneoscleral margin. The pupil appears to occupy the entire area of the cornea (Fig. 14–1). There is usually photophobia, poor vision and frequently nystagmus.[5] Other ocular manifestations associated with this anomaly are coloboma (in the family), hypoplasia of the macula, lens dislocation, and congenital cataract. Secondary glaucoma can also occur. Surgical treatment of the glaucoma associated with congenital aniridia, is the goniotomy procedure which attempts to release the adhesions of the iris stump. This is not always satisfactory.[6] Tinted contact lenses have been prescribed for cosmetic and therapeutic use. Systemic manifestations associated with aniridia include: cerebellar ataxia, Wilm's tumor, and unilateral aplastic kidney and other renal anomalies. Patterns of inheritance include dominant characteristics, but can also be sporadic.

NURSING INTERVENTION

Nursing intervention is supportive to the child's family, and to the adult who has struggled with this anomaly up to the point of encounter. It is necessary to be aware of the decreased visual acuity and photophobia suffered by patients with aniridia, so be cognizant of the need for dark glasses, and if the patient is admitted for hospital treatment, the need for a

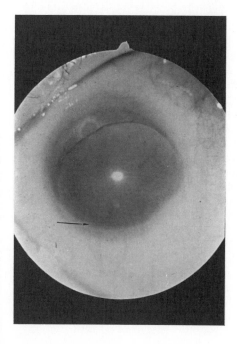

Figure 14–1. Aniridia, also showing subluxation of the lens.

darkened room. Assist as necessary with teaching and care of the contact lenses. Observe any unusual signs of discomfort which might be associated with an increase in intraocular pressure (see Chap. 17).

Coloboma

Coloboma manifests as a defect showing absence of the pigmented and vascular tunics of iris (Fig. 14–2A), which results from failure of closure of the embryonic fissure. The typical coloboma position is inferonasal, indicating its relationship to anomalous fetal cleft closure. A wide variety of colobomatous defects have been recorded. These range from a small notch in the pupil and a cleft in the iris (extending partially to the periphery), to associated defects involving lens, zonules, ciliary body, and choroid.[7] The lower portion of the disc is therefore involved in coloboma of the choroid (Fig. 14–2B) where the margins are usually noted to look sharp and pigmented on ophthalmoscopic examination. The macula may be eliminated by inclusion in the defect, and if the coloboma is unilateral it usually provokes strabismus soon after infancy.[6] Colobomas in the posterior fundus have also been known to cause leukocoria. Atypical coloboma may occur elsewhere in the iris. Coloboma is transmitted as a dominant characteristic.

Persistent Pupillary Membrane

Persistent pupillary membrane (Fig. 14–3) is a fairly common entity, and can be seen as thread-like strands running across the pupil. These are mesodermal remnants. It usually does not have any clinical significance nor does it interfere with visual acuity.

Albinism

Albinism is broadly defined is any congenital hypopigmentation. It is an inborn error of metabolism, illustrated by the fact that in the albino, the pigment melanin cannot be synthesized from tyrosine. Eye color varies from gray to blue with little or no visible pigment, red reflex is present at all ages and in all races. Albinos have a severe nystagmus detectable in the first few months of life, subnormal visual acuity, photophobia, frequent astigmatism, and significant myopia or hyperopia. At least four subtypes occur in humans, each inherited in a different manner.

Generalized or oculocutaneous albinism affects skin, hair, and eye color, and is inherited as an autosomal recessive trait. Two different forms can be identified using plucked hair bulbs: a) in the tyrosinase-negative type, a hair bulb when incubated with tyrosin, cannot form melanin, thus implying a lack of tyrosinase; and b) in the tyrosinase-positive type, melanin is formed in vitro by the hair bulb. It is thought that a defect might occur in a permease which transports tyrosine into the melanosome.[7,8] The significance of this is that hair color ranges from white to dark yellow, and iris color ranges from very light blue, with a pink reflex through an undilated iris, to light hazel. The skin may be without pigment or it may have some pigment, especially in nevi and freckles. Albinism, because of the affected person's appearance, poses psychological problems which must be considered. Such persons are also predisposed to actinic-induced cutaneous malignancies. Thus, someone with generalized oculocutaneous albinism should be advised to use sunscreens, and should be inspected for cutaneous neoplasms in sun-exposed areas such as the

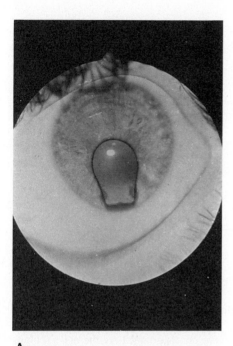

A

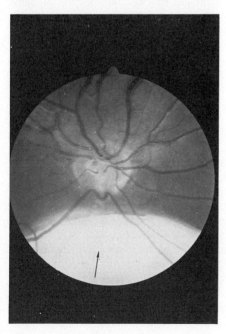

B

Figure 14–2A. Iris coloboma. **B.** Coloboma of choroid. (*Photographs courtesy of Hunter R. Stokes, M.D., Florence, S.C.*)

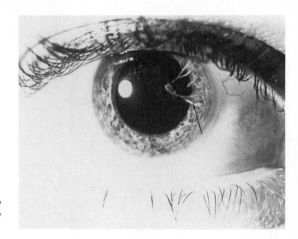

Figure 14–3. Persistent pupillary membrane. (*Photograph courtesy of Wills Eye Hospital.*)

eyelids, arms, and back of the hands, for later in life they can develop precancerous lesions and squamous cell carcinoma.[8]

In *ocular albinism* the pigmentary defect is limited to the eye and is transmitted in a sex-linked manner. Two simultaneous defects are present in the human albino, both of which help explain the typically severe photophobia. Like the normal blue-eyed individual, the albino has no melanin in the iris. In addition, the pigment epithelium layer of the retina also lacks melanin. As a result light passes through the pupil intact and that portion passing through the iris (the red end of the visual spectrum) impinges upon the retina. Normally, most of the light reaching the retina is absorbed in the pigment epithelium—but in albinos it is not. Light is then reflected from the choroidal layer and produces the red pupil and semi-transparent iris seen in the human albinos.

Partial albinism includes only the skin and hair and is inherited as an autosomal dominant trait.[7,8]

NURSING INTERVENTION

When assessing the albinotic patient be aware that a few of these people have a history of easy bruisability, epistaxis, or hemoptysis. Prolonged bleeding may occur following dental extractions and childbirth. Laboratory studies of this *albinism–hemorrhagic diathesis syndrome* as it is called, reveal that the hemostatic defect is due to platelet dysfunction—bleeding time is prolonged. Because of the variable clinical appearance of these patients with this syndrome, all patients should be asked about this possible hemorrhagic predisposition. Patients with this syndrome should be explicitly advised to avoid all aspirin-containing drugs, indomethacin, and other drugs blocking prostaglandin synthetase. A careful nursing history of hemostatic defects is the best screening method.[8]

PATIENT TEACHING

Patient teaching should include encouraging shielding of the skin from the sun, and the use of dark glasses to help reduce the photophobia.

ACQUIRED ANOMALIES

Uveitis

Inflammation of the uveal tract may involve one or all three portions simultaneously.[3] More often the inflammation is classified according to its position in the globe, namely *anterior uveitis* which most frequently presents as *iritis; cyclitis* can occur, but more often *iridocyclitis* (when both structures are involved together) is seen. *Pars planitis* results when inflammation of the pars plana (of the ciliary body) occurs. *Posterior uveitis* is classified depending upon the predominant cell layer involved. The inflammation can be termed *choroiditis* or *retinitis* if just the choroid or retina is involved, and *retinochoroiditis* or *choroidoretinitis* if both layers are involved. The first portion of the term denotes the more intensively involved layer.[9]

Patheogenesis of uveitis sometimes perplexes physicians, because often an etiology cannot be identified. The disease can take an acute, chronic, or recurrent course. Some etiological factors which can be responsible for the inflammatory response in the uveal tract are allergens, fungi, bacteria, viruses, and chemicals. Trauma, both accidental and surgical, can certainly be identified as a cause. Immunogenetic factors are probably important in the development of many types of uveal inflammation as well. Anterior uveitis can be associated with systemic diseases such as rheumatoid disease, ankylosing spondylitis, or Reiter's disease. Posterior uveitis can be caused by such systemic infectious entities as the protozoan parasite—toxoplasmosis (*Toxoplasma gondii*), histoplasmosis spores of the fungus (*Histoplasma capsulatum*), tuberculosis, syphilis, toxocariasis from the nematodes *Toxocara canis* and *Toxocara cati* to name just a few.

Anterior Uveitis. *Symptoms* of anterior uveitis include pain, referred to the periorbital region and described as a dull ache; photophobia or light sensitivity due to trigeminal irritation from cornea, iris, or ciliary body, and lacrimation or tearing. Blurred vision is due to media clouding from flare and cells in the anterior chamber, and to cells in the vitreous.

Signs of anterior uveitis include ciliary injection, seen as engorgement of episcleral vessels around the limbus (Fig. 14–4) or a small and often irregular pupil in the involved eye. Occasionally, an iris color change is suggestive of anterior uveitis. The hallmarks of uveitis, flare and cells, can only be seen using Slitlamp biomicroscopy. Flare is a milkiness of the aqueous humor. Keratic precipitates (KP) are inflammatory cell particles deposited on the back of the cornea. They tend to look "greasy" and are therefore described as "mutton-fat" KP.[10]

Differentiation of uveitis into *granulomatous* and *nongranulomatous* types originated from the work of Dr. Alan Churchill Woods. His original concept was that granulomatous disease was due to such agents as the tubercle bacilli, whereas nongranulomatous types were due to such agents as the streptococci. Unfortunately,

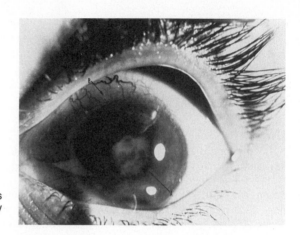

Figure 14–4. Anterior uveitis showing irregular pupil and ciliary injection.

this supposition turned out to be untrue, but the terms are still used in the literature. The most important features of granulomatous iritis or iridocyclitis are the presence of large mutton-fat keratic precipitates and nodules. Granulomatous uveitis tends to be insidious in onset, with little or no redness or pain. Granules (nodules) tend to develop in the iris, choroid, retina, ciliary body, or vitreous. However, it can also have many of the same features as nongranulomatous uveitis.

Nongranulomatous uveitis has an acute occurrence, many cells are seen in the aqueous and the flare grade (on the scale of 1 to 4), which is more intense than the cell grade. The attack lasts 3 to 8 weeks. Treatment is with topical cycloplegics and steroids during the acute stage.[10]

Posterior Uveitis. Many times the first inkling that a posterior uveitis is present is brought to the attention of the ophthalmologist by a patient's complaint of decreased or distorted vision in one eye. Ophthalmoscopic examination reveals a fundus lesion. Since it is known that posterior uveitis often has a systemic disease association, a variety of tests are performed to try to identify the specific disease which is responsible for the ocular inflammatory reaction.

Toxoplasmosis. Toxoplasmosis is one disease of the eye that is relatively common, and in varying studies accounts for between 16 and 70 percent of all posterior segment inflammations which can lead to permanent loss of vision.[11] *Toxoplasmosis gondii* is an obligate, intracellular parasite prevalent among various animals, but the excreta of cats has become the main suspect. Sources of infectious oocytes include materials subject to fecal contamination such as sand, dirt, and food. Ingested oocytes often lead to infection. Humans may also acquire infection by consuming undercooked meats. A history of eating undercooked meat such as steak tartare may be elicited from patients with acquired toxoplasmosis.

Trophozoites of *T. gondii* infect white blood cells when they enter the bloodstream via the intestinal wall. They seem to have a predilection for various organs including the brain, neural retinal elements, myocardium, skeletal muscle, and lymph nodes.

Congenital toxoplasmosis results after transplacental passage of trophozoites from a mother (with acute acquired toxoplasmosis) to the fetus, where the encysted organisms may lie dormant within the tissues for years or decades. Ocular toxoplasmosis results from reactivation of encysted forms of the congenital infection. Stimuli thought to potentiate cyst rupture include trauma, stress, seasonal variation, puberty, recent illness, and immunocompromise. This latter situation has been identified in patients with acquired immune deficiency syndrome (AIDS).[12]

Clinically, ocular toxoplasmosis is classic in its form, for on ophthalmoscopic examination a whitish-yellow focus of necrotizing retinochoroiditis will be seen adjacent to the edge of a pigmented scar (Fig. 14–5). Vitreous haze is due to inflammatory cells seen in the anterior and posterior vitreous. Inflammation, the hallmark of toxoplasmic retinochoroiditis results from the combination of rupture of infected cells, and cytoxic factors generated by cell-mediated and humoral immune mechanisms. Secondary iridocyclitis with granulomatous keratic precipitates may also be present. Intraocular pressure may be elevated, and therefore needs frequent monitoring. Other pathological manifestations which can occur include retinal and disc neovascularization, optic nerve edema, macula damage, loss of artery and vein patency through adjacent inflammation, nonresolving vitreous opacities, and retinal detachments. Diagnosis is made by laboratory tests such as the indirect fluorescent antibody and ELISA tests. Serological testing is of particular value in differentiating acquired versus reactivated toxoplasmosis.

Therapy is indicated when vision is threatened, and therapeutic modalities include oral triple sulfa, sulfadiazine, phyrimethamine, and tetracycline. Oral and/or subconjunctival injections of clindamycin and more recently, minocycline

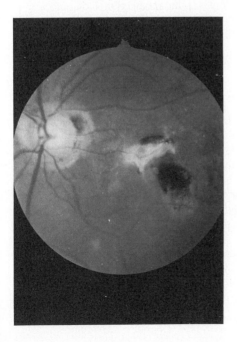

Figure 14–5. Posterior uveitis demonstrating a toxoplasmosis lesion.

have been prescribed. Topical, periocular, and oral corticosteroids will control secondary inflammation in the anterior segment and cycloplegics will prevent posterior synechia. Laser and cryotherapy have definite but limited roles in toxoplasmosis therapy. Vitrectomy may be indicated when vitreous opacities (which interfere with vision) persist after resolution of active retinochoroiditis.

NURSING INTERVENTION

Assess the patient who complains of a decrease in vision, acute pain, photophobia, and/or tearing, and note any pupillary changes if present. Be cognizant that symptoms differ from those of an acute glaucoma or conjunctivitis. Ask the patient if he or she has a history of allergy, rheumatoid arthritis, or any other systemic disease. Administer medications prescribed by the physician. A regimen of sulfadiazine and phyrimethamine includes a loading dose, followed by a maintenance dose for a prescribed number of days. Because of the possible side affects of phyrimethamine (Daraprim), a folinic acid supplement (Leucovorin) is given twice weekly to circumvent bone marrow suppression. Complete blood count (CBC) and differential may also be ordered and should be reviewed. If clindamycin is the treatment of choice, oral administration may alter normal bacterial flora of the intestinal tract and may result in pseudomembraneous enterocolitis.

PATIENT TEACHING

Patient teaching should include the correct self-administration of the medication. Development of an enterocolitis as a result of antibiotic therapy should prompt the patient to immediately stop the medication and contact the physician. Once treatment has started, patient compliance with self-medication and follow-up care is vitally important and should be stressed.

Sympathetic Ophthalmia. *Sympathetic ophthalmia* (SO) is a rare but devastating, bilateral, granulomatous panuveitis, which can develop anywhere from days to years after a perforating injury, following a retained foreign body or an operation. The cause is not known, but the disease is probably related to hypersensitivity to uveal pigment.[3] It has been hypothesized from an experimental model that SO is an autoimmune disease.[13]

Symptoms of SO may occur following injury, when the (exciting) eye becomes inflamed first, and then the fellow (sympathizing) eye becomes involved. The inflammatory process spreads from the uveal tract to the optic nerve, and then to the pia and arachnoid surrounding the optic nerve. This accounts for the papillitis that is sometimes observed. The patient complains of photophobia, blurred vision, and redness of the eye. Slitlamp examination may reveal KP and a flare in the anterior chamber of both eyes.[13]

Treatment of a severely injured, sightless eye (i.e., a penetrating injury through the sclera, ciliary body, and lens with loss of vitreous) will be the recommendation of enucleation to prevent SO. It is often a very difficult and devastating decision for the patient to make, therefore most times the eye will be sutured to give the patient some time to get used to the idea of the loss. When the inflammation is advanced, the ophthalmalogist will refrain from suggesting enucleation, because the injured eye may eventually prove to be the better of the two very bad eyes. Established SO lasts for weeks to years with exacerbations and remissions, which eventually lead to blindness without treatment. Medication of the acute diffuse, bilateral uveitis includes treatment with local corticosteroids and mydriatics, as well as systemic corticosteroids in high doses, e.g., prednisolone 40 to 120 mg every other day, which is gradually tapered off. In severe cases that fail to respond to corticosteroids, treatment with antimetabolites and alkylating agents has met with success. However, white blood cell count (WBC) and platelets must be monitored very carefully in these patients, and these drugs should not be used without careful consideration.[13]

NURSING INTERVENTION
Nursing assessment may reveal that the patient, suffering from a penetrating injury in one eye, is registering complaints of pain, photophobia, and decreased vision in the other eye. The nurse should seek early ophthalmological attention for this patient. Once the presumed diagnosis of SO is made, administering the prescribed systemic and topical medication regimen is a vital aspect of nursing care. Medicating for pain may be necessary. Shielding the eyes with dark glasses decreases the photophobia.

PATIENT TEACHING
Patient teaching will include an understanding of the importance of compliance with the medication regimen, and follow-up care once the patient is discharged from an inpatient setting.

Tumors of the Uvea
Benign and malignant tumors can be found in the iris, ciliary body, and choroid. Because the uvea contains melanocytes (pigmented cells), pigmented lesions are common, easily seen, but clinically difficult to classify without microscopic studies to determine cell type.

Benign Pigmented Lesions of Iris, Ciliary Body, and Choroid. These nevi cells vary in amounts of pigmentation, size, shape, and growth patterns. Lesions usually occur in the iris' inferior portion, and like nevi found elsewhere become pigmented at puberty. They should be observed and photographed to make sure they do not grow or undergo malignant changes. Choroidal nevi are considered the most common intraocular tumor. They are usually discovered on opthalmoscopic examination, and appear as distinct, flat, slate gray lesions which are nearly always found in the posterior portion of the globe. Occasionally, these lesions may become malignant and the best way to determine change is for the lesion to be followed with fundus photography and fluorescein angiography.[12]

Malignant Tumors. *Malignant tumors* with pigmentation occur in the iris and are called malignant melanomas. These slow growing tumors occur in white males and females equally, with the average age being about 45 years. Similar to nevi, these tumors are usually found in the lower half of the iris, but their growth is irregular with nodules. Seeding in the angles and on the iris' surface can occur or spread may be by direct extension.[14] These tumors should be studied, transilluminated, and photographed. Surgical excision of the iris is carried out if tumor growth is demonstrated and/or interferes with vision. If the angle is involved, an *iridocyclectomy* (surgical removal of a portion of the iris and the ciliary body) may be done; if a portion of the posterior ciliary body is involved, and *iridocyclochorioretinectomy* (surgical removal of a portion of the iris, ciliary body, and choroid) may be performed.

Melanomas of the ciliary body and choroid are noted for their size and may therefore cause rapid and serious symptoms (Fig. 14–6). They are composed of many cells growing in a tissue with a rich blood supply and the many vascular channels of the ciliary body and choroid facilitate the dispersion of malignant cells throughout the body. These are the most common malignant intraocular tumors. Tumor growth patterns vary with some growing inward, toward the center of the globe, which obstructs the visual axis. Others invade the ciliary body's circular muscles, following these fibers for 360 degrees, to form what is called a "ring melanoma." These are only detected if they break into the angle and produce glaucoma by blocking the canal of Schlemm. The tumor may also come through the sclera to the outside by means of the emissary vessels and nerve.[14] Malignant melanomas of the posterior choroid may extend inward, then when the tumor ruptures Bruch's membrane it takes on a mushroom configuration, so that the overlying retina is detached by serous fluid. Occasionally, these tumors become necrotic which produces an inflammatory reaction. The propensity for melanomas to extend and reveal their distant metastasis after years has been documented.

Management of malignant melanomas depends upon growth, size, age of patient, and condition of the fellow eye. Cell type might be established by *fine*

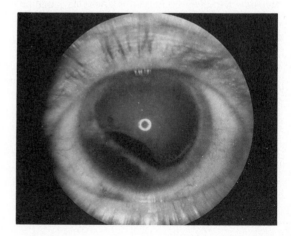

Figure 14–6. Melanoma of the ciliary body shown with iris transillumination. (*Photograph courtesy James J. Augsburger, M.D., Oncology Department, Wills Eye Hospital.*)

needle biopsy. Radioactive phosphorous (P-32) has been used to identify tumor activity. Treatment can be by photocoagulation, cryotherapy, radiation brachy-therapy, and enucleation.

Brachytherapy Treatment with Cobalt-60, Ruthenium-106, Iridium-192, or Iodine-125 Plaques for Ocular Tumors. Plaques are comprised of a sealed source of radioactive material which is surgically placed on, and sutured to, the posterior scleral surface over the tumor site. The conjunctival incision is then closed. The aim is to deliver a radiation dose between 4000 and 10,000 REMS to the tumor's base. The number of days that the plaque will remain in place is calculated taking into account the radiation dose to be administered, the strength of the plaque, and the size of the tumor. Cobalt-60 and Ruthenium-106 plaques are about the size of a dime and the radioactive source is enclosed in metal. Iodine-125 and Iridium-192 plaques are custom-made and the activity and number of seeds encased in the plastic depends upon the tumor size and the desired dose. The plaques are usually under the control of a nuclear medicine department.[16] The plaques are maintained in position for a calculated amount of time and then are removed, after which the patient can be immediately discharged from confinement and the hospital.

NURSING INTERVENTION
Patients are confined to their rooms during the period of plaque implanta-tion, and nurses must limit their amount of exposure to the radioactive source while these patients are being treated. It is therefore necessary to prepare the patient for the limited amount of contact which he or she will have while *Radiation Safety Precautions* are being observed. The patient will have discussed the pros and cons of such a treatment in detail with the physician, but the psychological aspect of anxiety still causes the patient to ask many questions and the nurse, in turn, can be very supportive during this stressful, but boring, period of treatment. Cycloplegic and steroid–antibiotic eyedrops are administered t.i.d. The eye may or may not be patched, depending upon the visual status of the other eye.

PATIENT TEACHING
Patient teaching should include the reasons for limited contact. The radia-tion is of no therapeutic benefit to anyone but the patient. Nothing but the plaque is radioactive. The precautions taken with linen and trash are so that there will never be a loss of the radioactive source. Visitors must keep their distance for the same reason that there is no therapeutic benefit to their being exposed. Patients may be taught to administer their own eye-drops. The most useful thing one can tell patients preoperatively is to bring some project that will keep them occupied for at least the full period of time they will be confined to the room on radiation precautions. Often patients are concerned about their artifacts being exposed to radiation. Once the radioactive source is removed from the patient's eye there is no need for further precautions. The only thing that is radioactive is the plaque.

Nursing Radiation Safety Precautions. Radiation exposure is dependent upon the *time* with and *distance* from a radioactive source. Employees may minimize their exposure by shortening the time they spend with the patient and by staying further away from the patient. Planning what needs to be done prior to entering the patient's room is a good means of reducing the exposure. Film badges are used to monitor staff exposure to radiation. Each person should have their own badge, and should never wear one belonging to anyone else. Pocket docimeters are also available which can monitor the exact amount of exposure of those who have to have extended contact with a patient, for example a baby (who has a retinoblastoma which is being treated with plaque therapy—see Chap. 17) who needs to be held and fed. Precautions for losing the source must be taken, and in order to meet this NRC (Nuclear Regulatory Commission) requirement, the linen and trash may not be discarded until after a survey meter (Geiger counter) has been passed over it. This is done to ensure that the radioactive source is not in either container. In the un- likelihood of a plaque becoming dislodged, a plaque should never be touched, only handled with forceps and then placed at least 7 feet away from anybody, until such time as the Radiation Safety Officer and oncology physician are notified and can take care of it.

Miscellaneous Primary Tumors. Other primary tumors of the uvea include: hemangiomata, epitheliomata, myomata, and those derived from neural and os- seous tissue.

Benign choroidal hemangiomata, occurs in two different patterns. A diffuse type is usually diagnosed at about the age of 10 years, and is associated with nonserous retinal detachments, glaucoma, and facial cutaneous hemangiomata. The localized type (always found in the choroid posterior to the equator) is diagnosed at about the age of 40, and must be differentiated from malignant melanoma, meta- static tumors, central serous chorioretinopathy, posterior scleritis, and choroidal osteoma. Visual field tests, fluorescein angiography, ultrasonography, and fine needle biopsy studies are used to help in diagnosis. These tumors are managed by repeated observation if there are no symptoms. For those tumors which produce symptoms of visual decrease, as a result of serous detachment of the fovea, pho- tocoagulation of the area with argon laser produces chorioretinal adhesion that will aid the retina in reattaching over the tumor, and facilitate reabsorption of subretinal fluid.

Metastatic Tumors of the Uvea. Choroidal vascularity makes it a logical target for the lodging of neoplastic emboli. This occurs where the vessels are most numer- ous at the posterior pole. In 85 percent of women, the breast is the original tumor site; lung carcinoma accounts for another 8 percent. The primary site in men is the lung; however, 24 percent of males have an unknown primary source. Metastatic lesions usually occur in patients over 40 years of age, and a past history of a malignancy is an ominous clue in diagnosis. Helpful tests are fluorescein angiogra- phy, ultrasonography, radioactive phosphorous uptake, and fine-needle biopsy. The treatment depends upon systemic symptoms and clinical findings, and is directed at the primary lesion. This would include chemotherapy, radiation with x-rays, or Cobalt-60 plaques for the eye tumor.

Uveal Injuries

Uveal injuries may be divided into those associated with mechanical causes and those that are nonmechanical.

Mechanical Trauma. *Mechanical trauma* produces a contusion effect on the iris and is the most common type of injury. The mildest degree of injury can be *traumatic miosis and spasm of accommodation* which occurs immediately after the contusion, may last for a considerable time, but is usually only temporary. A mild blow to the eye may not precipitate the secondary phenomenon of pupillary dilatation with cycloplegia, but it may cause a moderately dilated pupil with absent or diminished reaction to light and accommodation. Miotic drops may have no effect. Even after dilation subsides the pupil may be permanently irregular. This reaction may be due to nerve damage or sphincter muscle rupture. Tears in the iris and sphincter muscle also occur and can disrupt the pupil's size permanently. If the tear occurs at the iris base it is known as a *dialysis*. Symptoms which will bring the patient to seek attention are pain and blurred vision. Assessment will reveal any change in pupillary size, shape, and contour. The immediate treatment will be to obtain a visual acuity, then dilate the pupil to prevent iritis.

Iritis. *Iritis* may occur after contusion, and results from leaking of protein and cells from the iris' vessels as a result of the increased permeability of these vessels. If the trauma is severe enough there may be hemorrhage into the stroma of the iris, and if the concussion is sharp enough to rupture a larger iris vessel there may also be free blood in the anterior chamber which is known as *hyphema* (Fig. 14–7). If a hemorrhage occurs in the anterior chamber it usually disappears in about 5 to 7 days by being hemolysed, and is flushed out through the trabecular meshwork or is absorbed by the iris. If it does not disappear, the possibility of a more serious recurrence of a secondary hemorrhage can result. The hyphema may be severe enough to fill the entire anterior chamber, blocking the trabecular meshwork, and causing increased

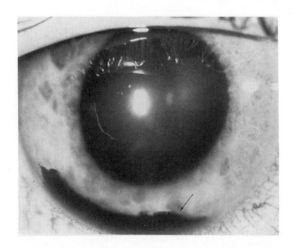

Figure 14–7. Hyphema—blood in the anterior chamber (*arrow*).

intraocular pressure. When a clot forms, it appears black and may obstruct all view of iris, pupil, and lens. The patient may experience delayed pain, photophobia, and tearing, and may therefore not seek medical attention until the day following the injury. Treatment for iritis includes pupillary dilatation with a short-acting cyclo-plegic to put the ciliary muscle at rest. Steroid drops and ointment decrease the inflammatory response. However, if there is a hyphema, the medication may be varied, ranging from nothing, to cycloplegics and steroids, to miotics.

NURSING INTERVENTION
Assess the visual acuity, note the time that the injury took place and the mechanism of trauma. If there is an obvious hyphema, keep the patient's head elevated so that it may settle by gravity into the lower portion of the anterior chamber (Fig. 14–7). Instill eye medications as prescribed. Shield the hyphema patient's eye to prevent any untoward accidents.

Contusion of the Choroid. *Contusion of the choroid* may cause hemorrhage with detachment of the choroid. There can also be a choroidal rupture which leaves a cleft in the choroid (Fig. 14–8). Most of these ruptures occur in the posterior pole on the temporal side and may interfere with the central vision. The pupil will be dilated to facilitate examination.

Perforating Wounds. *Perforating wounds* can cause serious disorganization of the globe with uveal incarceration into the site of perforation. Penetration of the iris can be difficult to see at first if the wound is small because of lack of reaction. However, wounds of the ciliary body and choroid are different. There is immediate reaction with hemorrhage, then later when the repairing process takes place there can be massive fibrosis with contraction followed by hypotony and phthisis bulbi. Penetration may be caused by a foreign body that may be retained in the choroid or ciliary body. Contamination may cause an infection and endophthalmitis.

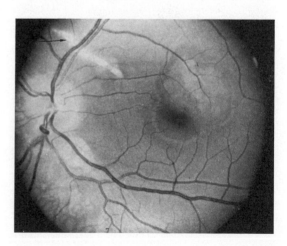

Figure 14–8. Fundus showing a choroidal rupture.

NURSING INTERVENTION

Taking an accurate history as to what the patient was doing at the time of injury is important and should be ascertained together with a visual acuity. If the lids are swollen, or uveal incarceration is suspected, great care should be taken not to cause further damage to the eyeball. Patch and shield the eye until medical attention can be obtained. Keep the patient NPO (nothing by mouth) until the time of surgery has been arranged.

Nonmechanical Trauma. *Nonmechanical trauma* to the uvea can be caused by radiation of light. The light source can be the sun, an atomic blast, or a laser beam. These burns cause damage immediately, and there is no way to prevent the damage once it has occurred.

NURSING INTERVENTION

Nursing intervention should be directed at prevention by encouraging people who are in situations where eye injuries can occur to wear safety glasses, visors, or protective glasses when dealing with today's technology.

REFERENCES

 1. Barsky D: Anatomy of the uveal tract, in Duane TD, (Ed.): Clinical Ophthalmology. Hagerstown, Md.: Harper & Row, 1983, pp. 1–10
 2. Barsky D: Color Atlas of Pathology of the Eye. New York: McGraw-Hill, 1966, p. 6
 3. Vaughan D, Asbury T: General Ophthalmology, 10th ed. Los Altos, Calif. Lange, 1983, pp. 110–119
 4. Jakobiek FA, Ozanics V: General topographic anatomy of the eye, in Duane TD, Jaeger E, (Eds.): Biomedical Foundations of Ophthalmology. Hagerstown, Md.: Harper & Row, 1983, pp. 1–9
 5. Knox DL: Disorders of the uveal tract, in Harley RD, (Ed.): Pediatric Ophthalmology, 2nd ed. Philadelphia: Saunders, 1983, pp. 515–548
 6. Walton DS: Glaucoma in infants and children, in Harley RD, (Ed.): Pediatric Ophthalmology, 2nd ed. Philadelphia: Saunders, 1983, pp. 585–598
 7. Spaeth GL, Auerbach VH: Inborn errors of metabolism affecting the eye, in Harley RD, (Ed.): Pediatric Ophthalmology, 2nd ed. Philadelphia: Saunders, 1983, pp. 1053–1143
 8. O'Donnell FE, Green WR: The eye in albinism, in Duane TD, (Ed.): Clinical Ophthalmology. Hagerstown, Md: Harper & Row, 1983, pp. 1–23
 9. Devron HC, Schlaegel TF: General factors in uveitis, in Duane TD, (Ed.): Clinical Ophthalmology. Hagerstown, Md.: Harper & Row, 1983, pp. 1–7
10. Schlaegel TF: Symptoms and signs of uveitis, in Duane TD, (Ed.): Clinical Ophthalmology. Hagerstown, Md.: Harper & Row, 1983. pp. 1–7
11. Schlaegel TF: Toxoplasmosis, in Duane TD, (Ed.): Clinical Ophthalmology. Hagerstown, Md.: Harper & Row, 1982, pp. 1–16
12. Naumann GOH, Yanoff M, Naumann JR: Pigmented nevi of choroid: Clinical study of

secondary changes in the overlying tissue. Trans Am Academy of Ophthalmol Otolaryn-gol, 75: 110–143, 1971

13. Schlaegel TF: Uveitis of suspected viral origin, in Duane TD, (Ed.): Clinical Ophthal-mology. Hagerstown, Md.: Harper & Row, 1983, pp. 1–11

14. Canny CLB, Shields JA, Kay ML: Stationary choroidal melanoma with extraocular extension. Archives of Ophthalmology, 96: 436–439, 1978

BIBLIOGRAPHY

Shields JA: Diagnosis and Management of Intraocular Tumors. St. Louis: Mosby, 1982

15

The Lens

NEW TERMS

Accommodation: the adjustment of the eye for seeing at different distances, accomplished by changing the shape of the lens through action of the ciliary muscle, thus focusing a clear image on the retina.[1]

Aphakia: absence of lens.

Iridodonesis: tremulousness of the iris seen in aphakic, dislocated, or subluxated lens patients.

Leukocoria: white pupil.

Presbyopia: physiologically blurred near vision, commonly evident soon after age 40.

Pseudophakia: eye which has an intraocular lens implant.

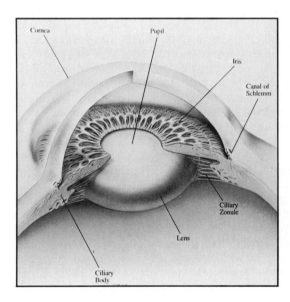

15–1. The lens is suspended from the ciliary body's ciliary processes by many fine zonular fibers radially attached at the equator. (*From Friedman AH, Desmarest RJ, Westwood WB: The Optyl Atlas of the Human Eye. Norwood, N.J.: Optyl, 1979, with permission.*)

The crystalline *lens* is a transparent, biconvex intraocular structure that, by altering its shape, contributes to one-third of the focusing power of the eye. It is enclosed in an elastic capsule and is suspended from the ciliary body's ciliary processes by many fine *zonular fibers* radically attached at the equator. Lying directly behind the iris, its anterior surface is in contact with the iris pigment epithelium at the pupillary margin (Fig. 15–1). The lens' posterior surface is supported by the vitreous (hyaloid) face where it lies in a small depression. The lens has no blood supply after fetal development. At birth, its diameter is 6.5 mm, and reaches 9.0 mm by age 15 years and thereafter. It is a living, metabolically active tissue whose needs must be met for the maintenance of transparency. Since it is avascular, nourishment for the cells must be obtained from, and waste products removed by, the surrounding aqueous and vitreous.[2]

The aqueous continuously flows from the ciliary body to the anterior chamber freshly bathing the lens' anterior surface. The area of contact with the iris depends upon the relative position of the iris–lens diaphragm and the pupil's size. Younger eyes with their smaller, more posterior lenses have less iris contact. As the lens enlarges with age, the iris is forced forward causing more surface contact and creating narrower anterior chamber angles.[2]

The lens is composed of an elastic *anterior and posterior capsule* which surrounds a cortex. The *cortex and nuclei* are made up of long concentric lamellas. In fetal life these lamellar fibers, by joining end-to-end, form Y-shaped suture lines. The anterior Y is erect, and posteriorly it is an inverted λ. After birth and throughout life the lens continues to increase in size through the addition of new, superficial fibers formed by epithelial cells at the equator. As newer cells are formed, older cells are displaced centrally and the nucleus migrates slightly forward (to form a lens bow) as the younger cells form more superficial layers.[1,2] The adult lens consists of 65 percent water, but this decreases with age. Its protein content (about 35 percent) is the highest of any tissue in the body. Electrolyte composition resembles the ions present in other body cells, with high potassium and low sodium and chloride concentrations, while aqueous closely resembles the ionic composition of the plasma, with high concentrations of sodium and chloride but low levels of potassium. This creates a concentration gradient between the inside of the lens and the aqueous, and maintains the lens in a relatively dehydrated state.

The sole purpose of the lens is to focus light rays upon the retina. In order to focus light from a distant object, the ciliary muscle relaxes, tautening the zonular fibers, flattening the lens, and minimizing the refractive power of the lens, thereby focusing the parallel rays upon the retina. To focus light from a near object, the ciliary muscle contracts, releasing tension on the zonules; the elastic lens capsule then molds the lens into a more spherical shape with correspondingly greater refractive power. The physiological interplay of the ciliary body, zonules, and lens which results in focusing near objects upon the retina is known as *accommodation*. As the lens ages, its accommodative power is gradually reduced, leading to mid-life presbyopia.[1]

DEVELOPMENTAL ANOMALIES

The size, shape, and opacification of the lens can be affected during the child's development. Congenital aphakia is extremely rare and is associated with underdevelopment of rudimentary eyes. The lens' shape may vary—in spherophakia it is more spherical than normal. Usually this condition is bilateral, it may be an incidental defect or seen in Marchesani's syndrome. Coloboma of the lens can also occur and usually the zonular fibers are absent in the region. When it occurs inferiorly, it may be found in conjunction with other ocular colobomatous defects. Cataracts in children may be developmental, acquired, or traumatic in nature.[3]

ACQUIRED ANOMALIES

Dislocated lenses (ectopia lentis) may be acquired with the rupture of the zonules caused by a blow to the eye. The lens may remain in the eye or even be forced through a rupture in the globe and may be under the conjunctiva. Usually, however, it is dislocated posteriorly into the vitreous, where it might be left undisturbed or may be removed using vitrectomy instruments. Occasionally it dislocates into the anterior chamber (Fig. 15–2).

Subluxated lenses are most frequently seen in Marfan's syndrome (arachnodactyly), which is characterized by an increase in skeletal length, spider fingers, scoliosis, and disturbances in the larger blood vessels;[3] homocystinuria, an inborn error of metabolism of the sulfur-containing amino acids; and Weill-Marchesani's syndrome, a hyplastic form of congenital mesodermal dystrophy. Those affected are usually short in stature and have short, stubby fingers. The displaced lens may be tilted, causing a significant myopia and astigmatism which are difficult to correct optically.

Trauma may precede the migration of a previously subluxated lens into the

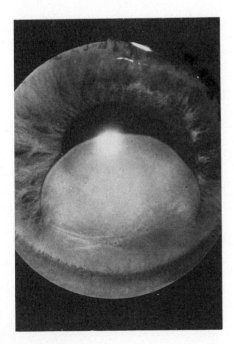

Figure 15–2. Dislocated lens in anterior chamber.

anterior chamber. A lens in the anterior chamber may be vigorously treated initially with cycloplegic and mydriatic agents to allow the lens to fall back behind the iris. The prognosis for vision varies with type and degree of dislocation and possible presence of other ocular complications. Associated complications include pupillary block glaucoma, cataract, uveitis, and retinal detachment.

NURSING INTERVENTION
Assessment information relating to any cardiovascular, skeletal, or ocular abnormalities which may be present in both patient and other family members should be noted. The patient's visual acuity may be poor without the aphakic correction often prescribed. Instillation of cycloplegic and mydriatic drops may be prescribed for repositioning the lens, as well as for breaking pupillary block glaucoma. Steroid eyedrops may be prescribed and will be instilled for uveitis.

PATIENT TEACHING
The patient who has the potential for dislocated lenses should be advised against participating in contact sports. Encourage medication compliance when prescribed. Encourage follow-up visits where appropriate.[4]

CATARACTS

Any opacity of the lens is called a *cataract*. Lens opacities are only important when they interfere with visual acuity.

Congenital Cataracts
Developing in utero, congenital cataracts may be described as *polar* and they occur at either the anterior or posterior pole of the lens. This type may be associated with the prenatal vascular network which surrounds the lens. Cataracts can also be categorized as *primary*—due to disturbance in development, and *secondary*—caused by noxious and/or toxic products which destroy the lens tissue. Sporadic, genetic, or hereditary causes must also be considered. In the genetic type, transmission is usually autosomal dominant. Recessive cataracts may be sex-linked. Cataracts may also be associated with other congenital anomalies.

Typical congenital types of cataracts are the *zonular* (lamellar) and *nuclear* cataracts. The zonular cataract is limited to a certain lens layer or zone, the embryonic nucleus may be normal, and some of the cortex is clear. The cortex laid down after the insult is also clear. This type of cataract accounts for 40 percent of all congenital cataracts. In a nuclear cataract, the embryonic nucleus and/or the fetal nucleus may be involved. If the embryonic nucleus has suffered some disturbance, the insult will have occurred in the first 3 months of development.

A leukocoria (white pupil) or a wandering, searching type of nystagmus may be the first symptom noticed by the child's parents which prompts them to seek the pediatrician's attention. For an infant suspected of developing a cataract from an intrauterine infection, antibody titers from the mother and from the patient may be obtained. Those entities that should be sought for with titers are covered by the acronym TORCH, which stands for toxoplasmosis, other viruses, rubella, cytomegalic inclusion disease, and herpes simplex.[5] Galactosemia is also a very rare cause of congenital cataract. Ultrasonography may be performed by the ophthalmologist to elicit if the other intraocular structures are functioning and intact. The pupil will need to be well dilated prior to surgery.

Surgical treatment is extracapsular cataract extraction using an irrigation and aspiration-type machine. Often an opening is made into the posterior capsule at the end of the procedure. One or two sutures close the 2- to 4-mm corneoscleral incision. Dilating and/or steroid–antibiotic drops are instilled postoperatively (depending upon the surgeons preference), and a patch and shield are applied over the eye. As soon as possible the child is fit with an aphakic continuous-wear soft contact lens or glasses to stimulate the use of the eye; however, amblyopia often becomes a problem which has to be dealt with. The insertion of intraocular lenses into the child's eye is still controversial at this point. In general, cataracts in children have a poorer visual prognosis than cataracts in adults.[5]

Senile Cataracts

The senile cataract is probably the most common type of lens opacity. Usually occurring after the age of 50,[6] and like gray hair, it is part of the aging process. Three main types of this cataract are *cortical, nuclear* (Fig. 15–3), and *posterior subcapsular*. As the patient ages, the lens fibrils undergo the changes of liquifaction—vacuoles are formed under the lens capsule and occasionally in the cortex. These cortical vacuoles may coalesce and form water clefts.

Another change which occurs is hardening of the nucleus. This sclerosing process begins at about 25 years of age and continues for the rest of one's life. It accounts for loss of elasticity of the lens which produces presbyopia. As these lens changes progress there is discoloration of the nucleus which becomes yellowish then brown. As the nucleus becomes hardened, pseudomyopia may result. Farsighted patients might find they are able to read without their glasses.[6] Eventually,

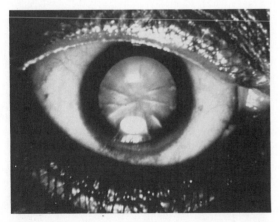

Figure 15–3. Nuclear cataract.

the hardening associated with opacification, discolorization, and vascularization leads to decrease in visual acuity and necessitates surgical intervention.

When the cataract is *posterior subcapsular,* the cortical material beneath the posterior capsule is involved because of its central location, and vision is usually impaired early, requiring early lens removal to restore sight.[6]

Metabolic etiology, such as diabetes, is another common cause for cataract formation. In the diabetic patient, senile cataractous changes frequently occur at an earlier age and with a much more rapid course to maturity than in nondiabetic patients. The clinical complaints for these patients are changes in vision—due to a change in refraction, and blurring of vision—due to the reflection and scattering of light rays which do not go through the lens.

Cataract formation can be associated with other ocular diseases such as heterochromic iritis, anterior uveitis of unknown etiology, and systemic diseases, e.g., thromboangiitis obliterans and hypoparathyroidism.

Traumatic Cataracts

Traumatic cataracts are caused by a number of mechanical, chemical, radiational, and toxic forces and substances. A contusion to the globe may cause rupture of capsule, interruption of blood supply to the anterior chamber, and/or dislocation of the lens (Fig. 15–4). Penetrating wounds of the cornea by foreign bodies from industrial accidents or gunshot wounds are not an uncommon cause of unilateral cataracts.

Toxic substances which include corticosteroids and anticholinesterase drugs, and industrial or accidental exposure to toxic chemicals such as naphthalene, dinitrophenol, paradichlorobenzene, thallium, and cobalt have also been implicated in cataract formation. Exposure to x-rays and other ionizing radiation, radar in communications, and recently microwaves used for cooking have also been implicated in cataract formation.

Cataract Extraction

There is no medical treatment for cataracts, the only treatment is surgical removal of the cloudy lens. Two methods of cataract removal are employed today. The most

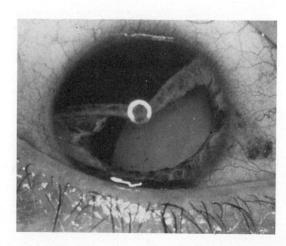

Figure 15–4. Traumatic cataractous and dislocated lens with large iris dialysis.

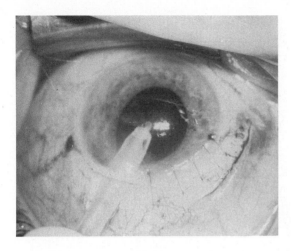

Figure 15–5. Extracapsular cataract extraction using I & A machine tip.

popular is the *extracapsular cataract extraction* (ECCE). Here an incision is made into the anterior capsule and the cataractous cortex and nucleus are removed by either expressing it or fragmenting it, using instruments such as phacoemulsification or irrigation and aspiration machines (Fig. 15–5). With this method the emulsified lens material is removed from the eye, through a fine infusion and aspiration tip, leaving the posterior capsule intact. Once the cortical substance has been removed a polymethylmethacralate *intraocular lens* (IOL) can be inserted into the eye. Most frequently the IOL is positioned in the posterior chamber (Fig. 15–6), although IOLs may also be placed in the anterior chamber (Fig. 15–7), and initially were held in place by the pupil. The incision is then closed with fine sutures. The operating room microscope is used for the procedure. The posterior capsule may cloud up at a future date, once again causing a decrease in vision, and will have to be removed surgically or by a noninvasive procedure using the Neodymium YAG (Nd:YAG) laser, before vision is restored.

Another technique is the *intracapsular cataract extraction* (ICCE). With this

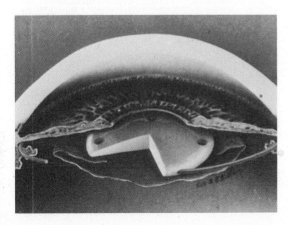

Figure 15–6. Intraocular lens placed in posterior chamber. (*From Abrahamson IA: Cataract update. American Family Physician, 24(4): 118, 1981. Photograph courtesy Don Keller, Columbus, Ohio.*)

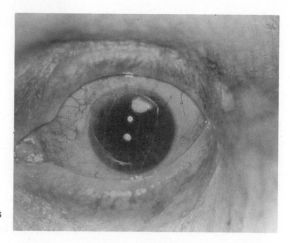

Figure 15–7. Intraocular lens placed in anterior chamber.

method, the intact capsule and lenticular substance is removed using a freezing (cryo) probe (Fig. 15–8). This may be done with or without implantation of an anterior chamber intraocular lens. If an implant is not used, then corrected vision must be obtained by postoperative contact lenses or aphakic glasses. The IOL usually has the power to correct the vision for distance, therefore, in order for the patient to read at near, reading glasses must be prescribed.

As with any surgical procedure, infrequent complications may occur. Among these in the immediate postoperative period are such things as hyphema, increased intraocular pressure (secondary glaucoma), and pupillary capture of the lens.

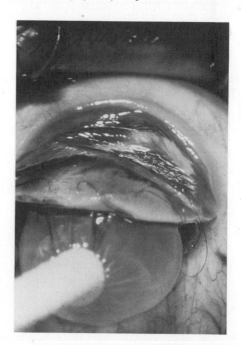

Figure 15–8. Intracapsular cataract extraction using cryo probe.

Endophthalmitis, infection inside the eye, would still be considered nosocomal if it occurred within the first postoperative 24 hours, even though the patient was not in the surgical setting. Two to 5 percent of patients develop retinal detachment as a later complication, and aphakic bullous keratopathy and pseudophakic bullous keratopathy can also occur. The development of a uveitis occasionally necessitates IOL removal.

Preoperative Preparation. Cataract surgery is performed on the same day that the patient is admitted for the surgical procedure, that is unless the patient has complicating ocular and/or medical problems. As a result of this, new methods of patient processing have become necessary. Preliminary laboratory testing, such as blood work (CBC and differential, FBS, BUN, and liver function studies), ECG and chest x-ray must be accomplished prior to admission (PAT—pre-admission testing) for surgery. In order to calculate the IOL, power ocular tests such as *keratometry readings,* to measure corneal curvature and *A and/or B scan ultrasonography,* to measure the axial length of the eyeball, as well as for identifying an intact retina (where a view of the fundus with Slitlamp or ophthalmoscope is obscured by a dense cataract), needs to be completed on an outpatient basis. Cataract surgery is an elective procedure, and since the patient population that undergoes it is one in which many other medical problems are to be found, patients will need to have medical clearance from their own physician prior to surgery under anesthesia. The surgical consent form should be discussed and signed. The type of anesthesia is also decided upon at this time. If the eye is to receive dilating drops, then the patient should be shown how to instill them, so that the pupil is dilated at the time of admission and ready for surgery. Patient teaching should be done at this time also. Ideally, completed papers should accompany the elective cataract patient on admission to the hospital or surgicenter.

NURSING INTERVENTION
The process of assessing the well-being of patients who are admitted for the procedure of cataract extraction becomes the important part of the total nursing care. In taking the history, astute questioning will sometimes intercept a discrepancy between a patient's knowledge of a medical condition and medication being taken for that condition. Physical problems can also be identified at this interview. A laboratory study may have an abnormal value on it which must be brought to the physician's attention, so that corrective action can be taken if possible prior to surgery under anesthesia.

A telephone call to the patient prior to admission, requesting allergy, medication, and physical complaint history may be a time-saving way of obtaining this information. It can also be the perfect way to decrease presurgical apprehension by answering questions which may predispose to patient anxiety. Patients should be requested to bring their systemic medications in with them, so that their medication routine may remain uninterrupted, and also to ensure that there will be no possible conflicting drug interactions.

A reminder to the patients to have nothing by mouth for 6 hours prior to surgery should be included in the conversation.

PATIENT TEACHING

The correct method of instillation of cycloplegic and mydriatic eyedrops, given to the patient by the physician for pupillary dilatation, should be reinforced by the nurse as part of patient teaching.

Discharge planning and patient teaching should begin in the office before the patient reaches the surgical arena. It is important to stress that a responsible person accompany the patient at discharge, following recovery from anesthesia. Planning ahead ensures that all the necessary paperwork and information is available to the nursing staff to facilitate the patient's safe passage through the surgical procedure. Written discharge instructions should accompany the patient on leaving the hospital (see Figure 15–9).

Implementing the care according to the rules and regulations which make for smooth running of the operating room is a major challenge for the nurse dealing with patients on a short-stay, surgical basis. Prior to going to the operating room (O.R.), the patient must empty his or her bladder; remove dentures (if the patient is undergoing general anesthesia) and earrings, and don a hospital gown. The patient should also remove glasses or contact lenses. If the physician requests that extended wear lens be left in the eye, the nurse should make a note of this fact so that the O.R. nurse is careful not to damage it with betadine scrub solution. The patient must receive the premedication and osmotic agents at the appropriate time, and further dilating drops may have to be instilled into the eye if the pupil is not fully dilated. If the surgery is scheduled to be under local anesthesia, then the patient should be aware that the blood pressure will be monitored throughout the procedure, as will the heart rate, and that the O.R. sounds will be heard throughout the operation. The patient should be encouraged to remain still during the surgical procedure, and not move out of curiosity of an awareness of these sounds. Intraoperative procedures were discussed in Chapter 8.

Postoperative Care. Management of the patient's safe recovery in the immediate postoperative period is a definite nursing concern. The patient is monitored until the effects of anesthesia have worn off. Often the patient is able to be helped to the bathroom upon recovery from local anesthesia. He or she might even be hungry enough to eat breakfast or lunch.

The eye will be carefully patched and shielded, ensuring that the eyelids are properly closed and to prevent possible corneal abrasion. Sometimes this will cause a decrease in vision in the other eye if the patient wears glasses, and cannot get them on properly over the shield. When the patient is fully recovered from anesthesia, he or she is able to take fluids and ambulate, and discharge instructions should be given to both patient and accompanying friend or relative. Discharge instructions (Fig. 15–9) require the patient to return to the physician's office the next day so that the eye can be dressed, examined at the Slitlamp, and medicated accordingly. Sometimes, however, the patient may be required to remove the eye patch later on the same day as the surgery and begin instillation of eyedrops. Guidelines for safety in the immediate postoperative period are also reviewed by the nurse (Fig. 15–10).

Evaluating the patient the day after surgery by a follow-up telephone call is a

JJJ Wills Eye Hospital

DISCHARGE INSTRUCTIONS

DATE OF DISCHARGE: _____

FOLLOW-UP APPOINTMENT:

Return to: _____ Service   PHONE: _____

_____ Office   DATE : _____

Location _____   TIME : _____

Clerk/R.N. _____

In case of Emergency Call: _____ or 928-3080
If unable to contact M.D., return to Wills Eye Hospital Emergency Room.

SPECIAL EYE INSTRUCTIONS: No Restrictions ( )   ACTIVITY INSTRUCTIONS: No Restrictions ( )

Patch	- Left	- Right	- Day/Night
Shield	- Left	- Right	- Day/Night
Glasses	( )	- Day
Compresses ( )	- Yes

Shower ( ) NO ( ) YES
Shave ( ) NO ( ) YES
Wash hair with head held back . ( ) NO ( ) YES
Bending and/or Lifting .... ( ) NO ( ) YES
Driving .... ( ) NO ( ) YES
Return to Work............. ( ) NO ( ) YES
When _____

DIET: _____
OTHER SPECIFIC INSTRUCTIONS:

_____
_____
_____
_____

MEDICATION INSTRUCTIONS:
( ) Use eye and other medications as prescribed on discharge and as labeled by hospital or local pharmacy.

MODE: ( ) Ambulatory ( ) Wheelchair ( ) Stretcher/Ambulance
Accompanied By: _____
( ) Home medications returned to patient/family.

I hereby acknowledge receipt of these instructions
I understand the instructions and will arrange for follow-up care.

_____   Signature of Physician   Date
Signature of Patient/or Responsible Party

   Signature of Resident/Fellow   Date

I HAVE REVIEWED THE ABOVE INSTRUCTIONS WITH THE PATIENT   Signature of Nurse   Date

WEH No. 37 Rev. 10/83

PATIENT'S COPY

Figure 15–9. Ophthalmic Discharge Instructions. (*Reprinted courtesy of Wills Eye Hospital.*)

really nice nursing touch. It can preempt anxiety relating to postsurgical symptoms, such as tearing, running nostril on the surgical side, and ascertaining any level of discomfort which is unrelieved by mild analgesics. The patient's general well-being can also be inquired after at this time. Vision may or may not be improved at this time, and should be asked about.

PRINTED BY THE STANDARD REGISTER COMPANY U.S.A. ZIPSET ®

))) Wills Eye Hospital

Phone Number: _____

Date & Time Called: _____

Procedure: _____

Date of Surgery: _____ Age: _____

Signature: _____

DISCHARGE INSTRUCTIONS

Surgical Procedure:

1. Do not drive or operate hazardous machinery for 24 hours.

2. Do not make important personal or business decisions for 24 hours.

3. Eat light foods as you can tolerate them. (water, jello, soups, cola, 7-up, etc.)

4. No alcoholic beverages should be taken for 24 hours.

5. Because you will have periods of sleepiness or feeling tired, it is not advisable to engage in strenuous activities. Rest when you are tired.

6. Tylenol may be taken every 4 hours for pain. Follow prescribed dosage on bottle.

7. Call your surgeon if you should become ill or develop a high fever. If a child, call pediatrician. If he can't be reached, Dr._____from the anesthesia department will be available tonight at phone #:_____.

PATIENT POST-OP FOLLOW-UP

Nausea	☐ severe	☐ moderate	☐ slight	☐ none
Pain	☐ severe	☐ moderate	☐ slight	☐ none
Fever	☐ severe	☐ moderate	☐ slight	☐ none
Sore Throat Hoarseness Cough	☐ severe	☐ moderate	☐ slight	☐ none

If so, is it getting better?_____

RED	DRAINAGE	USE OF EYE MEDS

Condition of eye: _____ _____ _____

Were there any muscle aches? ☐ severe   ☐ moderate   ☐ none

If so, where? _____

Was pain medication helpful? (if prescribed)_____

General Condition of Patient: ☐ excellent ☐ good   ☐ fair   ☐ poor

Patient General Comments:_____

_____

Unit Response:_____

_____

WEH 192 10/84

Figure 15–10. Discharge instructions for same-day surgery. (*Reprinted courtesy of Wills Eye Hospital.*)

PATIENT TEACHING

Patient teaching should include:

1. The correct instillation of eyedrops and compliance with the eye medication regimen.

2. Cleansing the eye should be done gently, and may be necessary first thing in the morning when the lids are stuck together.
3. The eye should be shielded for a month at night after the surgery. Glasses should be worn during the day to protect it. Sunglasses maybe suggested to patients who now find that bright lights bother them.
4. An understanding that there will be tearing after the procedure and that care should be taken not to rub the eye, but rather mop tears from the cheek.
5. Heavy lifting (articles over 15 to 20 lbs) should be avoided.
6. Discomfort can be relieved by taking mild analgesic medications such as acetaminophen.
7. Any increased discharge, pain, and/or a decrease in vision should be reported to the physician immediately.
8. Follow-up care is as important as the surgery itself.
9. Patients may shower, as long as they do not get the eye wet.
10. Men will want to know when they can shave. Usually this is permitted the day after surgery.
11. Hair may be washed as long as the head is bent backwards, away from the water.
12. The sexually active patient should abstain until after the first postoperative visit, and at this time discuss this activity with the ophthalmologist. Restrictions may be imposed when ocular complications are found to be present.

REFERENCES

1. Vaughan D, Asbury T: General Ophthalmology, 10th ed. Los Altos, Calif. Lange, 1983, pp. 120–128
2. Olson L: Anatomy and embryology of the lens, in Duane TD, (Ed.): Clinical Ophthalmology. Hagerstown, Md.: Harper & Row, 1983, pp. 1–8
3. Calhoun JH: Disorders of the lens, in Harley RD, (Ed.): Pediatric Ophthalmology, 2nd ed. Philadelphia: Saunders, 1983, pp. 549–567
4. Nelson BL, Maumenee IH: Ectopia lentis. Survey of Ophthalmology, 27(3): 143–160, 1984
5. Calhoun JH, Hiles DA: Cataracts and intraocular lens implantation, in Harley RD, (Ed.): Pediatric Ophthalmology, 2nd ed. Philadelphia: Saunders, 1983, pp. 549–567
6. Abrahamson IA: Cataract update. American Family Physician, 24(4): 111–119, 1981

BIBLIOGRAPHY

McKoy K: Cataracts and intraocular lenses, in Boyd-Monk H, (Ed.): Nursing Clinics of North America, 16(3): 405–14, 1981
Stark LA: Treating vision loss. Today's O.R. Nurse, 6(3): 9–13,44, 1984

16

The Vitreous

NEW TERMS

Siderosis: degenerative eye toxicity caused by an iron intraocular foreign body.
Syneresis: degenerative process of liquifaction of the vitreous.

The clear, avascular, gelatinous *vitreous* body comprises two-thirds of the volume and weight of the eye. This vitreous gel fills the space bounded by the lens, retina, and optic disc. Because of its inelasticity and imperviousness to cells and debris, it plays an important role in maintaining the transparency and form of the eye. If the vitreous were removed (without being replaced), the eye would collapse.[1]

The *hyaloid membrane,* the outer surface of the vitreous, is normally in contact with the posterior lens capsule, the zonular fibers, the pars plana epithelium, the retina, and the optic nerve head.

The *vitreous base* is firmly attached to the pars plana epithelium, and the retina immediately behind the ora serrata. The lens capsule and the optic nerve head attachment are firm in early life, but soon disappear. This is the principal reason that intracapsular cataract extraction without vitreous prolapse or ''loss'' is possible in adults and not in children.[1] Vitreoretinal adhesions can occur at retinal sites of lattice degeneration, meridional retinal folds, vitreoretinal scars, and new retinal blood vessels, such as those found in diabetes and central retinal vein occulsion.

The *hyaloid canal (Cloquet's canal),* which in the fetus contains the *hyaloid artery,* passes from the lens to the optic nerve head. The hyaloid artery usually disappears soon after birth, but the hyaloid canal remains throughout life. It is not visible ophthalmoscopically unless certain eye maneuvers are made.

The vitreous is approximately 99 percent water. The remaining 1 percent is made up of macromolecules which include solid proteins from the vitreous itself, hyaluronic acid, and proteins from the blood. The hyaluronic acid is arranged with vitreous collagen fibers in a network fashion which gives it its specific physical character. The vitreous gel then owes its form and consistency to a loose syncytium of long-chain collagen molecules capable of binding large numbers of water molecules, which help to increase its rigidity.[2]

CONGENITAL ANOMALIES

Persistent Hyaloid Artery and Persistant Hyperplastic Primary Vitreous

The hyaloid artery of the embryo—going from the optic nerve to form a vascular network around the lens—may not totally atrophy. When this occurs, it may produce severe and even total visual impairment. The cause for this lack of atrophy is unknown. It does not seem to be a genetic defect, and it is not passed on by heredity. It is probably due to an arrest in development.

Many variations of the remnant artery may occur. Varying amounts of glial tissue may be present and/or the artery may be patent with blood flowing through it. In some cases, just the posterior end of the artery may persist and may be attached to the optic disc. Other cases may just present the anterior end of the artery, and this may be extensive or a mere dot attached to the posterior surface of the lens (called a Mittendorf dot).

When the *persistent hyaloid artery* is associated with other defects it is considered to be *persistent hyperplastic primary vitreous.* In a recent study from the Massachusetts Eye and Ear Infirmary in Boston,[3] the average age of diagnosis was found to be 6 years. Five-sixths of the patients with this condition had only one eye involved. Most of the children had a visual acuity of 20/200 or less, and strabismus was present in two out of three of the patients studied. Other congenital anomalies associated with the persistent hyperplastic primary vitreous were microophthalmus, microcornea, "juvenile" angle, congenital lens opacity, and vitreous membrane. Complications that may occur include retinal detachment, vitreous hemorrhage, and open angle glaucoma.[4] Reports are beginning to appear on treatment of these cases using microsurgical vitreous techniques. Even if the surgery is successful, the other ocular anomalies, and the development of amblyopia may prevent useful visual acuity.

NURSING INTERVENTION

Nursing intervention includes administering dilating drops to facilitate fundus examination which may have to be performed under anesthesia (EUA) if the patient is a small child. Vitrectomy care will be discussed in detail in the following entry.

ACQUIRED ANOMALIES

Vitreous Hemorrhage

There are several causes of vitreous hemorrhage. It may be spontaneous, usually occurring from the retinal vessels, or it may occur secondary to trauma. In the spontaneous type of hemorrhage, the retinal vessels may rupture, spilling the blood into the vitreous. Sometimes these hemorrhages can be seen beneath the internal limiting membrane of the retina, only to rupture into the vitreous at a later date. If the retina should tear due to vitreoretinal traction, a retinal vessel may be severed and bleed into the vitreous. Retinal tears and detachments should be suspected in all spontaneous vitreal hemorrhages. If a large vessel should rupture, then a severe hemorrhage may obscure vision, and cause irreparable damage to the internal ocular structures.

The seriousness of those hemorrhages into the vitreous occurring after trauma depends upon the force exerted to the eye, as well as other damage to the retina and globe. With minimal bleeding, absorption may be fairly rapid. A solid blood clot in the vitreous has a poorer prognosis than hemorrhage in a liquified vitreous. If membranes form around the clot, this reduces the chances of rapid and complete absorption. *Fibrosis and siderosis* are complications that may occur with vitreous hemorrhage. When clots become organized, fibroblasts can grow into the clot and when these contract the retina is detached. Siderosis occurs with the breaking down of hemosiderin in the hemorrhage. The iron ions are toxic to the capillary bed of the retinal circulation and cause atrophy and gliosis of the retina. Other conditions beside the spontaneous or traumatic tearing of the retinal vessels that can be responsible for vitreous hemorrhages are the retinal neovascularization of proliferative diabetic retinopathy, hypertensive retinopathy, retinal vasculitis, occlusion of retinal veins, neoplastic erosion of retinal vessels, and occlusion of the vessels such as that which occurs in leukemia, polycythemia, sickle-cell disease, and anemia.

Diagnosis of vitreous hemorrhage is made by visual examination of the vitreous using a direct or indirect ophthalmoscope, the Hruby lens with a Slitlamp, or ultrasound A and B scans. This latter method provides an excellent way of following the absorption of a hemorrhage and/or the formation of membranes. If there is absorption and no membrane formation, then watchful waiting is considered for 6 months to 1 year. If patients have dense hemorrhage and/or membrane formation, then vitrectomy is performed through a pars plana approach.[5]

NURSING INTERVENTION

Assess the patient with the symptom of sudden loss of vision for a history of trauma, systemic disease (diabetes, hypertension, blood dyscrasia etc.), or ocular disease (amourosis fugax—previous transient ischemic attacks, diabetic retinopathy, glaucoma). Sudden loss of vision should be considered an ocular emergency, for it might be caused by a retinal artery occlusion which with early treatment may show visual improvement.

PATIENT TEACHING

When the diagnosis is established that a vitreous hemorrhage is present, it is appropriate to reinforce the physician's instructions to the patient to observe a sedentary period, with the head elevated, in the hope that the hemorrhage will settle by gravity. Emotional support should be given, and reassurance that vitreous hemorrhages have been known to resolve with time should also be offered. Some patients are placed on a daily aspirin (salicilic acid) regimen. Encourage patient compliance.

Vitreous Opacities

Vitreous opacities may be the congenital remnants of the embryonic vascular system, or the structural elements and fibrils of the vitreous. These are nonpathological entities known as *muscae volitantes*, and are described by the patient as "specks seen floating before the eyes." The pathological vitreous opacities may be divided into *degenerative, hematogenous, neoplastic, and inflammatory* causes.

Degenerative opacities include the golden yellow crystals of *synchesis scintalans*, cholesterol crystals, which can be observed in patients who just present with it, as well as those patients who have had surgical trauma; and the white snowballs of *asteroid hyalitis*. With aging, the vitreous becomes liquified due to biochemical degeneration. This liquification is referred to as syneresis. When the vitreous shrinks with aging, it pulls on its posterior attachment at the optic nerve, and when it tears free, a ring of condensed tissue is drawn forward into the vitreous and appears as a fly or a ring in the vision. Occasionally, this *posterior vitreous detachment* is associated with flashes of light as the unstable vitreous rubs the retina. It may also be associated with vitreous hemorrhage, retinal breaks, and vitreoretinal detachment. Blood in the vitreous has been previously discussed. Tumor cells may break into the vitreous from tumors of the retina, choroid, ciliary body, iris, or the hematogenous system. The inflammatory group includes chorioretinitis, optic neuritis, and iritis. Inflammatory cells from the area of involvement usually enter the vitreous and produce vitreous opacities and a hazy view of the fundus.

NURSING INTERVENTION

Nursing intervention will include assessing the visual acuity and identifying if there is just an occasional floater or if there are showers of spots associated with light flashes. Patients who have degenerative changes in their vitreous become very distressed at the decrease in the vision which often affects their reading ability. Support can be offered, but there is little reassurance that can be given that the situation will change. The underlying cause for vitreous inflammations will need to be identified by the physician, and the nurse will then teach the patient to administer the prescribed dilating drops to the affected eye, and systemic steroids and/or antibiotics. It is important to encourage compliance with the medication regimen and follow-up care.

Trauma

Intraocular foreign bodies (IOFB) (Fig. 16–1) are usually caused by trauma. Occasionally, they are seen following surgery. Steel on steel (hammer on nail) is a common cause. These IOFBs must be localized, and the amount of trauma done to the eye by their arrival must be evaluated. The best way for these to be diagnosed in the vitreous, while the media is still clear, is by direct vision using the direct or indirect ophthalmoscope, Hruby lens and Slitlamp. Ultrasound A and B scans, x-ray—localization with Comberg contact lens or the Sweet technique, and/or CAT scan are other methods frequently used to identify just where the IOFB is to be found. Removal depends upon the nature and location of the foreign body and any associated blood and fibrosis.

If the IOFB is magnetic metal, then removal is attempted with a magnet. If it is

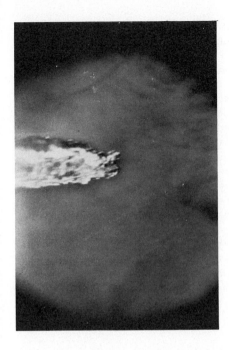

Figure 16–1. Intraocular foreign body in vitreous.

nonmagnetic, then vitrectomy may be attempted. In some cases it may be left in place if it is nonmetalic, nontoxic, without blood clot or fibrosis, and is a noninfectious material such as glass. The site of entrance must be repaired and if the lens has been damaged and a cataract has formed, this should also be removed.

NURSING INTERVENTION
Often the nurse is the first person to be told by the patient that "something flew in my eye." The most important assessment question then, is "What were you doing?" Patients make the same statement when the wind has blown a foreign body on to the cornea. The symptoms of pain, photophobia, and decreased vision may be elicited, and conjunctival redness noted. Treated as an ocular emergency, the patient with an IOFB history will need to have a fundoscopic examination through a well-dilated pupil as soon as possible. Care must be taken not to place any pressure on the eye, for there may be a small rupture in the globe where the IOFB entered. The patient should be warned not to eat or drink anything until the operating room time is established for IOFB removal. Diagnostic studies will have to be completed prior to surgery. A patch and shield is applied to the eye to prevent further injury prior to surgery. Systemic intravenous antibiotics will be initiated as a prophylactic measure to prevent infection.

Endophthalmitis
Endophthalmitis is an infection and/or inflammation inside the eye. If all three coats of the eye as well as the vitreous are involved by an inflammatory process, the

condition is known as *panophthalmitis*.[1] Bacterial or fungal infections can be introduced into the eye by perforating or penetrating injury, or they can be brought via the bloodstream to such ocular structures as retina or choroid. Occasionally, this can be seen in those individuals who inject street drugs using dirty needles. A severe inflammatory reaction to toxic substances or necrotic tumors can give the same intraocular picture of hazy vitreous, hypopion, and a red, angry, painful eye (Fig. 16–2). Unless the etiology of the infection and/or inflammation can be determined and appropriate therapy instituted, the results can be disastrous. For example, a pseudomonas corneal ulcer can produce a severe, rapid endophthalmitis, with destruction of the globe in a matter of several hours. Fungal and viral agents may take longer, but the final result may be as severe.

Corneal scrapings, anterior chamber tap, and vitreous tap are used as a means of identifying the invading organisms. Smears may give a preliminary bacterial diagnosis, but cultures and sensitivity results will take at least 24 to 48 hours. The patient is initially treated with intensive systemic antibiotic therapy. At least two antibiotics are given to ensure covering all organisms. Topical and subconjunctival eye medications are also given in an attempt to "save the eye." Recently, vitrectomy with antibiotic used to replace vitreous, has been helpful in saving globes which would otherwise have been lost. Visual results depend upon the severity of the endophthalmitis.

NURSING INTERVENTION

Patients with endophthalmitis may first seek attention for a throbbing, painful eye. Visual acuity testing will reveal poor vision in the affected eye; the patient may only have light perception. Purulent discharge which crusts on the lid margins and mats the eyelashes together may be observed. Nurses responsible for administration of intravenous medications will find a heparin lock works well for this type of situation. Eyedrops prescribed will include a cycloplegic to decrease the associated iridocyclitis and two different antibiotic eyedrops to be given hourly or

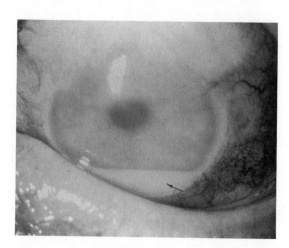

Figure 16–2. Endophthalmitis, showing hypopion, hazy media, and conjunctival injection.

every 2 hours. The times should be alternated for best results. This places a great burden on the nurse whose time must be used to give an eyedrop every 30 minutes. If there is a purulent discharge, the eye will need frequent cleansing before eyedrops are instilled. Patients can become very irritable because they are deprived of complete rest when the drops are given around the clock. They also tend to be anxious, frightened, and depressed because of the unknown outcome of their ocular disease, so great patience, understanding, and gentleness is necessary to support these patients through this difficult time.

An *endophthalmitis* patient admitted as an inpatient is considered infectious, and should be cared for using "Isolation" or "Protective Care" precautions. Handwashing before entering, and upon leaving the area, ensures that the patient incurs no secondary infection.

PATIENT TEACHING
Patient teaching includes the nature of the intensity of the treatment. A request should be made that separate tissues be used (to prevent cross-contamination of the uninfected eye) if there is a need to wipe drainage from the cheek. Explain the reason for confinement to an "Isolation Room" (to prevent cross-contamination of the hospital population) and reinforce the necessity for the intravenous medication route of administration. Constant emotional support will be necessary.

Vitrectomy
Modern vitrectomy started early in the 1970s and was pioneered by Robert Machemer, who used fine mechanical cutters combined with suction and infusion systems. The instrumentation became smaller and more sophisticated, with light and lasers being delivered into the eye by fiberoptic probes. Today, removal of dense, nonclearing, vitreous hemorrhage is done routinely. Five year follow-up from the first series of patients showed 77 out of 164 had 6/60 or better visual acuity at the 6-month examination, and 64 continued to have good or better vision than they had prior to the surgery at the 6-month examination. There were no increases in iris rubrosa (new blood vessels on the iris) among those treated. The maculae of 94 percent that were attached, remained attached. Later figures should be better.[7]

Closed vitrectomy (see Chap. 8) is achieved by placing three instruments (an infusion, a light, and a cutting/suction tip) into the eye through the pars plana region, while maintaining a closed system. At the same time as the vitreous is being removed, it is replaced at the same rate by an infusion of a basic salt solution. As the hazy media is cleared, and if a retinal detachment is found, then a scleral buckling procedure will also be performed to repair it. At the end of the procedure, gas SF^6 (sulfhexafluride) or air may be introduced into the eye to keep the retina in place as it expands. Silicon oil is used in some cases. Upon completion of the procedure, a pressure patch is placed on the eye. Even after the vitrectomy surgery has been done successfully, and some vision restored, there is still the possibility that another blood vessel might bleed at a later date. Postoperative complication can also include corneal erosion and cataract if a lensectomy is not performed.

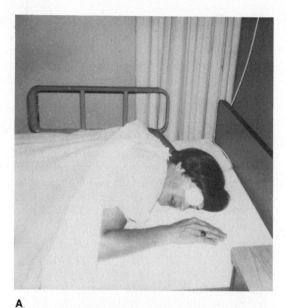

Figure 16–3. Vitrectomy postoperative positions. **A.** Face down. **B.** Head down—resting on bedside table.

NURSING INTERVENTION

Initial assessment of patients who are to undergo vitrectomy includes identifying if the reason for the surgery is due to a systemic disease such as diabetes mellitus. The associated systemic disease will need careful monitoring during the time the patient is hospitalized.

Before surgery, the eyes will receive cycloplegic drops which the physician has ordered. The patient's own medication regimen will be maintained.

After the surgery is complete, positioning the patient on the abdomen (Fig. 16–3A), in order *to allow the gas or air to float against the retina,* will often be ordered by the physician. Maintaining patients in this position becomes quite a nursing challenge, for patients find it a rather uncomfortable position to be in constantly. As an alternative the patient is permitted to sit up and lean forward (Fig. 16–3B), placing the head on the bedside stand. This at least relieves the pressure on the back. The "face down" position is maintained until the gas has been absorbed, which takes about 4 to 5 days. With early discharge this positioning may have to be continued at home.

Cycloplegic and steroid–antibiotic combination drops will be instilled in the eye four times daily postoperatively, and for up to a month after surgery. Ice compresses will help to decrease lid swelling. A light patch may be placed on the eye after treatment. However, if the patient has the use of only one eye, then the patch might be removed and glasses should be worn for protection.

When silicon oil is used as a vitreous replacement agent, no special positioning is usually ordered, but the nurse should still request the patient to lie only on the back or the unoperative side when in bed.

Postoperative pain and nausea should be medicated as soon as they are complained about. The patient will express mixed emotions, and will show signs of anxious hope that there will be improvement in the vision. Since it is often months before this is truly evident, it is difficult for either physcian or nurse to predict the visual outcome of the surgery in this immediate postsurgical period. However, there are people who can see 20/20 with correction after this surgery, and this can be offered as reassurance to the patient.

REFERENCES

1. Vaughan D, Asbury T: General Ophthalmology, 10th ed. Los Altos, Calif.: Lange, 1983, pp. 129–136
2. Tasman W: The vitreous, in Duane TD, (Ed.): Clinical Ophthalmology. Hagerstown, Md.: Harper & Row, 1983, pp. 1–21
3. Pruett RC: The pleomorphism and complications of posterior hypoplastic primary vitreous. American Journal of Ophthalmology, 80(10): 625, 1975
4. Laatikainen L, Tarkkanen A: Microsurgery of persistent hypoplastic primary vitreous. Ophthalmologica, 185: 193–198, 1982
5. Coleman DJ, Franzen LA: Vitreous surgery. Archives of Ophthalmology, 92(11): 375–381, 1974
6. Blankenship GW: Stability of pars plana vitrectomy: Results for diabetic retinopathy complications. Archives of Ophthalmology, 99(6): 1009–1012, 1981
7. Benson EW: Vitrectomy, in Duane TD, (Ed.): Clinical Ophthalmology. Hagerstown, Md.: Harper & Row, 1982, pp. 1–23

17

The Retina

NEW TERMS

Drusen: concretions produced by the pigment epithelium of the retina.
Operculum: flap or free floating piece of retina.
Optic disc: optic nerve head (papilla).
RPE: retinal pigment epithelium.

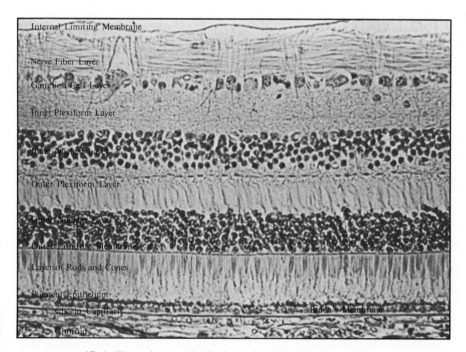

Internal Limiting Membrane

Nerve Fiber Layer

Ganglion Cell Layer

Inner Plexiform Layer

Inner Nuclear Layer

Outer Plexiform Layer

Outer Nuclear Layer

Outer Limiting Membrane

Layer of Rods and Cones

Pigment Epithelium

Chorio Capillaris

Bruch's Membrane

Choroid

17–1. The retina—a histologic section showing the ten layers.

The *retina,* the innermost coat of the eye, is derived from two embryonic layers, the outer pigment epithelium, and the inner multilayered sheet of neural tissue which varies in thickness from 0.2 to 0.4 mm. Three types of tissue are identified. The first is the *neuronal component,* consisting of photoreceptor cells. These convert light signals into nerve impulses, then transmit the impulses via the nerve fiber layer, optic nerve, and the optic tract to the visual cortex in the brain. The second type of tissue is the *glial component* which synthesizes and stores glycogen and thus provides glucose for the nutritional support of the sensory retina. The third component is *vascular.* The retina receives its blood supply from two sources, the choriocapillaris—the microvascular network of the choroid which nourishes the *retinal pigment epithelium* (RPE) and the outer one-third of the retina; the inner two-thirds of the sensory retina receives its blood supply from branches of the central retinal artery.

The ten layers of the retina (Fig. 17–1) are identified as the RPE, *retinal pigment epithelium* a single layer of cells attached to Bruch's membrane, which extends from the optic disc to the ora serrata. Photoreceptors, the *rod and cone layer,* are highly-specialized cells which absorb light within a mass of densely packed molecules containing visual pigment. The *external limiting membrane* separates the photoreceptor layer from the *outer nuclear layer.* This layer is composed of the photoreceptor cell bodies with their nuclei and cytoplasm. The axons of these cells synapse with the horizontal and bipolar cells in the *outer plexiform layer,* a junctional zone between the photoreceptors (rods and cones) and the first order neuron (bipolar cell). The *inner nuclear layer* consists roughly of four layers of cell bodies. From within outward, these are the nuclei of the amacrine, Müller, bipolar, and horizontal cells. The bipolar cells transmit the nerve impulse from the photoreceptors to the ganglion cells. The *inner plexiform layer* is the zone in which synapse between the first order neuron (bipolar cell) and second order neuron (ganglion cell) occurs. The *ganglion cell layer* contains the cell bodies of the second order neurons, the ganglion cells. Signals generated in the photoreceptors are transmitted through the bipolar cells to the ganglion cells whose axons form the *nerve fiber layer,* optic nerve and tract, and ultimately synapse in the lateral geniculate body (in the brain). The *internal limiting membrane* (ILM), for the most part, is derived from the Müller cells.[1]

The thinner *macula,* with a 1.5-mm diameter, is a clinical landmark and is identified as a capillary-free zone located on the temporal side, slightly below the center of the other major landmark, the *optic nerve head (optic disc).* In the macula's center is the *fovea.* The tiny, central foveal reflex identifies the *foveola.* Consisting exclusively of cone photoreceptors, the fovea is responsible for color and sharp discriminating vision.

The peripheral retina is composed mainly of rods. It ends at the ora serrata with the ILM becoming thinner as it interweaves with collagenous filaments of the vitreous base. The external limiting membrane meanwhile continues forward between the pigmented and nonpigmented epithelia into the ciliary body. The RPE is continuous with the pigment epithelium of the ciliary body.[1] Peripheral retina has better capability to recognize light intensity and also rapid movement.

The function of the retina is to transform information present in light to a form acceptable to the brain. Processing of retinal information proceeds from photoreceptor layer through the retinal microcircuitry to the optic nerve.

When a photon strikes a photoreceptor it initiates a biochemical change in the visual pigment molecule. Molecules of *rhodopsin* (visual purple) are composed of a protein known as opsin and a chromophore group known as 11-*cis*-retinal, a form of vitamin A. A single photon of light energy causes the isomerization of the 11-*cis* form of retinal to the all-*trans* form. The rhodopsin alterations that take place are known collectively as "bleaching." For this all-*trans* form to again become light sensitive it must be reisomerized to the 11-*cis* form. After a relatively total bleach, it takes approximately 5 minutes for one-half of the rhodopsin to be regenerated (in the rod) but only approximately 1 minute to reisomerize one-half of the cone pigments. Illumination of the rods temporarily decreases their sensitivity in a process known as *light adaptation*. Conversely, the subsequent return of the rod to its maximum sensitivity is known as *dark adaptation*.[2]

FUNDUS EXAMINATION

Direct Ophthalmoscope

The *direct ophthalmoscope* makes use of a strong light reflected into the interior of the eye by a small mirror located within the instrument. The light from the interior of the patient's eye is reflected back to the examiner's eye through a hole in the mirror. The direct ophthalmoscope permits monocular examination of the illuminated interior of an eye directly and closely. The images seen using this method are magnified about 15 times their normal size. This magnification is accomplished by the refractive components of the patient's eye—the cornea and the lens—and together with vitreous, must be clear if fundus ophthalmoscopy is to be achieved.

1. The head of the direct ophthalmoscope has a graduated series of lenses mounted on a wheel, which enables the examiner to bring objects at different distances into sharp focus. The 0 on the disc is a plano lens and is used when both examiner and patient have no refractive error.
2. The graduated lenses, numbered from 1 to 20, are either black or red on a white background. (Sometimes the numbers will be white on a black background.) The black numbers designate *convex,* plus (+) lenses. Convex lenses converge light rays. The higher the number of the convex lens, the more the rays are converged, thus the closer the focal point. This type of lens is used for the *farsighted, or hyperopic,* patient.
3. The red numbers are designated to *concave,* minus (−) lenses. Concave lenses diverge light rays. The higher the number of the concave lens the more the rays are diverged, thus the focal point is brought into focus at a greater distance. Concave lenses are used for *nearsighted, or myopic,* patients.
4. The second rotating wheel on the head of the ophthalmoscope has an assortment of openings through which the light can be projected. There is a small and a large aperture to vary the size of the beam, a grid, for use to measure the size of a lesion, a slit beam, and a green disc for filtering out the color red.
5. To facilitate pupillary dilatation, direct ophthalmoscopy is best performed in a dimly-illuminated room. The best fundus view will be obtained when the pupils have been dilated with mydriatic and/or cycloplegic drugs, however, a physician must prescribe these eye medications since they have the potential to produce glaucoma in a patient with anatomically narrow angles.
6. Seat the patient so that both examiner and patient are at the same eye level.

The patient is now asked to fix his or her gaze on a point on the wall straight ahead. The ophthalmoscope is turned on—the small white light is best used for the pupil not dilated by mydriatics. The dial is set at 0, and with the index finger positioned on the disc for easy lens changes, the examiner begins the examination.

7. To examine the patient's right eye, the examiner holds the ophthalmoscope in the right hand and must use his or her right eye to avoid rubbing noses (Fig. 17–2). The left eye is examined in the same way.

8. The examiner places his or her eye directly behind the viewing aperture, and from a distance of about 12 inches moves in toward the patient's eye, until the red reflex is observed, and until both foreheads almost touch.

9. Fundus landmarks are looked for as the lens wheel is rotated to bring them into focus. A blood vessel might be identified first, and should be followed to the *optic disc,* located slightly nasally. *Note the disc margins.* In the center, the physiological cup, a yellowish-white depression, is about one-third of the size of the optic disc. *Note the cup–disc ratio.* The "disc diameter" size is used to measure distances of lesions from the disc.

10. The vascular elements—the *central retinal artery* and the *central retinal vein*—will be observed in the center of the optic disc. Each vessel divides into four main branches—the superior and inferior, nasal and temporal vessels (Fig. 17–3). Retinal veins appear darker than the arteries. *Note their caliber at the crossings, and any variations which might be evident.* Each vessel should be followed to the periphery.

11. To inspect the general background of the fundus the patient is asked to look up, down, and to each side. Darkly pigmented individuals will have a dark-colored fundus, while lightly pigmented or blond individuals will have a lighter fundus.

12. The macula region is about two disc diameters temporal to, and slightly below, the optic disc. It is examined last, and will be seen as a deeper red than the surrounding retina. The blood vessels seem to stop at the periphery of this spot which suggests that the area is avascular. The darker point

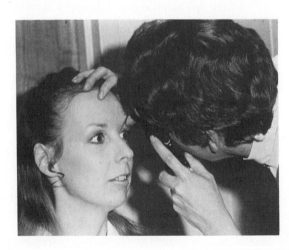

Figure 17–2. The direct ophthalmoscope.

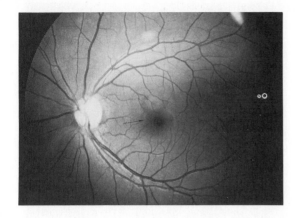

Figure 17–3. The fundus.

in the middle is the fovea. One way to examine the macula is to ask the patient to look directly at the ophthalmoscope light. Sometimes the patient being examined complains that the light hurts his or her eyes. These patients may also claim that they see a dark spot (scotoma) in the center of their field of vision—this will gradually change color, and shortly, this "after image" will disappear.

Findings should be documented noting which eye was observed. The landmarks are described in terms of the face of a clock, and the distance expressed in disc diameters.[3]

Indirect Ophthalmoscope
The *indirect ophthalmoscope* offers the physician an opportunity not only for stereoscopic observation, but also for binocular vision with a slight difference in the angle of observation between the images of the two eyes. It requires great skill and much time to be used correctly. Interpretation of the images is also necessary as they are inverted when visualized (Fig. 17–4). Pupillary dilatation with cycloplegic is necessary prior to examination because of the intensity of the head light. Two other components necessary for examination are a magnifying lens and a scleral depressor used for indentation to facilitate viewing the peripheral retina at the ora serrata.

Fundus Photography
Photography of the fundus has come to play an integral part in identifying and documenting changes which take place in the retina, choroid, and optic disc. These changes can be due to local or systemic disease, and the satisfactory and unsatisfactory effects of medical intervention. Photography plays a definitive part in assessing the retinal vasculature through the test known as *Intravenous Fluorescein Angiography* (IVFA). Prior to the procedure, the patient's pupils must be widely dilated. For this photography a "fundus camera" (Fig. 17–5A) is mounted on a stand similar to that used for Slitlamp biomicroscopy. The patient is seated in front of the camera, chin in chinrest, and forehead against a bar, as if being examined at the Slitlamp. The photographer focuses a lens so that the posterior portion of the eye comes

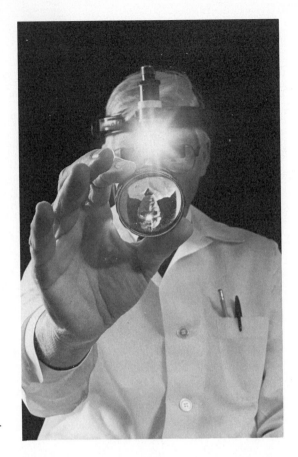

Figure 17-4. The indirect ophthalmoscope.

clearly into view, and takes a picture. The photographs may be colored polaroids, 35-mm slides, or black and white slides for contact prints.

When the retinal vasculature is to be studied, flurescein dye is injected intra-venously through a peripheral vein; serial photographs are then taken at 2-second intervals, using a blue cobalt filter. The patient sits back, and 10 to 20 minutes later the final photograph is taken. In this manner the arteries, veins, arteriolar-venous capillaries, and any new vessels are studied. Fluorescein dye, as it passes through the blood vessels, fluoresces and "lights up" the lumen (Fig. 17-5B). If the blood vessels leak, then a hyperfluorescent patch will appear on the photograph. Where there are no viable blood vessels, there will be patches of hypofluorescence.

NURSING INTERVENTION

The nurse, administering the intravenous fluorescein dye under a pro-tocol, assesses the patient's general health status, including diabetes, heart disease, or hypertension, and identifies any allergies. He or she will ask the patient if he or she has had any similar dye test previously, and were there any side effects from it, such as itching, hives, or nausea. Since anaphalactic shock is a remote possibility whenever a foreign pro-

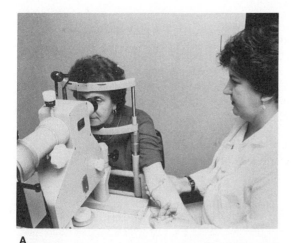

A

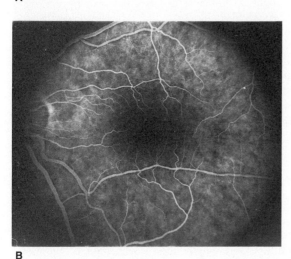

B

Figure 17–5. **A.** Patient seated at a fundus camera receiving intravenous fluorescein dye. **B.** Normal Intravenous Fluorescein Angiography (IVFA).

tein is injected into the body, the blood pressure will be measured as a baseline. (Emergency equipment should be immediately available in the event that this situation is precipitated.) Assessment of the past ocular history will include open and closed angle glaucoma, medications being used, and whether there is an intraocular lens or contact in place. A consent form should be signed and witnessed before this procedure is initiated. The eyes will be checked for adequate dilatation, and one or two "sets" of dilating drops (phenylephrine hydrochloride 2.5 percent and tropicamide 1 percent gtts. i of each) will be instilled. When the pupils are well dilated the patient will be seated at the camera, and the nurse will rapidly inject (at about 1 cc per second) 3 cc of IV sodium fluorescein 25 percent or 5 cc of sodium fluorescein 10 percent dye (amount depends upon the concentration) through a peripheral vein, and the photographer will begin taking the photograph series.

PATIENT TEACHING

Patients are told to listen for a clicking sound as each photograph is taken; this will be accompanied by the flash from the camera. As the dye is injected some patients feel a warm sensation. About 10 percent feel transitory nausea, and a small percentage of those vomit. During the next 24 hours patients will notice that their urine will be a fluorescent yellow or orange. Patients are encouraged to increase fluid intake to hasten the dye's excretion from the system. Light-complected patients should be told that their skin may be tinted yellow for the next 4 to 6 hours, but as the dye is excreted it will return to its normal color. Dark glasses may be necessary, for the pupillary dilation will make the patient sensitive to sunlight.

Electroretinography

The technique of electroretinography (ERG) essentially is a means of measuring the electrical response of the retina to a flash of light. The test which is performed most successfully in the dark takes about 20 minutes, and is conducted by placing a contact lens electrode over the cornea and conjunctiva (after it has been anesthetized with a topical anesthetic eyedrop). The ERGs component parts include a recorder with pickup, amplifier, and readout equipment.

ERG is a mass response of the retina. The test is used to differentiate between the cone-mediated (photopic) portion of the response which functions only in daylight or artificial light, from the much larger rod-mediated (scotopic) portion of the system which functions best at night-time or in moon-light.

Two electrical waves originating in the outer retinal layers can be identified; these are called *a* and *b* waves. Photoreceptors produce the *a* wave: Müller cells produce the *b* wave. Ganglion cells do not contribute to the ERG, an important point used in differentiating eye diseases. Only the *b* wave is affected by anoxia—it diminishes or disappears within minutes after onset of the lack of oxygen. This reflects the retina's similarity to the brain and, like the brain, the retina suffers irreversible damage if the anoxia is not promptly corrected. Retinal ischemia can result from many different disease processes e.g., arteriosclerosis, giant cell arteritis, occlusion of a retinal artery or vein, and carotid artery insufficiency. All result in diminished *b* wave and a proportionately large *a* wave due to "unmasking" of the process responsible for the *a* wave.

The electroretinograph's clinical application is its usefulness in the study of hereditary and constitutional retinal disorders. These include partial and total color blindness (achromatopsia), night blindness, and retinal degenerations. The ERG will show corresponding abnormalities when the disorders involve either the rod system or the cone system exclusively. For example the ERG is "extinguished" in patients with retinitis pigmentosa. It may be nonrecordable in chorioretinal degenerations or inflammations which may result in complete destruction of the photoreceptors. While in other retinal degenerative states such as Tay-Sachs' disease (in which the lesion is located in the ganglion cells) the ERG may be normal.

Electroretinography changes also occur in:

1. Toxic states of the retina such as siderosis and those known to result from the administration of many drugs which may produce retinal damage, such as chloroquin and quinine.

2. Retinal detachment—the ERG may completely recover following surgical reattachment of the retina.
3. Systemic diseases such as vitamin A deficiency—the ERG may be restored to normal after treatment; mucopolysaccharidosis, e.g., Hurler's disease; hypothyroidism—the altered retinal metabolism reflects that of the whole body; the anemias—the lower ERG response is usually, but not always, proportionate to the Hbg level.[4]

Ultrasonography

Ultrasound plays an essential part in ophthalmologic diagnosis because of its ability to detect, outline, and characterize soft tissue of the eye and orbit, regardless of intervening opacities of cornea, lens, or vitreous. Ultrasonography of soft tissue is analogous to radiographic diagnosis of bone. As the high frequency soundwaves pass through soft tissue, acoustic differences between two tissues and the differential reflection of these waves by tissues in the path of the beam is recorded. In this manner, ultrasound can document changes such as neoplasm, intraocular foreign bodies, retinal detachment, and vitreous hemorrhage undetectable or measurable by other methods.

Graphic recording of these reflections can give a two-dimensional cross section of the eye (B-scan), or can take the form of a one-dimensional tracing (A-scan) resembling an electrocardiogram. Ultrasonography gives specific comparisons of tissue reflectance as well as accurate measurements of tissue dimensions.

Three ultrasound modes are used in ophthalmology:

- The *A-mode* (A-scan) provides the most accurate way of relating the echo amplitude of different tissues and thus allows deductions of tissue components to be assessed. It is also used in determining *axial length measurements by measuring the time intervals between echoes along optic axis of the eye* (Fig. 17–6A).
- The *B-mode* (B-scan) presents a two-dimensional outline or cross-section of the globe and is the technique most commonly used for graphic display (Fig. 17–6B). The amplitude of the echoes is brightness modulated as dots on the oscilloscope face.
- The *M-mode* provides a two-dimensional means of studying the motion of tissues, as the display moves up and across the oscilloscope in real time.[5]

CONGENITAL ANOMALIES

Retinoblastoma

Retinoblastoma is the most common primary intraocular malignancy of childhood, occurring in about one out of 17,000 live births. This tumor has a tendency to spread locally, can undergo distant metastasis, and if not treated promptly is invariably fatal. The mortality rate in the United States is less than 10 percent. Most children with retinoblastoma have no history of an obvious ocular abnormality at birth. They usually develop strabismus and/or leukocoria between 6 months and 2 years of age.[6]

The fact that children with retinoblastoma now survive into adulthood, and are

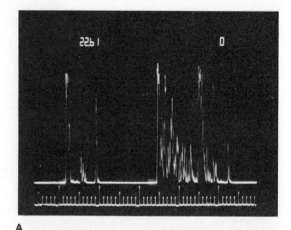

A

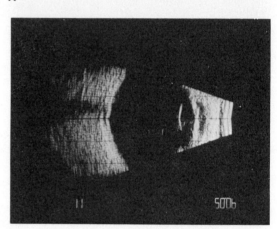

Figure 17–6. A. A-scan. **B.** B-scan.

B

reproducing, appears to support the fact that there is an increased number of the abnormal genes in the gene pool. Retinoblastoma also occurs in a nonfamilial form as a spontaneous mutation. In about 5 percent of retinoblastoma patients with an associated mental retardation, a deletion of the long arm of chromosome 13 has been identified. One-third of the retinoblastoma cases are bilateral; these tumors are due to independent origins in both retinae, and not to extension from one eye to another.[6] The tumor can be inherited as an autosomal dominant characteristic trait, with an extremely high penetrance.

The tumors arise from the photoreceptor elements in the outer layers of the retina. The abnormal cells have a similarity to primitive retinal elements which should become rods and cones.[6] Histologically, they are characterized by abnormal cells arranged radially around a central cavity to form spherical clusters called Flexner-Wintersteiner rosette formation.

Retinoblastomas are divided into two groups. The *endophytic* type which can be seen with an ophthalmoscope, extend into the vitreous cavity. As this type enlarges within the eye, peripheral portions can break away from the parent mass to float freely in the vitreous, and produce "seedings." The *exophytic* type grows into the subretinal space causing the retina to detach. On rare occasions spontaneous regression has been known to occur.

A detailed history is taken from the parents, prior to the patient having a complete blood count, skull x-rays, long bone x-rays, spinal fluid examination, and bone marrow evaluation in an effort to detect extraocular tumor spread. CT scan may also be performed to rule out the presence of brain tumor, since it is now recognized that some patients with bilateral retinoblastoma have a tendency to develop a concurrent brain tumor, particularly a pinealoblastoma.[6]

The external examination may show a white pupillary "cat's eye" reflex (Fig. 17–7), strabismus, or heterochromia. Slitlamp biomicroscopy and binocular indirect ophthalmoscopy is deferred until the child can be examined under anesthesia. Fundus photographs and drawings document the tumor. Fluorescein angiography is not widely used in young children, but is useful in providing clinical information regarding the tumor's blood supply and viability. A-scan and B-scan ultrasonography is a valuable adjunct in the differential diagnosis of children with leukocoria. (The transducer of some systems can be placed on the child's eyelids without anesthesia.) CT scan, though less practical and more expensive than ultrasonography, facilitates detection of optic nerve enlargement due to posterior extension of the tumor, or a possible brain tumor.

Management of a patient with retinoblastoma is complex, each case being individualized according to the extent of involvement. The traditionally accepted methods include enucleation, external beam irradiation, episcleral plaque irradiation, photocoagulation, cryotherapy, and chemotherapy when metastases are suspected.

Enucleation is probably indicated for all unilateral cases in which the tumor fills most of the globe and in which there is little hope of salvaging any viable retina or useful vision. In bilateral cases, the eye with the more advanced tumor is usually enucleated and the less involved eye is managed with irradiation or other methods. If both eyes have far advanced tumors and there is no hope of any vision, bilateral enucleation may be necessary. At surgery an attempt is made to obtain as long a

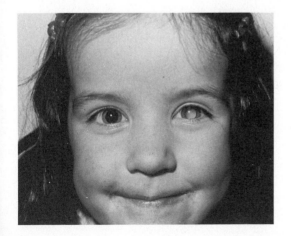

Figure 17–7. "Cat's eye" reflex seen in a child with retinoblastoma.

section of the optic nerve as possible. A pressure patch is applied for 24 to 48 hours to minimize postoperative ecchymosis of the eyelids. Ice compresses will also decrease the swelling. Long-term complications such as a sunken orbit may be managed by adjustments of the prosthesis by the ocularist or by orbital reconstructive plastic surgery.

External beam irradiation may be indicated for treatment of the second eye after the eye with the more advanced tumor has been enucleated, or following enucleation when the tumor is found histologically to extend into the optic nerve to the line or surgical transection. It may also be used when there is orbital recurrence of the tumor. The therapeutic dose is about 3500 to 4000 rads, delivered in divided doses over a 3-week period. Complications that affect some patients include a dry eye, a sunken orbit with atrophy of the temporal fossa, and optic atrophy. External irradiation may also be responsible for the development of such radiation-induced tumors as orbital sarcomas.

Cobalt [60] *plaque irradiation* is an alternate treatment modality (see Chap. 14) and appears to offer fewer complications. This treatment may be used for unilateral tumor cases, or it may be used to treat the second eye in bilateral cases. Tumor size and plaque strength are used as parameters to calculate the amount of time that the plaque will be left in place. After 3000 to 4000 rads have been delivered to the apex of the tumor, the plaque is surgically removed. Most tumors show a dramatic response to irradiation within the first 3 weeks after plaque removal.[6]

Photocoagulation and/or cryotherapy may be the treatment of choice for selected small retinoblastomas.

Chemotherapy for matastatic disease is administered by pediatric oncologists experienced in the use of chemotherapeutic agents. Vincristine 0.05 mg/kg and cyclophosphamide 30 mg/kg are given intravenously every 3 weeks for 1 year.

Many combinations of these therapy modalities may be used to bring the tumor under control.[6]

Genetic counseling is a most important part of management of this disease. Parents should be encouraged to tell their child the reason for the eye's removal. If a child with no family history of retinoblastoma presents with unilateral involvement, the parents should be informed that they have about a 1 percent chance of having a subsequent child with a retinoblastoma. However, if a child with bilateral sporadic retinoblastoma survives to adulthood, there is a 40 to 50 percent chance that each of his or her children will have the tumor. Bilateral cases invariably represent the hereditary type. Another aspect of genetic counseling concerns the development of new, unrelated cancers in survivors of bilateral retinoblastoma, regardless of whether irradiation treatment has been used.

A follow-up plan devised for each patient, includes examination under anesthesia every 4 months until 3 years of age, and then every 6 months until 5 years of age. After 5 years of age, the examination should be conducted every 6 to 12 months, without anesthesia. Examination includes inspection and palpation of the anophthalmic socket and indirect ophthalmoscopy of the opposite eye, looking for evidence of new tumors and for the response to therapy of previously treated tumors.[6]

Visual prognosis is excellent for the uninvolved eye in patients with unilateral disease. The occurrence of new tumors in a previously normal eye is rare and most children grow up to have good vision in the remaining eye. The prognosis for vision in bilateral cases depends upon the extent of involvement and the effectiveness of treatment in the remaining or less involved eye. Prognosis for life has improved and can be attributed to early diagnosis and prompt treatment.

NURSING INTERVENTION

The nurse who notices a child with a leukocoria or a newly acquired strabismus should refer him or her to a pediatrician for evaluation.

1. Prior to examination under anesthesia, the pupils will have to be well dilated with a mydriatic and/or cycloplegic drops.
2. Enucleation care was discussed in Chapter 9. The large pressure patch will be irritating to the small child. Head rolling or banging might indicate the young patient has pain, and medication should be administered. The comfort measure of holding the child is as important as pain medication.
3. Cobalt^{60} plaque irradiation presents a nursing problem when the child is small, for the child will need to be held while being fed and to allay crying. *Remember radiation exposure is decreased by limiting the amount of contact time and maintaining an adequate distance from the source.* A rotation schedule should be devised to limit the amount of contact time for each person looking after the child. Film badges to monitor exposure should be worn at all times by the nurses, and may also be assigned to parents. Pocket dosimeters can also make individuals attending the child more aware of their radiation exposure.

PATIENT TEACHING

Patient teaching should be directed to the parents of the child. Discharge planning includes a demonstration of irrigation and instillation of ointment or drops to the enucleation site which will be necessary once the patch is removed. Compliance with follow-up appointments should be encouraged. The parents great sorrow and guilt feelings will need to be talked about if the nurse is to be supportive to the parents of these children. If there is a support network available, this information might be offered to the parent.

Retinopathy of Prematurity

Retinopathy of prematurity (ROP) (*retrolental fibroplasia*) is a bilateral retinal disease found in 25 to 30 percent of infants who have a birth weight of 1700 g or less and/or are premature. Risk factors identified are low birth weight and length of time in and oxygen concentration given to those infants with respiratory distress syndrome. Even with careful blood gas monitoring, using a conservative estimate, about 500 infants are blinded from ROP annually in the United States.[7]

Up until the 4th month of gestation, no blood vessels are present in the retina. Retinal vascularization proceeds slowly until the retinal vessels reach the ora serrata nasally at 8 months gestation. The temporal retinal periphery is completely vascularized only shortly after the full-term infant's birth.[7]

With the increased use of oxygen, particularly in closed incubators, the incidence of ROP rose, reaching epidemic proportions by 1950. When rigid restriction of oxygen's use was imposed in the premature nursery (a decade later), pediatricians found an associated increase in infant mortality and morbidity (i.e., brain damage) from hyaline membrane disease, and from the resultant severe oxygen deprivation in infants with respiratory distress syndrome.[7] When a high oxygen concentration was maintained, it was discovered that the retinal blood vessels developed spasms. It is now known that if elevated arterial PO_2 levels are sustained significantly, then some of the more immature peripheral vessels become permanently occluded. This leads to retinal neovascularization which extends forward into the vitreous in a manner similar to the fibrovascular proliferation seen in other retinopathies. Hemorrhages into the vitreous and vitreoretinal adhesions occur ultimately leading to total retinal detachment.

The clinical classification ranges from the acute stage where there is vascular vasoconstriction and occlusion, through five other stages, each one being a little more damaging to visual potential. In advanced cases, a white retrolental membrane containing blood vessels might be seen in both eyes, this is caused by detachment of the entire retina. A shallow anterior chamber may be present. High myopia and strabismus are common.[7] Spontaneous regression takes place in approximately 80 percent of infants with Stage I and II ROP. Vision varies depending upon the involvement of the damage to the retina generally, and the macular particularly (Fig. 17–8).

Retinopathy of prematurity management has included such treatment techniques as xenon-arc photocoagulation and/or cryotherapy to the peripheral retina. Peripheral neovascularization has also been treated with argon-laser photocoagulation. A scleral buckling procedure for repair of retinal detachment, closed vitrectomy, and open-sky vitrectomy techniques have all been used with varying degrees of success. Experiments conducted by Hittner and co-workers have shown that vitamin E (Alpha-tocopherol) administered orally reduces the severity, but not the incidence of ROP in the nursery population.[8]

NURSING INTERVENTION

The fact that these premature and smaller neonates with poor pulmonary function are placed in oxygen puts them at risk, and the more prolonged the oxygen therapy, the greater the chance the infant has of developing ROP. However, infants not placed in oxygen have also been known to develop ROP. Oxygen administration should be controlled by blood gas measurements—not by percentage flow rates—and the arterial oxygen concentration should be maintained at the range of 60 to 80 mm Hg (never exceeding 100 mm Hg). If blood gas measurements are not available, the oxygen concentration should be kept below 40 percent and the infant transferred as soon as possible to a facility where such measurements can be made.[7]

When the premature infant is to be examined, one drop each of tropicamide (Mydriacyl) 0.5 percent or cyclopentolate (Cyclogyl) 0.5 percent followed by phenylephrine (Neo-Synephrine) 2.5 percent is instilled in the cul-de-sac of each eye and may be repeated after 10 minutes. The nurse administering these medications should be aware of their side

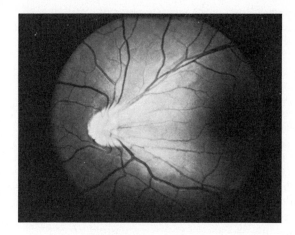

Figure 17–8. Cicatricial retinopathy of prematurity—dragged disc.

effects, for it is important to avoid the use of excessive drops in the premature infant.

PATIENT TEACHING

Children with arrested ROP should be cautioned to avoid contact sports because of their increased susceptibility to retinal breaks and detachments.

ACQUIRED ABNORMALITIES

Hypertensive Retinopathy

Approximately 22 million Americans have hypertension, but half are unaware of it. Hypertension is a condition of the blood pressure elevation only; hypertensive disease suggests the development of vascular lesions in the kidneys, brain, heart, and eyes. Hypertensive disease occurs in approximately 5 percent of the population.

Varying degrees of hypertensive retinopathy can be identified using the Wagener and Keith classification which placed patients into four groupings, and although this 1939 study has been somewhat modified since then it is still used. The appearance of the fundus in hypertensive retinopathy is determined by the degree of elevation of the blood pressure and the state of the retinal arterioles. There is a definite relationship between the arterioles narrow caliber and the height of the diastolic pressure. Accurate documentation of these microcirculatory changes is made possible by fluorescein angiography. A patient with hypertension for which no specific basis can be found is said to have "essential hypertension" (chronic, benign, and "arteriosclerotic" are other terms which describe it). The following findings might be present when the fundus of the eye is examined with an ophthalmoscope:

- Grade I—Hypertensive retinopathy reveals minimal narrowing and sclerosis of the arterioles. This relatively mild hypertension with moderately elevated blood pressure can be reduced by rest.
- Grade II—Hypertensive retinopathy reveals localized and generalized narrowing of the arterioles giving the appearance of "copper" or "silver" wiring. Changes described as "A–V nicking" (widening of the apparent arteriovenous crossing spaces, with almost complete invisibility of portions of the veins which underlie the crossing arterioles) are evident (Fig. 17–9).[9] The blood pressure prevails at higher, more sustained levels. The patient complains of headaches and some increased nervousness.[9]
- Group III—Not only is there arteriolar narrowing and focal constrictions, but the retinopathy includes small, soft exudates (cotton-wool spots) which are areas of focal ischemia due to occlusion of the supplying arteriole. Extensive microvascular changes are also occurring, particularly around the cotton-wool spots. Hard exudates (edema residues which are seen as yellowish white deposits) assume the appearance of a "macular star," and scattered, round, or flame-shaped hemorrhages may also be seen. The blood pressure is higher and usually more sustained. Symptoms include headaches, vertigo, and nervousness. There may be mild impairment of cardiac, cerebral, and renal function. Successful hypertensive therapy can produce resolution of the cotton-wool spots and arteriolar changes.[9,10]
- Group IV—In addition to all the findings seen in group III there is the additional feature of edema of the optic disc. General arteriolar narrowing with severe focal constriction and chronic arteriolosclerosis can also be identified. In accelerated or malignant hypertension, the blood pressure is persistently elevated. Symptoms include headaches, asthenia, loss of weight, dyspnea, and visual disturbance. There is impairment of cardiac, cerebral, and renal function. Severe retinopathy may be seen in advanced renal disease, in patients with pheochromocytoma, and in toxemia of pregnancy. All such patients should have a complete medical work-up.[9,10]

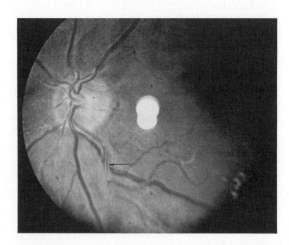

Figure 17–9. Hypertensive retinopathy showing "A–V nicking."

Young patients with accelerated hypertension who have extensive retinopathy, with hemorrhages and retinal infarcts may occasionally develop serous detachment of the retina. Elderly patients with arteriosclerotic vessels are unable to respond in this manner, because their vessels are protected by the arteriosclerosis. (These underlying changes are irreversible.) It is for this reason that elderly patients seldom exhibit florid hypertensive retinopathy.

It has been found that there is a definite relationship between the severity of retinal changes and the survival rate and the incidence of cardiac and renal complications of hypertension.[10]

NURSING INTERVENTION
Nursing intervention should include taking the blood pressure as a method of screening as well as monitoring patients. There is a tremendous nursing role to be played in patient education since the treatment of hypertension includes general hygiene measures and drug therapy. Assessing the patient's general condition, ascertaining drugs given for other disease entities, and identifying adverse effects of newly prescribed drugs can contribute to the patient's well-being.

PATIENT TEACHING
Patient teaching should include encouragement of entertaining all encompassing programs which include weight control, sodium restriction, exercise, relaxation, and control of lifestyle. Compliance with drug therapy which includes diuretics, adrenergic inhibitors, and vasodilators should also be encouraged. If potassium replacement is necessary because of loss from taking diuretic medications, appropriate replacement through diet or medication should be reinforced.

Diabetic Retinopathy
The retinovascular complications of diabetes mellitus are collectively called diabetic retinopathy.[11] As one of the leading causes of blindness in the United States, this disease causes approximately 10 percent of new cases of blindness each year. Both juvenile onset (Type I) and maturity onset (Type II) diabetics are prone to develop diabetic retinopathy. At present there is no evidence that diabetic retinopathy occurs in insulin-dependent juvenile diabetics who have had diabetes for 5 years or less. However, of those patients who have had diabetes for longer than 10 years, some will develop diabetic retinopathy. The incidence of retinopathy rises to 90 percent after 30 years.

In noninsulin-dependent diabetics, the incidence of diabetic retinopathy is harder to determine because in some cases the diagnosis of diabetes mellitus is made for the first time by the ophthalmologist who finds diabetic retinopathy in patients who are completely unaware that they have elevated blood glucose. It is known that the incidence and severity of retinopathy increases with the duration of the diabetes, and is worse if control of the diabetes is poor in the early years after onset. The 5-year mortality rate for patients blind from diabetic retinopathy is 36 percent, usually from cardiac or kidney complications.[11]

Diabetic retinopathy has been divided into background (nonproliferative) retinopathy and proliferative retinopathy. Proliferative diabetic retinopathy patients have a higher incidence of systemic hypertension than do patients with background retinopathy. Pregnancy can accelerate diabetic retinopathy; blacks have a 20 percent higher risk of blindness than whites, and women have a 23 percent higher risk than men. Complications of diabetic retinopathy which result in loss of vision and ultimately cause blindness are macula edema, vitreous hemorrhage, traction detachment, dense vitreous or preretinal membranes, and macula dragging.[11,12]

Background Retinopathy. The earliest change in *background retinopathy* at the microscopic level, is loss of mural cells and thickening of the retinal capillary walls *Microaneurysms* (Fig. 17–10A) are the first ophthalmoscopically detectable change in diabetic retinopathy—these are intraretinal budding of new capillaries. The retinal blood vessels and the retinal pigment epithelium form a barrier, and together prevent large molecules from passing from the blood into the retina. If there is a breakdown of this blood-retinal barrier because it is significantly damaged, fluid accumulates in the retina, especially in the macula region, causing the *macula edema* that leads to decreased visual acuity and decreased color discrimination. Yellow lipid deposits (*hard exudates*) collect where the fluid is being resorbed. Blood ceases to flow through some capillaries (*capillary nonperfusion*); and irregular *venous dilation*, referred to as "beading" might also be seen. Rupture in the capillaries causes small *intraretinal ("dot or blot") hemorrhages. Superficial ("flame-shaped") hemorrhages* in the nerve fiber bundles are indistinguishable from hemorrhages seen in hypertensive retinopathy. If these hemorrhages are seen, it is an indication that the blood pressure should be checked. Background diabetic retinopathy can cause legal blindness, although patients with it usually maintain ambulatory or better vision.

Preproliferative Retinopathy. One common denominator shared by all proliferative retinopathies is retinal hypoxia which precedes the new vessel formation. Important signs of hypoxia are the nerve fiber layer microinfarcts, which are caused by occlusion of precapillary arterioles, they look like tufts of cotton (soft exudates). Other signs of hypoxia are engorged, irregularly dilated (beaded) veins, and intraretinal microvascular abnormalities (IRMA) or shunts which bypass focal obstructions. When intravenous fluorescein angiography (IVFA) is performed, large areas of capillary nonperfusion, vessels that leak, and microaneurysms which look like light bulbs can be identified (Fig. 17–10A). These signs collectively categorize the preproliferative retinopathy stage and these eyes are at risk of developing proliferative retinopathy.[11]

Proliferative Retinopathy. Proliferative diabetic retinopathy on the other hand may result in severe vitreous hemorrhage or retinal detachment with hand movements vision or worse. Proliferative vessels usually arise from veins, and begin as collections of the fine (IRMA) intraretinal microvascular abnormalities already referred to. Later, extraretinal new vessels develop *on* the retina or the optic nerve head. When new vessels arise on or within 1 disc diameter of the optic disc they are referred to as *NVD* (neovascularization on the disc). When these vessels arise further than 1 disc diameter away, they are called *NVE* (neovascularization elsewhere).

As the posterior vitreous face detaches, it also becomes a frequent site of growth for new vessels. These new vessels are then pulled into the vitreous cavity by the contracting vitreous to which they are adherent. It has long been assumed that sudden vitreous contractions tear the fragile new vessels, causing vitreous hemorrhage. However, 60 to 80 percent of diabetic vitreous hemorrhages occur during sleep, possibly because of an increase in blood pressure secondary to early morning hypoglycemia or to rapid eye movement (REM) sleep.

As proliferative diabetic retinopathy progresses, fibrovascular changes begin to occur. Traction is transmitted not only to the adherent new blood vessels, but also on the retina itself. A focal concentration of fibrovascular tissue may create stria involving the macula area leading to actual dragging of the macula itself, causing decreased visual acuity. Two types of diabetic retinal detachments occur, those caused by traction alone (nonrhegmatogenous) and those caused by retinal break formation (rhegmatogenous). Repair of retinal detachment is achieved with combined vitrectomy and scleral buckling procedure, and offers a newer and preferred method of treating traction retinal detachments.[1]

Medical Therapy. A current study called the ETDRS (Early Treatment of Diabetic Retinopathy Study) is evaluating the role of aspirin in slowing the progression of diabetic retinopathy. It should be stressed that aspirin therapy is experimental and is not recommended for all diabetics.

Photocoagulation is the basic mechanism of the energy of well-focused, intense light, when absorbed by pigment cells (such as erythrocytes or pigment epithelial cells) is converted to heat which coagulates the cells and surrounding tissues.

Pan retinal photocoagulation (PRP) (Fig. 17–10B) burns, when scattered throughout the retina, decrease the retina's need for oxygen and thereby cause neovascularization to regress. The National Institute of Health's sponsored *Diabetic Retinopathy Study* (DRS) proved that PRP not only prevented decreased visual acuity from established neovascularization, but also seemed to prevent neovascularization from developing in eyes with severe background diabetic retinopathy.

Pars plana vitrectomy (PPV) is indicated for a long-standing vitreous hemorrhage and tractional retinal detachments. Retinal breaks in the posterior pole can be treated with external cryotherapy and intraocular gas injection. Following vitrectomy, recurrent corneal erosion, striate keratopathy, and corneal edema are more common in diabetic patients.

Other ocular complications of diabetic retinopathy include glaucoma and rubeosis iridis which is the growth of new vessels on the iris, usually seen in eyes with proliferative, rather than background, diabetic retinopathy. This occurs slightly more frequently in those patients who have not received PRP than in those patients who have. Pan retinal photocoagulation appears to have some protective value against rubeosis iridis. Rubeosis iridis resulting in *neovascular glaucoma* is the most common cause of failure following otherwise successful vitrectomy.

Ischemic optic neuropathy is another complication of diabetic retinopathy. The patient reports a sudden decrease in visual acuity or sudden visual field loss. The main ocular finding is a "pale swelling" of the optic nerve. Adult patients with diabetes, and even teenagers, appear to be susceptible to ischemic optic neuropathy, and many of the reported cases have been found in patients with uncontrolled blood sugar.

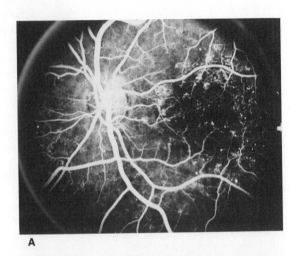

A

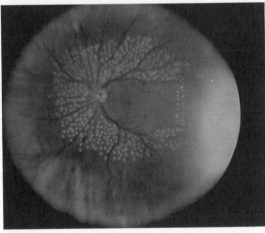

Figure 17–10. A. Microaneurysms seen in background retinopathy as seen on intravenous fluorescein angiography. **B.** Pan retinal photocoagulation. (*Photograph B courtesy Wills Eye Hospital.*)

B

Another complication of diabetic retinopathy is cranial nerve neuropathy. Extraocular muscle palsies may occur in diabetes secondary to neuropathy involving the third, fourth, or sixth cranial nerves. Pain may or may not be experienced, and not infrequently an extraocular muscle palsy may be the initial symptom due to a latent diabetic condition. When the third cranial nerve is involved, pupillary function is usually normal. This pupillary sparing in the diabetic third nerve palsy is an important diagnostic feature, distinguishing it from other causes of oculomotor involvement such as intracranial tumors or aneurysm. Recovery of function takes place over a period of months.[11]

NURSING INTERVENTION

Assessing the patient's visual acuity and visual field should be done first. One of the earliest symptoms of macula edema is the patient's complaint of difficulty driving at night. Blood pressure should also be checked. Since increased blood pressure is known to cause retinal arteriolosclerosis with resultant retinal hypoxia, it seems prudent to counsel all diabetics to rigorously control their blood pressure. Reinforcement of the necessity of good control of the blood glucose to prevent hypo- and hyperglycemia is essential. For fundus examination, IVFA, and PRP, the eyes will need to be dilated with a cycloplegic medication such as tropicamide 1 percent or cyclopentolate hydrochloride 1 percent, and a mydriatic, e.g., phenylephrine 2.5 percent, prior to the procedure being performed. Nursing care of the retinal detachment surgery can be found in the section on Retinal Detachments.

PATIENT TEACHING
Encourage patient compliance with a diet which will work toward better blood glucose control. Encourage decreased salt intake, exercise, and relaxation as a means toward controlling hypertension. Reinforce the need for at least annual visits to the ophthalmologist. If photocoagulation is performed, ensure that the patient understands that his or her vision will be blurred from the eyedrops immediately following treatment. Dark glasses may be necessary to decrease light sensitivity. Pan retinal photocoagulation helps to prolong the vision that the patient has, and prevents vessels from further bleeding.

VASCULAR OCCLUSIONS

Retinal Artery Obstruction
The blood supply to the internal layers of the retina is through the circulation from the central retinal artery. Any interruption of the blood flow causes a sudden, dramatic, but painless loss of vision. The vision may never return, it may partially return with residual impairment, or it may return to normal. Recurrent transient loss of vision is called *amaurosis fugax*.

The ophthalmoscopic picture of occlusion of the central retinal artery is typical. The large retinal arterioles are reduced to threads or are collapsed and nearly invisible. Occasionally, an emboli might be seen occluding a vessel (Fig. 17–11A). The blood in the veins is fragmented or beaded. These multiple fragments (referred to as "boxcars") may have no motion, they may move slowly toward the optic disc, alternately they move very jerkily back and forth or even away from the nerve head toward the periphery of the retina. The retina quickly becomes pale and milky, while the macula appears quite red. Swelling of the retina's ganglion cells causes the milky appearance, and since these ganglion cells are more numerous around the fovea, and absent in the macula, the intact choroidal circulation is easily seen and appears as a "cherry-red spot." In a few cases, central vision is preserved by the presence of the cilioretinal artery which supplies the ganglion cells of the fovea.[13] If the obstruction occurs in a branch of the central retinal artery, then only the retinal segment supplied by the occluded branch or branches will become milky. Of the four branches, the superior temporal is the most frequently involved.

If the blockage is spontaneously relieved, there may be leakage and bleeding through the damaged vascular walls. Eventually, the milky appearance and edema will subside and circulation in the retina may appear normal on ophthalmoscopic examination, however, the inner layers, especially the ganglion cell layer, will atrophy and the optic nerve may become white and atrophic.

The effect of treatment depends upon whether the occlusion has just happened or whether it is several hours old.[14] In either condition, a visual acuity should be quickly obtained. Emergency measures to lower the intraocular pressure of the globe by a paracentesis is the first step taken by the physician.[15] A #27-gauge needle on a tuberculin syringe is inserted at the limbus, into the anterior chamber and a small portion of aqueous is withdrawn (Fig. 17–11B). This procedure is performed with the illumination and magnification of Slitlamp biomicroscopy. Gentle intermittent massage of the globe is then performed using a goniolens, or just the fingers. Intravenous acetazolamide 500 mg per 5 cc is given to decrease aqueous humor production. Ophthalmoscopy of the fundus should be performed to see if circulation has returned, and the patient should be asked if the vision is returning. The massage and fundus examination should be performed with the patient in a reclining position with the head on the level with, or a little lower than the heart. This will increase the flow and pressure of the blood to the head and eye. Breathing and rebreathing air from a paper bag for 10 minutes will cause mild vasodilation. If available, 95 percent oxygen and 5 percent carbon dioxide (Carbinogen) given by mask for 10 minutes is even better. The higher oxygen content will supply the oxygen-deficient tissue and the carbon dioxide will produce vasodilatation. If it is possible to restore circulation rapidly there is less chance of visual impairment.

If after 1 hour circulation has not fully returned, the visual acuity should be rechecked. The oxygen/carbon dioxide inhalations will be continued for 10 minutes every hour while awake and every 4 hours during sleep for the next 48 to 72 hours. Acetazolamine 250 mg q.i.d. and asprin 65 mg b.i.d. for the next 2 to 3 weeks is also prescribed.

A complete history and physical examination stressing the cardiovascular condition of the patient is indicated. Laboratory studies should include a complete blood count (CBC), erythrocyte sedimentation rate (ESR), a serum lipid profile, fasting blood glucose (FBS), an electrocardiogram (ECG), and a chest x-ray. Ophthalmological studies such as intravenous fluorescein angiography (IVFA) and electroretinogram (ERG) are indicated. If medical work-up indicates, or if a bruit is heard over the carotid artery, further studies such as the noninvasive Doppler ultrasonogram or the invasive digital substraction arteriogram (DSA), as well as a CAT scan may supply a clue to the etiology and lead to direct treatment.

The important factor as to the prognosis of final visual usefulness seems to be the initial visual acuity.[16] From personal experience we feel that starting treatment minutes after the onset of symptoms, if possible, will help in the final visual outcome of these patients.

NURSING INTERVENTION
When a patient presents with a sudden loss of vision, this is truly an ophthalmologic emergency, and should be brought to the attention of the physician immediately. A baseline visual acuity is taken. After examination, and identification of the problem, treatment is immediately begun with the administration IV or IM of acetozolamide 500 mg as prescribed. After the physician has completed the anterior chamber tap (paracentesis)

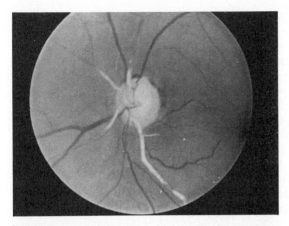

A

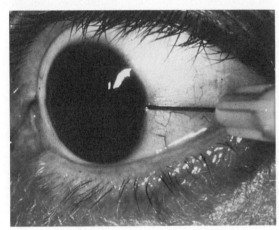

B

Figure 17–11. A. Retinal artery obstruction. **B.** Anterior chamber tap (paracentesis).

and the ocular massage, the nurse will administer the Carbinogen. As a precaution, the patient's vital signs will be monitored pre- and posttreatment: any variation above 15 mm Hg to 20 mm Hg in either diastolic or systolic pressure is brought to the physician's attention. The patient is requested to hold the inhalation mask over his or her face and nose while the treatment is administered. This acts as a safety measure in the event that the patient becomes agitated or disoriented, in which case he or she will immediately remove the mask from the face. Treatments should also be stopped if erratic pulse rate or cardiac arrhythmia develops. The patient must be closely observed at all times during Carbinogen treatment.

PATIENT TEACHING
Patient teaching should include the reason for the treatment. A request should be made that the patient hold the mask over the face for the period that the Carbinogen is being administered. Compliance with follow-up

medical care once the acute episode has been resolved should also be stressed.

Retinal Venous Occlusion

Unlike arterial occlusions, the symptoms of venous occlusions are usually gradual in onset unless there is a hemorrhage into the macula. The vision gradually becomes impaired and decreases to hand motions; light perception always remains. Vision may improve, but this depends upon the circulations' return with recanalization of the veins or formation of a collateral circulation. If the occlusion of the vein is *incomplete,* vision may be retained.

The picture seen on ophthalmoscopic examination is quite dramatic with hemorrhages throughout the retina (Fig. 17–12) and edema of the internal retinal layers. The optic nerve head appears red with indistinct borders, but without measurable elevation. The veins are engorged, dark red in color, and tortuous, while the arteries are narrowed and difficult to recognize in the edematous inner layer. Flame-shaped radial hemorrhages are seen in all quadrants of the retina. Hemorrhages in the deeper layers appear round. When the hemorrhages rupture into the vitreous it may appear quite smokey. Later, after some of the hemorrhages have absorbed, exudates may be seen between the hemorrhages. These may be hard exudates, or some may be fluffy. Hemorrhages may be less severe and fewer in number in partial central retinal vein occlusions.

Incipient venous occlusion may show signs of impending occlusion, with engorged veins and edema along the veins and nerve head months before the occlusion really occurs. Pulsations of the veins of the nerve head are also absent and there may be formation of small new veins.[17] The site of the central vein occlusion is usually behind the lamina cribosa where the central retinal artery and vein share the same fibrous adventicial sheath. If the artery is sclerotic and the sheath is fibrosed, the vein is easily compressed with resulting diminution and stagnation of blood flow, and thrombus formation. When occlusion of a branch vein occurs it is usually distal to an arterial vein crossing, (another site where there is shared adven-

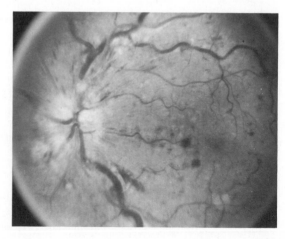

Figure 17–12. Retinal vein occlusion.

ticia). Other causes for venous thrombosis may be glaucoma, polycythemia vera and polycythemic syndrome, sickling hemoglobinopathies and macroglobulinemia, as well as hypertension and diabetes.

When *branch vein occlusions* occur, hemorrhages and edema are limited to the sector drained by the occluded branch. The upper temporal branches are most frequently occluded. The supertemporal quadrant hemorrhages and edema may gravitate inferiorly and cause permanent damage to the macula.

Resolution of central and branch vein occlusions are similar with absorption of hemorrhages, subsidence of the retinal edema (which leaves a residue of deposits and exudates in the retina), and the formation of thin-walled collateral veins. The dreaded complication following venous thrombosis is a secondary hemorrhagic glaucoma which can occur as a result of neovascular tissue formation in the anterior chamber angles, resulting in permanent closure of the angles. This occurs in approximately 20 percent of central retinal vein occlusions usually within 2 to 5 months of the occlusion.[18,19]

Treatment of the acute venous occlusions may include asprin and dicumarol for their anticoagulation effect. Administration of these drugs should be monitored carefully. Intravenous fluorescein angiography can demonstrate the degree of perfusion and drainage of the retina as well as the ischemic tissue. Pan retinal laser photocoagulation ablation of the ischemic retinal area is believed to decrease the angioblastic substance which stimulates the neovascular proliferation in the angle, thereby reducing the complication of secondary hemorrhagic glaucoma.[20] Once glaucoma has occurred, pan retinal photocoagulation may reduce the neovascularization. If this is not successful in reducing the glaucoma, cyclocryotherapy over the ciliary body may be of benefit. Chapter 20 will discuss glaucoma.

If vitreous hemorrhage occurs and obscures the retina, then vitrectomy may be performed to permit observation and retinal photocoagulation.

NURSING INTERVENTION
Nursing intervention begins with concern about the patient's general health status. Any patient who presents with a decrease in visual acuity should have his or her vision checked. If the patient is to be treated for an established neovascular glaucoma, medications to decrease the intraocular pressure and inflammation will be prescribed and will need to be administered (see Chap. 20). Vitrectomy nursing care was discussed in Chapter 16.

DYSTROPHIES AND DEGENERATIONS

Retinitis Pigmentosa
Primary retinal degeneration or the retinitis pigmentosa group are rare conditions which have intrigued ophthalmologists for the past century and a half. The degenerations first manifest as a narrowing of the retinal arterioles. Associated with this vascular change is a disturbance of the pigment epithelium. Atrophy of the pigment epithelium releases pigment granules which migrate to the perivascular spaces or clump forming irregular-shaped, bone corpuscular deposits in the midperiphery and

anterior retina. The pigment epithelium atrophy is secondary to the atrophy of the adjacent photoreceptor layer of the neuroretina. Rods atrophy first in the midretina; this accounts for loss of the peripheral vision and dark adaptation.

As the degeneration progresses, there is loss of central vision as the cones become involved. Electroretinography shows a decreased or absent response. The electro-oculogram shows absence of light rise.

These are hereditary degenerations and can be autosomal recessive, autosomal dominant, or sex-linked (which may be of an intermediate type with the female carriers showing ophthalmologic signs without loss of visual function). About 39 percent of the cases are spontaneous without a known pedigree and these are usually considered as autosomal recessive. With this type of inheritance onset is delayed, with milder symptoms than in the autosomal dominant type.

There are variants of retinitis pigmentosa in which only a sector of the retina is involved, and another type which is without the pigment dispersion. These degenerations may be associated with metabolical disorders, such as amaurotic familial idiocy and Hurler's mucopolysaccharide abnormalities, or neurological disorders such as Laurence-Moon-Bardet-Biedl syndrome and Friedreich's hereditary ataxias.

There is no treatment to arrest this degeneration at this time.

Retinal Detachments

The term ''detachment of the retina'' is a misnomer, for the whole retina is not involved. The ''detachment'' is actually a *separation of the sensory layers of the retina* from the *retinal pigment epithelium* (RPE), whose outer surface is bonded to Bruch's membrane and the choroid. These two retinal layers are lightly glued together by an acid mucopolysaccharide. When a separation occurs, the space created between the retinal pigment epithelium and sensory retina is referred to as the *subretinal space;* fluid which accumulates in this space is called *subretinal fluid.*

Retinal detachments are commonly classified as either primary, those occurring as a result of spontaneous degenerative changes in the retina or vitreous, or secondary, those directly attributable to mechanical trauma, intraocular inflammation, or another problem. A more useful classification divides the retinal detachment on the basis of their mechanisms of development.

Rhegmatogenous detachments represent the most common type of retinal detachment encountered. By definition they are all associated with a hole or tear in the retina which permits vitreous to seep into the subretinal space (Fig. 17–13A and B). These breaks may be trophic holes, tractional tears which may be combined with a retinal flap of free operculum, or a product of both of these entities.

Tractional detachments occur when contraction of fibrous tissue in the vitreous pulls the retina away from the RPE. Patients affected by this type of detachment are those with proliferative retinopathy secondary to diabetes mellitus, sickle-cell hemoglobinopathy, or retinopathy of prematurity. Traction detachments can also occur secondary to trauma such as an intraocular foreign body (IOFB), or as a result of uveitis.

Exudative detachments present with an accumulation of fluid beneath the retina and are caused by such processes as intraocular inflammation, e.g., posterior uveitis; circulatory abnormalities, e.g., leaking vessels, or secondary to systemic disease, such as accelerated hypertension or toxemia of pregnancy; and tumors of the choroid or retina. Exudative detachments are not characterized by a tear in the

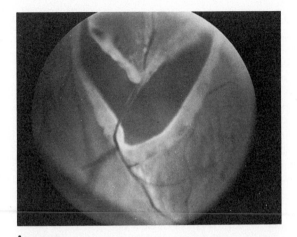

A

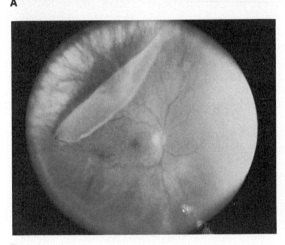

B

Figure 17–13. A. Retinal horseshoe tear showing intact blood vessel. **B.** Giant tear in the peripheral retina (wide angle photograph). (*Figure B from Boyd-Monk H: Retinal detachment and vitrectomy: Nursing care. Nursing Clinics of North America, 16(30): 440, 1981, with permission.*)

retina, and thus if the underlying abnormality can be managed effectively, the retina will reappose itself spontaneously as the subretinal fluid is absorbed.

Visual prognosis in retinal detachment depends upon the type of detachment which occurs and the area involved. If the macula is damaged, then central acute vision will be lost.

Characteristically, retinal detachment is a relatively rare condition in infancy and childhood. The incidence of affected patients increases after the fourth decade with a peak being reached between 50 and 60 years of age.

Predisposing ocular conditions which contribute to this condition, are *aphakia* (following cataract extraction), *lattice vitreoretinal degeneration* characterized by elongated, excavated troughs in the peripheral retina (an etiological factor found in about one-third of all cases of rhegmatogenous retinal detachment);[21] and *high myopia* which is found in roughly two-thirds of retinal detachment patients.

Historical perspectives in management of patients with retinal detachment include the contribution made in 1918 by Jules Gonin, a Swiss ophthalmologist who discovered that by cauterizing the sclera in the area of a retinal hole or tear, several cases of retinal detachment could be cured. However, diagnostic problems prior to development of modern diagnostic techniques and instruments were a major stumbling block to retinal surgery. With the advent of the binocular indirect ophthalmoscope, retinal holes in the periphery could be identified. The Slitlamp biomicroscope with fundus contact lenses permitted examination of the posterior pole.

Prior to development of modern scleral buckling materials and techniques, only the holes that could be sealed by diathermy were amenable to treatment. Different types of sutures, to change the shape of the globe, were also tried. With the advent of silicone sponges, bands, plates, etc., spatula needles, diathermy, and cryotherapy, the scleral buckling technique offered greater success for repair of retinal detachment. Patient management problems before and after surgery, such as prolonged immobilization with binocular patching, were also eliminated.

Preoperative Care. Examination of both fundi through widely dilated pupils is accomplished by the physician using the indirect ophthalmoscopy and/or Slitlamp biomicroscope with the fundus contact lens. A retinal drawing is made of the fundus identifying normal retina and any pathology. If the macula region of the retina is still attached but threatened, or if there is a large superior retinal break, then severe restrictions which impose limitation of patient activity and ocular movement are accomplished by binocular patching of the eyes, and placing the patient on bedrest with or without bathroom privileges.

Moderate to no restrictions—ranging from no vigorous activity to normal activity, and a uniocular or no patch—may be imposed on patients who have small peripheral detachments not threatening the macula; retinal detachments involving the macular and causing profound visual impairment; or retinal detachments with fixed folds.

Both mydriatics (sympathomimetics, pupillary dilators) such as phenylephrine 2.5 percent (occasionally 10 percent is used) and cycloplegics (parasympatholytics, inhibitors of pupillary constriction and accommodation) such as tropicamide 0.5 percent or 1.0 percent; cyclopentolate hydrochloride 1.0 percent and 2.0 percent eyedrops are prescribed preoperatively to achieve dilatation. (Other cycloplegics such as scopolamine 0.25 percent; homatropine hydrobromide 2 and 5 percent and atropine sulfate 1 percent can also be used.) One drop of each is administered to the eyes for the initial dilatation, and then just prior to surgery the administration is repeated q.5.min × 2 or 3 times.

Postoperative Care. Limitations of activity are usually restricted to the immediate postoperative period, when the patient is recovering from anesthesia. The patient soon proceeds from bedrest to ambulatory activities. The marked periocular congestion which occurs is contained by a pressure patch over the operative eye. This is removed in 12 to 24 hours and the physician examines the eye to assess the status of the retinal break(s), and the presence and amount of subretinal fluid. The surgical eye continues to receive eyedrops for the next 2 to 6 weeks. These may include a single antibiotic, e.g., chloramphenicol or gentamycin, or a combination of antibiotics, e.g., Neosporin, followed by a corticosteroid eyedrop such as prednisolone sodium phosphate, or dexemethezone. Antibiotic–steroid combination drops such as Maxitrol and Vasocidin are also available. Cyclopegics such as scopolamine 0.25 percent and/or tropicamide 1 percent, and the mydriatic phenyl-ephrine 2.5 percent will continue to be prescribed. A light patch replaces the pressure patch. Ice compresses applied to the ocular area at least q.i.d. and then as needed, help to decrease the lid swelling (and pain). Discharge from the hospital takes place in 3 to 5 days in uncomplicated cases. Follow-up appointments are necessary during the next 4 to 8 weeks, after which the patient may resume normal activities.

NURSING INTERVENTION
See Table 17-1.

MACULAR DEGENERATIONS

Because the macula area is the site of fine visual acuity and color vision, a small defect can cause severe visual deficit. The study and treatment of macular lesions has been expanded considerably with the advent of fluorescein angiography. With this technique it is possible to determine if the trouble is in the retinal vascular system or if it is located within the choriocapillaris, pigment epithelial, and Bruch's membrane complex. Mascular degeneration and disease can be due to hereditary, traumatic, inflammatory, senile, and miscellaneous causes.

Hereditary Macular Disorders
Hereditary macular disorders are rare and progressive with no known treatment. *Fundus flavimaculatus* degeneration is the most common hereditary disorder which is inherited as an autosomal recessive trait. Onset of symptoms occur in childhood (occasionally include slow dark adaptation) and progress to loss of central vision, usually within the first two decades of life.[21] The retina contains yellowish, fuzzy-margined flecks of various sizes and shapes, which are probably deposits in the retinal pigment epithelium. Similar flecks are seen in *Fundus albipunctatus* except that the periphery and not the macula is involved, so neither visual acuity nor color perception is disturbed, but it does produce *stationary night blindness*. Also placed in this category of flecked retinal disorders is the autosomal dominant inherited degeneration known as *familial drusen*. Round or oval, yellowish lesions occur at the retinal pigment epithelium level with pigment clumping around the lesions. These are most numerous in the central macular area and they increase in size and number and eventually lead to atrophic or hemorrhagic macular degeneration.

Traumatic Macular Lesions
Blunt trauma to the globe can cause traumatic macular lesions. *Retinal edema* called *Berlin's edema* may result. When this occurs there is generalized whitening of the retina and a cherry-red spot in the fovea. Retinal vascular perfusion is intact and relatively good visual acuity is maintained. Ophthalmoscopic examination reveals patent arteries filled with blood, and this establishes the difference between traumatic retinal edema and central retinal artery occlusion. The edema usually subsides with time.

TABLE 17–1. NURSING STANDARDS OF CARE FOR RETINAL DETACHMENT AND VITRECTOMY

Teaching Guidelines	Potential Problems	Expected Outcomes	Deadlines
Preoperative Management			
At the time of the initial interview, and during each shift thereafter, explain general preoperative and postoperative routines of the unit	Anxiety over impending surgical procedure and possible visual loss	Patient should be able to verbalize concern	Day of surgery
Explain specific procedures relating to the patient's type of surgery; for example:	Need to reinforce information	Patient should:	Day of surgery
Preoperative preparation		1. Be able to express an understanding of what to expect	
Activity levels such as bedrest, ambulation ad lib,		2. be able to comply with activity restriction	Day of surgery
Dietary restrictions (NPO or clear liquids, if permitted)			Day of surgery
Time of surgery			
Frequency of eyedrop administration and action			
Clipping of eyelashes, if ordered	Acute blepharospasm may occur when lashes are being clipped	3. Know that the lashes will grow back in 6–8 weeks	
Types of patches (light or pressure)		4. Have a restful preoperative night	
Preoperative sleeping medication may be ordered at bedtime			
Explain general postoperative mangement; for example:		1. Vital signs should be stable	Postoperative period and throughout the patient's hospitalization
Check vital signs of patient upon his or her return to the unit after surgery			
Monitor any coexisting medical problems such as diabetes or hypertension		2. Preexisting medical problems should be stable	
Monitor intravenous infusion if *in situ*			
Assist patient to the bathroom the first time he or she is ambulatory			
Evaluate patient's need for assistance thereafter			
Immediate Postoperative Management			
Note the frequency of urination	Patient tries to go to the bathroom without assistance and falls	Patient should:	Every 8 hours postoperatively and during the entire hospitalization
Note any restlessness in the immediate postoperative period and during the night (may indicate full bladder)		1. Void a sufficient quantity	
Encourage patient to use the call bell for assistance		2. Not sustain any falls or injuries	

Nursing Interventions	Potential Problems	Expected Outcomes	Timing
Position the patient on the nonoperative side immediately postoperatively in case of possible active emesis, unless contraindicated by doctor's orders Offer anti-emetic for nausea, in conjunction with pain medication, if needed Chart effectiveness Hold fluids until after nausea subsides	Potential nausea and vomiting secondary to anesthesia	1. Prevention of emesis by administration of anti-emetic if patient is nauseated 2. No emesis or aspiration occurs	Every 4–6 hours as needed during hospitalization
Instruct patient: To lie on the nonoperative side or on his or her back. (Or, if air or sulfahexafluoride-6 has been inserted at surgery, the patient should be positioned according to the doctor's instructions; this may be on the abdomen, or sitting up with the patient's head over the bedside table) Not to bend, strain, lift heavy objects, sneeze too heartily, or make jerky movements. To ambulate with assistance when necessary	Potential for pain or headache Patient lies on operative side. An air bubble may be displaced if the position is not maintained	3. Relief of pain is achieved Air bubble or gas absorbs Headache does not persist There is no sudden or persistent eye pain	Immediately postoperatively During every shift
Care of operative eye: Expect the patient to have mild discomfort after the pressure patch has been removed Clean the eye and eyelashes very gently Instill dilating and combination steroid–antibiotic drops as frequently as ordered Apply cold compresses to decrease swelling	Potential for accidents as a result of decreased alertness, decreased vision, or both Patient may have: Slightly swollen lids Serosanguinous drainage on eye dressing Difficulty cooperating initially	No falls or injuries occur during hospitalization Drops should be given very gently, as ordered	During hospitalization
Keep the light in the room to a minimum Apply a light patch to the affected area as ordered	Light sensitivity when patch is removed	Patient should verbalize reasonable comfort	

General Care of Ophthalmic Patient

Nursing Interventions	Potential Problems	Expected Outcomes	Timing
Identify oneself upon entering the patient's room Orient the patient to the placement of foods on the tray if bilateral functional vision is poor	Patient may express frustration because of necessary	Patient should: 1. Demonstrate an ability to do partial to complete self-care	During entire hospitalization

(continued)

TABLE 17-1. (Continued)

Teaching Guidelines	Potential Problems	Expected Outcomes	Deadlines
Stress to the patient that the nursing staff is there to assist him or her as necessary	dependence on others and restricted activities	(bathing, eating, etc.)	
Allow the patient to verbalize personal concerns while receiving treatment		2. Verbalize his or her ability to cope with temporary restrictions	
Permit the patient to utilize diversional activities (radio, knitting, games, crafts, T.V.) if permitted by doctor			
Psychosocial Support	Anxiety secondary to unknown outcome of surgery	Patient should be able to:	During hospitalization
Work with patient to devise a method for coping with anxieties or situational problems		1. Verbalize concerns and fears	
Encourage family participation in the patient's care		2. Identify potential problems for own care, and work toward resolution of these problems	
Arrange a social service consult if necessary			
Refer the patient to an extended care facility if warranted			
Discharge Care	Noncompliance with home care due to poor instruction	Patient should be able to:	Prior to discharge
Nurse will instruct patient/family in the correct method for eyedrop instillation		1. Verbalize importance and understanding of home care instructions	
Stress handwashing before starting procedure		2. Verbalize knowledge of signs and symptoms of complications (such as flashing lights, sudden loss of vision, excessive pain, or purulent discharge from the eye)	
Retract the lower lid and instill eyedrops (only one drop unless otherwise ordered)			
Close the eye gently (do not squeeze)			
Apply pressure to the inner canthus of the eye (at the tear duct) to prevent systemic absorption			
Do not contaminate the eyedrop bottle with the patient's lashes			
Instruct the patient regarding the importance of keeping clinic or doctor's appointments for follow-up care			
Provide teaching aid upon discharge			

(From Boyd-Monk H: Retinal detachment and vitrectomy: Nursing care. Nursing Clinics of North America, 16(30):444–446, 1981, with permission.)

Severe blunt trauma may cause immediate visual impairment as a result of a choroidal tear through the macular, subretinal hemorrhage or a round, irregular macular hole without any identifiable operculum. With the hole formation, visual acuity and color perception is severely impaired. The reason the macular is so sensitive to the traumatic force of blunt trauma at the front of the eye is that the contra-coup effect of the energy is being focused at the posterior pole from all directions.

Solar burns can occur as a result of viewing an eclipse without the protection of appropriate glasses. This type of burn can also occur when a person "sun gazes" or stares at the sun while on a trip from using drugs such as marijuana or LSD. The macula can be damaged in this manner.

NURSING INTERVENTION

Preventative health care is the best course of action, and persons engaged in contact sports should be encouraged to wear safety goggles or glasses so that these types of injuries can be avoided. Appropriate protection for the eyes should be worn when viewing a solar eclipse. Should blunt trauma have occurred, the injured patient is immediately assessed to ascertain the degree of damage. Visual acuity is checked. Shield the eye to prevent further damage until the patient is seen by an ophthalmologist. At this time, the pupil will be dilated with a mydriatic to facilitate ophthalmoscopic examination.

Inflammation

Inflammatory lesions in the choriocapillaris and pigment epithelium which result from organisms such as histoplasmosis or presumed viruses can also involve the macula. In histoplasmosis infection, macular involvement begins with a focal lesion involving the choriocapillaris and Bruch's membrane which produces atrophy of the pigment epithelium. Eventually, a scar forms and results in development of a neovascular membrane under the pigment epithelium. If this bleeds, then the sensory retina above the scar will become detached and show cystic change. If the blood is below the retinal pigment epithelium it will appear green on ophthalmoscopic examination. When it breaks through the pigment epithelium it will appear red. As the blood organizes and fibrosis sets in, a fibrous disciform scar in the macula will destroy the sensory cells and severely reduce the visual acuity.

Retinal pigment epithelitis is considered to be a viral infection of the retinal pigment epithelium beneath the neurosensory cells of the macula. Fluorescein angiography demonstrates it as a window defect. Ophthalmoscopically, it appears as an atrophic retinal pigment epithelium. Both eyes are usually involved and visual acuity is only slightly reduced. These lesions may resolve without visual loss, but recurrences may sometimes occur.

Senile Macular Degeneration

Two types of senile macular degeneration can occur. These are described as *atrophic (dry) and serous (exudative)*. The atrophic type has retinal pigmentary epithelial damage, choriocapillaris drop out, and loss of retinal photoreceptors occurs. There need not have been an exudative stage, and/or if a retinal pigmentary epi-

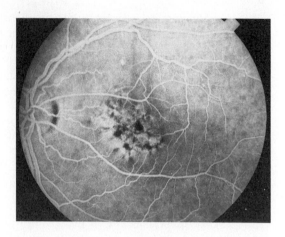

Figure 17–14. Senile macular degeneration.

thelium detachment has occurred it may have flattened out spontaneously without a trace. Laser therapy or other treatments are not indicated.

The exudative form of senile degeneration starts with a serous detachment of the pigment epithelium (Fig. 17–14). This can be identified on fluorescein angiography. There is early hyperfluorescence (as the vessels leak the dye) and even after the choroid has cleared the dye, fluorescent pools remain beneath the detached pigment epithelium. Following serous detachment of the retinal pigment epithelium, the fluid may be absorbed or it may be invaded with neovascular tissue which forms a net. The neovascular tissue hemorrhages easily, and if hemorrhage occurs then fibrous tissue invades and a scar forms with resultant atrophy and destruction of the overlying retina. It is in this latter type of senile macular degeneration that laser treatment is effective. The object is to "close" the neovascular net and not destroy the macula. Treatments are achieved with great care, for there is the risk of damaging central vision permanently. If the net is eliminated, then central vision should be maintained.

However, 165,000 new cases of macular degeneration occur in the United States each year, and many of these patients lose reading vision and fall into the category of being legally blind. They may be helped by using hand-held magnifiers, using large letter books, and retraining to use peripheral vision. These patients' lifestyles are changed considerably by the loss of acute vision.

Miscellaneous

The most prominent entity in the miscellaneous category which must be considered is *central serous choroidopathy or retinopathy.* This relatively common condition occurs most commonly between the ages of 25 to 50. There is an acute decrease in central vision with the development of metamorphopsia and distortion of letters and objects. The sensory retina is elevated. A fluorescein angiogram will show leakage of dye through the pigment epithelium which is usually detached. With time, the visual acuity improves spontaneously but the metamorphopsia remains. The leak through the retinal pigment epithelium heals but there is formation of a window defect. Amsler grid self-testing should be carried out by all patients with early macular degeneration to check if there is progression of this problem.

NURSING INTERVENTION
Initial assessment may reveal a central scotoma which can be identified by the history and on checking the visual acuity. Assess for systemic diseases.

PATIENT TEACHING
These patients are followed, and should be shown how to check the metamorphopsia with an Amsler grid several times a week (see Chap. 4).

Macular Hole. *Macular hole* may occur in elderly patients without any known cause. In these cases the pigment epithelium beneath the retinal hole becomes atrophic and the pigment is dispersed leaving a transparent area through which the choroidal vasculature may appear quite red. Central vision is decreased. There is no treatment for this problem.

Photocoagulation and Cryotherapy
Retinal holes and/or tears can be sealed when a chorioretinal scar is produced by *diathermy,* which causes a heat burn, *photocoagulation, or cryotherapy.* These latter two methods are also used to treat ischemic retina caused by new blood vessel growth. Photocoagulation treatments are directed at pathology located in the posterior pole, while cryotherapy, which causes a freeze, is usually reserved for anterior holes or pathology in the peripheral retina. If cryotherapy is to be used for pathology in the posterior portion of the eye, then the conjunctiva must be cut so that the eye can be rotated with exposure of the sclera, and this will be performed as a sterile surgical procedure.

Thermal photocoagulation or light coagulation as a treatment of ocular disease depends upon the absorption of light by the pigmented tissues, and the conversion of light energy into heat which enables the light to coagulate or denature the protein, as a burn is produced. Most of the light is absorbed by the pigment epithelium of the retina, but melanin is also present in the melanocytes of the choroid. Other pigments include xanthophyll, present in the macula, and hemoglobin which is normally confined to the red blood cells. Modern photocoagulation started when the xenon arc photocoagulator, with incoherent white light was designed in the 1950s by Meyer-Schwickerwrath. Xenon photocoagulation has been replaced by the laser photocoagulation.

The process by which *light is amplified by the stimulated emission of radiation,* is referred to as LASER.[22] The Argon blue–green and Krypton red lasers are most frequently used and have been adapted to the Slitlamp delivery system. (Newer lasers which are being used in ophthalmology include the CO_2, and Argon yellow and orange and the Nd:YAG, laser.) The Argon laser produces a spot size of 50 or 100μ, with short exposure time. The smaller spot sizes enable the physician to treat closer to the macular region. The intensity of the burn is variably affected by the

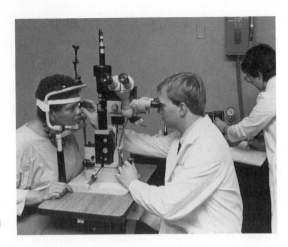

Figure 17–15. Nurse assisting with a laser treatment.

spot diameter, the power setting, the wavelength, and the duration. These are controlled from a panel, set on a table apart from the laser, and the physician will require assistance with changing the settings while the procedure is being performed (Fig. 17–15).

Before the procedure can be accomplished, the patient's pupils must be well dilated with one drop each of 1 percent tropicamide, 1 percent cyclopentolate hydrochloride, and 2.5 percent phenylephrine hydrochloride.

The patient is seated comfortably at the laser (Slitlamp) with the head secured in place, in the headrest, by a strap.

A proparacaine hydrochloride eyedrop is administered for topical anesthesia. A viscous solution such as Gonio-sol (methylcellulose) is placed on a goniolens, as the photocoagulation procedure is achieved through a contact lens placed on the eye. The procedure is now ready to begin. The patient will hear a clicking as each burst of energy is "pulsed," and will be aware of a bright flash of light. This procedure is not painful, but if the patient cannot keep the eye still, or complains of pain, then a retrobulbar anesthetic injection of 5 cc, 2 percent Carbocaine might be used prior to or even during the treatment. Most times this is not required. However, when it is used, the eye will be patched until the anesthesia wears off (about 6 hours). The patch may then be removed.

Clinical photocoagulation is used in the treatment of diseases of the retina and choroid, and most treatments are performed on an outpatient basis.

Cryotherapy can be performed if the patient's eye is well dilated, so that the physician can observe the retinal pathology while applying the cryoprobe to the external eye. A topical anesthetic eyedrop is also given. If the hole is a large one, anesthesia is achieved by administration of either a subconjunctival injection of 2 percent carbocaine hydrochloride or a 4 percent cocaine "pledget" (small wisp of cotton placed in the cul-de-sac), prior to placing the probe over the affected area. The eye is patched until anesthesia has worn off. These patients do experience a large degree of pain, and as a result of this will need to be given a prescription for pain medication following this outpatient treatment.

REFERENCES

1. Kozart DM: Anatomic correlates of the retina, in Duane TD, (Ed.): Clinical Ophthalmology. Hagerstown, Md.: Harper & Row, 1982, pp. 1–18
2. Charles S: Physiology of the retina, in Duane TD, (Ed.): Clinical Ophthalmology. Hagerstown, Md.: Harper & Row 1982, pp. 1–9
3. Boyd-Monk H: How to use a direct ophthalmoscope. Occupational Health Nursing, 31(8): 13–16, 1983
4. Weinstein GW: Clinical visual electrophysiology, in Duane TD, (Ed.): Clinical Ophthalmology. Hagerstown, Md.: Harper & Row, 1982, pp. 1–10
5. Coleman JD, Dallow RL: Introduction of ophthalmic ultrasonography, in Duane TD, (Ed.): Clinical Ophthalmology. Hagerstown, Md.: Harper & Row, 1983, pp. 1–5
6. Shields JA, Augsburger JJ: Current approaches to the diagnosis and management of retinoblastoma. Survey of Ophthalmology, 25(6): 347–372, 1981
7. Patz A, Payne JW: Retinopathy of prematurity (retrolental fibroplasia), in Duane TD, (Ed.): Clinical Ophthalmology. Hagerstown, Md.: Harper & Row, 1983, pp. 1–19
8. Hittner HM, Godio LB, Rudolph AJ, et al.: Retrolental fibroplasia: Efficacy of vitamin E in a double-blind clinical study of pre-term infants. New England Journal of Medicine, 305: 1365, 1981
9. Vaughan D, Asbury T: General Ophthalmology, 10th ed. Los Altos, Calif. Lange, 1983, pp. 137–157
10. Becker RA: Hypertension and arteriolosclerosis, in Duane TD, (Ed.): Clinical Ophthalmology. Hagerstown, Md.: Harper & Row, 1983, pp. 1–21
11. Benson WE, Tasman W, Duane TD: Diabetic retinopathy, in Duane TD, (Ed.): Clinical Ophthalmology. Hagerstown, Md.: Harper & Row, 1983, pp. 1–24
12. Kahn HA, Hiller R: Blindness caused by diabetic retinopathy. American Journal of Ophthalmology, 78: 58, 1974
13. Brown GC, Shields JA: Cilioretinal arteries and retinal arterial occlusion. Archives of Ophthalmology, 97: 84–92, 1979
14. Younge BR, Rosenbaum TJ: Treatment of acute central retinal artery occlusion. Mayo Clin Proc, 53: 408–410, 1978
15. Margargal LE, Goldberg RE: Anterior paracentesis in the management of acute non-arteritic central retinal artery occlusion. Surg Forum, 28:518–521, 1977
16. Augsburger JJ, Magargal LE: Visual prognosis following treatment of acute central retinal artery obstruction. British Journal of Ophthalmology, 64: 913–917, 1980
17. Magargal LE, Donoso LA, Sanborn GE: Retinal ischemia and risk of neovascularization following central vein obstruction. Ophthalmology, 89: 1241–1245, 1982
18. Zegarra H, Gutman FA, Conforto J: The natural course of central retinal vein occlusion. Ophthalmology, 86: 1931–1939, 1979
19. Magargal LE, Brown GA, Augsburger JJ, Parish RK: Neovascular glaucoma following central retinal vein obstruction. Ophthalmology, 88: 1095–1101, 1981
20. Hayreh SS, Rojas P, Podhajsky P, Montague P, Woolson RF: Ocular neovascularization with retinal vascular occlusion—III incidence of ocular neovascularization with retinal vein occlusion. Ophthalmology, 90: 488–506, 1983
21. Eagle RC, Lucier AC, Bernadino JB, Yanoff M: Retinal pigment epithelial abnormalities in fundus flavimaculatus. Ophthalmology, 87: 1189–1200, 1980
22. Swanson DE: Photocoagulation of the ocular fundus, in Duane TD, (Ed.): Clinical Ophthalmology. Hagerstown, Md.: Harper & Row, 1984, pp. 1–12

BIBLIOGRAPHY

Boyd-Monk H: Retinal detachment and vitrectomy: Nursing care. Nurs Clin North Amer, 16(3): 433–451, 1981

Deutman AF: The Hereditary Dystrophies of the Posterior Pole of the Eye. Netherlands: Assen, 1971

Smith JF, Nachazel DP: Ophthalmological Nursing. Boston: Little Brown, 1980

18

Optic Nerve and Visual Pathways

NEW TERMS

Anisocoria: unequal pupils.
Bitemporal hemianopsia: blindness occurring on the temporal side of both visual fields.
Contralateral: opposite side.
Decussate: term used for crossing of optic chiasm nerve fibers.
Homonymous hemianopsia: blindness in the opposite half of both visual fields.
Ipsilateral: same side.
Peripapillary: surrounding the optic disc.
Retrobulbar: behind the eyeball.
Scotoma: a blind or partially blind area in the visual field.

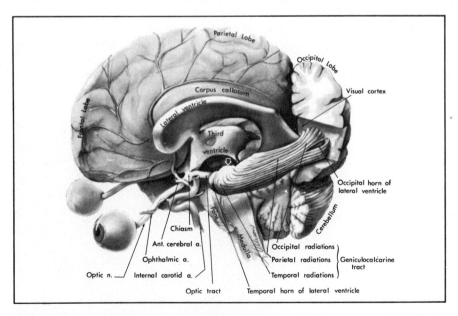

18–1. The visual sensory system. (*From Glaser JS: Anatomy of the sensory system, in Duane TD, (Ed.): Clinical Ophthalmology. Philadelphia: Harper & Row, 1984, p. 2, with permission.*)

THE OPTIC NERVE

The axons of the ganglionic cells of the retina leave the eyeball at the posterior pole and form a large multiaxonial nerve called the *optic nerve*. This is the second cranial nerve and is the initial pathway of the visual sensory system (Fig. 18–1). Eighty percent of this nerve is made up of visual fibers, while the remaining 20 percent are afferent pupillary fibers. Before the optic nerve leaves the globe, it appears as a round, orange area called the *optic disc* or the *optic nerve head* (Fig. 18–2). This nerve head is approximately 1.5 mm in diameter and is the easiest landmark to distinguish on ophthalmoscopy. There are no photoreceptors in the optic disc, and this is projected as an absolute scotoma, known as the "blind spot." From the center of the nerve head, branches of the *central retinal artery* radiate to the periphery, while the peripheral retinal veins converge toward the disc's center to form the *central retinal vein*.

The optic nerve head usually has an orange hue, but may vary from grayish red to red. If the nerve head is chalk white or waxy yellow it may signify optic nerve atrophy. Normally the anterior contour of the optic disc has a slight indentation or cup, referred to as the *physiological cup*. This cup should be about one-third the size of the optic disc. If this cup on the disc is deep, it will expose the white scleral wall with its many perforations through which the ganglion cells' axons pass. This perforated scleral wall is known as the *lamina cribrosa*. As the axons pass the lamina cribrosa they become myelinated, increasing the diameter of the optic nerve to 3 to 4 mm. While the optic nerve looks like a white peripheral nerve, it acts like a tract of the brain in that if it is cut it will not regenerate. The meninges form the sheaths of the nerves. The dura of the nerve and periosteum of the bones are fused, but the subarachnoid space communicates with the intracranial subarachnoid and contains cerebrospinal fluid. As the nerve leaves the orbit it passes through the *optic foramen* and bony canal into the cranial cavity where it meets the optic nerve from the other eye. At this junction of the optic nerves, called the *optic chiasm*, there is a *crossing of the axons from the nasal retina* and these fibers now run together with

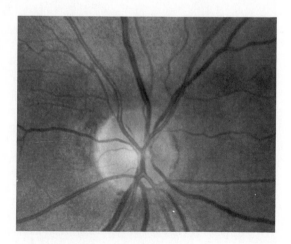

Figure 18–2. Normal optic disc.

the *uncrossed axons of the temporal retina* of the other eye. These crossed and uncrossed axons form the *optic tract* in the brain which permits the left half of the visual field to be represented by the right half of the central visual cortex and vice versa.[1,2]

EXAMINING THE OPTIC DISC

The shape and size of the optic nerve head is usually the same in each eye or there may appear to be a variation on ophthalmoscopic examination. Distortion of the ophthalmoscopic image may be due to refractive error. Hypermetropic eyes have a smaller appearing disc, while the disc appears quite large in myopic eyes. Astigmatism may distort the optic nerve head so that it will appear oval. The nerve head may slant, depending upon the axis and amount of the astigmatic refractive error. In high hypermetropia, the nerve head may have a smaller diameter. The nerve may enter the globe at a slanting angle and there may be an inversus of the retinal vessels with a slanting of the vessels nasalward instead of along customary temporal paths.

A bare scleral area known as conus, may partially surround the nerve head. In myopia this is usually due to stretching of choroid with peripapillary atrophy exposing sclera. The pigment epithelium of the choroid may proliferate at the edge of the optic nerve giving it a dark collar made up of clumps of pigment.

The vasculature of the nerve head may also vary with the vessels forming different patterns. The presence of the *cilioretinal artery* running from the temporal nerve head to supply the macula may be seen. The importance of this artery is demonstrated when there is a central retinal artery occlusion and this vessel maintains the circulation to the macula.

CONGENITAL ANOMALIES

The optic nerve may have congenital anomalies, which vary from a pit (a little depression) to coloboma and cyst.

Coloboma results when failure of the optic fissure to close may leave a gaping white scar in the inferior and infero temporal optic nerve. *Cyst* formations may occur in the nerve and the adjacent retina may be folded into the cyst. When the fusion of the coloboma is nearly, but not quite completed, there is a deep depression or absence of optic nerve tissue which forms a *pit*. These pits may adversely affect vision.

ACQUIRED ANOMALIES

Amblyopia is a name given to reduced vision in an apparently normal eye and optic nerve. This may be due to toxic chemicals, such as accidental methanol (methyl alcohol) poisoning or drugs, e.g., quinine compounds used in the treatment and prevention of malaria. The amblyopia can be nutritional due to alcohol and tobacco where there is an associated deficient diet. In *amblyopia exanopsia,* central vision loss occurs when the eye is not used. This occurs in children with crossed or deviated eyes—when one eye is used for seeing and fixation, the deviated eye is not used for fixation—and the child is able to suppress central vision. Patching of the good eye under ophthalmologic supervision is initiated to stimulate useful vision in the amblyopic eye.

NURSING INTERVENTION
Nurses responsible for visual screening of children should refer any child who has a difference of two or more lines in his or her vision when reading the visual acuity chart to the ophthalmologist.

PATIENT TEACHING
Compliance should be encouraged for any treatment regimen prescribed for the patient who is identified as having amblyopia due to poor nutrition resulting from chronic alcoholism.

Optic Nerve Pathology
Pathology of the optic nerve can occur as a result of many different diseases and can be seen on ophthalmoscopic evaluation in varying forms.

Atrophy of the optic nerve can be induced by trauma such as cutting, evulsion, and contusion. Glaucoma destroys the ganglion cells and produces atrophy of the axons. Circulatory problems produce hemorrhage and ischemia. Multiple sclerosis, which is a demyelinating disease, may also produce atrophy. Severe malnutrition, as was seen in prisoner of war camps, can cause optic atrophy and blindness. No effective treatment is available once optic atrophy has developed.

Papilledema (chocked disc) (Fig. 18–3) is the swelling of the nerve head and is most frequently caused by an increase in intracranial pressure. It is nearly always bilateral and can be due to brain tumor, malignant hypertension, or thrombosis of the central retinal vein. In the beginning, papilledema has little visual loss but visual field examination might reveal enlargement of the blind spot. Later however, depending upon the cause, the patient may have marked visual deterioration. A thorough neurological examination is indicated. Treatment is directed at the cause which can result in complete resolution of the papilledema, however, unresolved long-standing papilledema may result in optic atrophy. *Pseudopapilledema* occurs in small or hypermetropic eyes and resembles papilledema ophthalmoscopically, but is stationary and causes no visual loss. *Drusen of the optic nerve head* may also resemble papilledema with few symptoms and rarely causes visual loss.

Other signs and symptoms with papilledema are related to the basic pathological process which has caused the increased intracranial pressure. Headache, nausea and vomiting, and lateral recti (muscle) weakness may be evident and can be associated with raised cerebrospinal fluid (CSF) pressure. Visual field defects, specific ocular motility disturbances, hemiparesis, and seizures all help to localize the lesion.

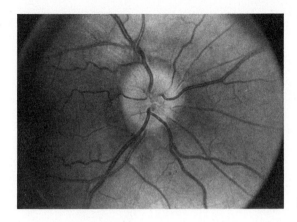

Figure 18–3. Papilledema.

Optic Neuritis

The term "optic neuritis" is best reserved for primary inflammation of the nerve, including that accompanying demyelinating disease or contiguous spread of inflammation from meninges, orbital tissues, or paranasal sinuses. Papillitis is the typical form of optic neuritis in childhood, while unilateral retrobulbar neuritis is the common form in adults. The more general term of "optic neuropathy" is used where the nerve is damaged by vascular, compressive or unknown mechanisms.[2]

Papillitis is disc swelling caused by local inflammatory process of the nerve head.[2] It resembles all of the findings described in papilledema, but has visual loss early and may be associated with retinal edema, exudates, or hemorrhages around the disc. Often there is also an associated orbital neuralgia which is increased by rotating the globe. In children, papillitis is the common form of neuritis, though etiology is infrequently determined. Severe cases should be treated with systemic corticosteroids. Papillitis is also found in intraocular diseases such as vitritis, retinitis, and endophthalmitis.

Retrobulbar neuritis is an inflammation of the nerve that can cause rapid visual reduction without intraocular signs or changes. This acute impairment of vision progresses rapidly for hours or days, reaching its lowest level by 1 week after onset. In the majority of cases visual function begins to improve in the second or third week. Many patients enjoy normal or near-normal vision as it continues to improve over the next several months. In adults, the typical episode involves one eye only. Visual field defects usually involve the central field with the diminution of acuity. The leading cause of this is probably multiple sclerosis, and the episode may be an isolated incident. However, a small number of patients have exacerbations and remissions of the disease which may eventually produce pallor and atrophy of the optic nerve head. The largest proportion of cases of optic neuritis present without identifiable underlying cause. Such cases may follow a nonspecific upper respiratory infection, and therefore a viremia may be implicated.[2] Corticotropin therapy may or may not be prescribed.

Ischemic optic neuropathy occurs with infarction of the anterior portion of the optic nerve and results in sudden, painless loss of vision. Usually the patient is elderly. In this disease, there is usually no inflammation, demyelinization, or lesion which causes the compression. In the *nonarteritic* type, the majority of patients will

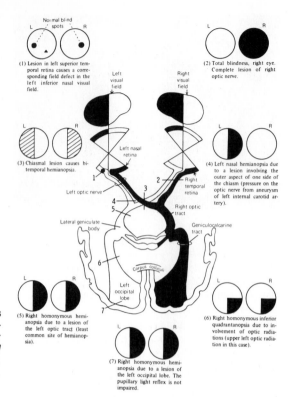

Figure 18–4. Visual field defects associated with lesions of the visual system. (*From Chusid JG: Correlative Neuroanatomy and Functional Neurology, 19th ed. Los Altos, Calif.: Lange, 1985, p. 204, with permission.*)

have hypertension, though arteriosclerosis, carotid artery disease, or postoperative occurrence following cataract surgery may be elicited. Treatment is directed at the hypertension, and at the underlying cause if possible.

The *arteritic* disease occurs equally in patients between 60 and 70 years of age, both male and female, and the visual loss is devastating. (This disease rarely occurs in blacks.) Headache, scalp tenderness over the tortuous, pulseless, nodular temporal artery, precludes them from brushing their hair or lying on a pillow on that side; myalgias and malaise are the main symptoms. The patient may have a central scotoma or other visual field defect (Figure 18–4). When the fundus is examined, there is pale swelling of the optic nerve head, with the edema being profuse or localized; peripapillary streak hemorrhages and retinal arteriole narrowing may also be seen. Optic atrophy ensues as disc edema resolves. One-half to one-third of these patients will have an occurrence in the other eye, and when this occurs, a "pseudo-Foster-Kennedy syndrome" may be present. This is described as disc edema in one eye and optic atrophy in the other.[2] Laboratory studies show that the erythrocyte sedimentation rate (ESR) is increased. Although it has been found that ESR increases with age and is "elevated" (greater than 20 mm per hr) in apparently healthy elderly subjects.[2]

The patient is hospitalized for diagnositc studies which includes a *temporal artery biopsy* and treatment which ranges from steroids 60 to 100 mg given orally, daily to *pulse therapy* of corticosteroids 250 mg given intravenously over 30 minutes every 6 hours for 12 doses. Then the steroid is changed to oral administration of Prednisone 80 mg daily, which is gradually tapered off as the ESR rate returns to normal.

NURSING INTERVENTION
Initial assessment of visual acuity will need to be taken. The vision loss may have been sudden or the patient may describe having had occasional amaurosis attacks. Symptoms of discomfort or headache or tenderness over the temporal artery may be elicited. The patient will need to be prepared for diagnostic studies which will include a skull x-ray or CT scan; a tuberculosis (Tb) skin test such as the TINE or PPD will be given prior to starting the steroids. The patient should be observed closely during the administration of the *pulse therapy* for symptoms of disorientation which certainly can be a problem. Note any petechiae spots which may appear. Check the blood sugar values which have been ordered, for there is often an increase in blood sugar. Notify the physician of any changes as they occur and document the findings. The patient's temporal scalp area may need to be shaved if a biopsy is planned when *giant cell arteritis* is suspected.

Tumors
Tumors of the optic nerve are fortunately rare. Gliomas can cause visual impairment, and as they grow larger can also proptose the globe. Unfortunately, most of these grow within the optic nerve and the nerve must be sectioned for removal which blinds the eye. Optic nerve gliomas can also occur in association with systemic disease such as neurofibromas (von Recklinghausen's disease).

Meningiomas grow from the covering of the optic nerve and may impair vision by compression. Some of these can be removed without sectioning the nerve.

NURSING INTERVENTION
Nursing intervention for orbital surgery was discussed in Chapter 9.

THE VISUAL PATHWAYS

The primary visual–sensory system in man comprises the *retina* and the *optic nerves,* which decussate at the *chiasm* and continue on to the *lateral geniculate body*. These visual neurons synapse to form the *geniculocalcarine tract,* then proceed to the *calcarine cortex* in the occipital lobe. The pupillary motor fibers leave the optic tracts anterior to the lateral geniculate bodies en route to the *midbrain's pretectal area via the brachium of the superior colliculus*.

Examination of the Pupils
The examination of the pupils and their reactions is simple, quickly done, and gives important information about the visual pathways. Normal pupils are round, equal in

diameter, and will constrict in bright light and accommodation. Pupils should be looked at in both dim and bright illumination. There is an anisocoria in 20 to 25 percent of people, which is normal.

In order to examine a patient's pupil:

1. The patient should fixate at a distance and then a light is shone into one eye from an oblique angle (Fig. 18–5). The normal pupil should constrict and if the reaction is normal, the opposite pupil will behave in similar fashion. These reactions are known as the *direct and consensual* pupillary reflexes. Normal pupils should constrict briskly to become miotic and then gradually escape from the constriction and become an intermediate size.
2. There is a constriction of the pupil when the patient *accommodates* or fixates at near. For this, the light or an object is held about 13 inches from the eyes, and the patient is asked to look at the object.
3. The amount of miosis for near should be compared with the amount of miosis occurring when a direct light is shone into the eye. The latter miosis should be equal to or greater than the miosis which occurs with accommodation. Pupillary diameter is measured in millimeters.

Abnormal Pupillary Reactions.   The *Marcus Gun pupil* (afferent pupillary reaction) is an asymmetric pupillary reaction to light. The affected optic nerve prevents the direct light stimuli from producing full constriction, but maintains the consensual reflex when the light is shone in the normal eye. This demonstrates that the damaged optic nerve *does not* transmit the light stimuli, while the intact nerve *does* transmit light stimuli.

In order to elicit this pupillary reaction, the *swinging light test* is performed. The light is shone in one eye, and the size of the pupils are observed in both eyes (if there is no pupillary defect both pupils will constrict consensually). The light is "swung" across to the other eye, and the pupils are observed (if there is an afferent pupillary defect neither pupil will constrict).

Argyll Robertson pupils are small irregular pupils that do not react to light but do constrict when looking at near. These pupils neither dilate well in the dark, nor do mydriatics produce dilation. This type of pupillary reaction occurs in neurosyphilis.

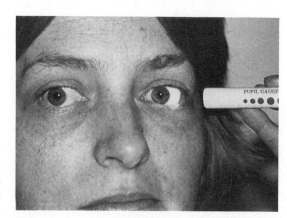

Figure 18–5. To examine the pupils, the light should be shone at an oblique angle.

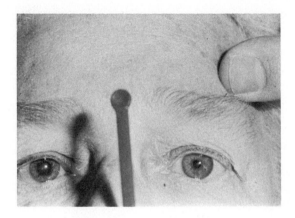

Figure 18–6. Adie's pupil will not constrict on accommodation. (*Photograph courtesy of Wills Eye Hospital.*)

Adie's pupil (Fig. 18–6) is usually a unilateral and dilated pupil which shows no rapid constriction to bright light but may slowly constrict under continuous bright light stimuli. Most frequently, the Adie's pupil is seen in young females with depressed deep tendon reflexes. The significance of this is not known, but the patient who has this type of unequal pupillary reaction should wear a "meditag" identifying the entity in case its presence should be misconstrued as being the result of an injury.

Horner's syndrome consists of ptosis of the upper lid and miosis of the affected eye. The apparent enophthalmos is caused by the ptosis and narrowing of the palpebral fissure. Absence of sweating on the face and neck on the same side comprise the complete syndrome. It is caused by a superior cervical sympathetic ganglion lesion, and may occur as a result of trauma, tumor, or systemic disease.

CRANIAL NERVES ASSOCIATED WITH THE EYE AND THE ADNEXA II, III, IV, V, VI, AND VII

The cranial nerve that plays a role in the coordination and maintenance of the health of the eyes is the *II nerve (optic),* and as previously discussed, any insult on this nerve produces a decrease in vision.

III nerve (oculomotor) paresis occurs as a result of many causes and both site and/or causes may be difficult to locate. However, the nerve does split into two divisions before entering the orbit. The *superior branch innervates the levator superioris muscle of the upper lid, and superior rectus muscle. The interior branch of the third nerve innervates the following extraocular muscles: the interior rectus, the medial rectus, inferior oblique, and the intrinsic pupillary and ciliary body musculature which controls the lens' shape in accommodation.* In a large series of III nerve palsy, undetermined cause accounted for 24 percent; aneurysm 21 percent; ischemia 18 percent; head trauma 13 percent; neoplasms 12 percent; and miscellaneous 12 percent.[1]

Assessment reveals a divergent strabismus, the pupil is dilated and fixed, accommodation is absent, and there is ptosis of the upper lid (Fig. 18–7).

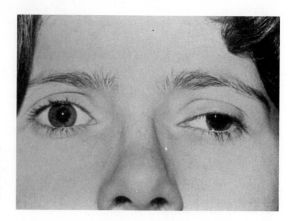

Figure 18–7. Assessment of the III nerve palsy will reveal a divergent strabismus, a dilated pupil, and a ptosis of the upper eyelid. (*Photograph courtesy of Wills Eye Hospital.*)

The *IV (trochlear) cranial nerve* palsy produces vertical muscle imbalance, due to its *innervation of the superior oblique masculature.* There are other causes of verticle deviation and the antagonists have to be carefully examined before a definitive diagnosis of IV nerve palsy is made. Trauma can be a cause of damage to this nerve. The patient may complain of diplopia, which can be relieved by tilting the head.

The *V (trigeminal) cranial nerve* is a *sensory nerve the first division of which can be involved in local corneal disease,* i.e., herpes simplex keratitis and after cataract extraction. Other involvement of intracranal nature can produce referred pain. Trigeminal neuralagia (tic douloureaux) with its lightning-like flashes of hemifacial pain is well-known.

The *VI (abducens) cranial nerve innervates the lateral rectus muscles.* Thirty percent of the VI nerve palsies are of undetermined etiology, and these are transient and benign. Because of its long, anatomical course, many causes for the palsy must be investigated. Cerebrovascular accidents are a common cause. Lesions in the brain stem, elevated intracranial pressure producing tugging on the nerve, contact with an inflamed petrous pyramid produced by an otitis media, cavernous sinus disease or lesions, orbital involvement with tumor, and inflammation or thyroid disease round out the cause of VI nerve palsy associated with other cranial nerve problems.

If nothing previously mentioned can be identified, then the isolated VI nerve palsy is probably due to an ischemic mononeuropathy. Esotropia is present in the primary position and increases upon gaze to the affected side.

The *VII (facial) cranial nerve* is a motor nerve which innovates the musculature of the face and runs with the *nervus intermedius* which produces tearing, salivation, and taste as well as the nerve to the stapedius muscle of the middle ear. This nerve also innervates the *obicularis oculi muscle* whose function is to close the lids. The most common facial palsy is seen in Bell's palsy. This is due to swelling of the nerve in the Fallopian canal. There is total ipsilateral facial palsy with ptosis and loss of obicularis tone. Complete recovery may occur in 75 percent of patients within 60 days. However, these patients must be checked for exposure keratitis.

Nystagmus is seen as involuntary rhythmic to and fro oscillations of the eyes. It is important to note the direction of the component, the amount or amplitude, the occurrence or rate, whether it is jerky or pendular and whether it is horizontal, vertical, circular, or rotatory elliptical. The etiologies are varied from congenital, poor vision to brain tumors. Downbeat nystagmus usually indicates a brainstem lesion.[1]

NURSING INTERVENTION

1. Observe the overall appearance and attitude of the patient as he or she presents for attention. Note degree of distress, anxiety, and coherent or incoherent ability to describe symptoms.
2. Elicit the patient's *chief complaint* by asking "What is troubling you?"
3. Observe the overall *appearance of the lids and the eyeball.*
4. Check the *visual acuity* using a Snellen Chart and ordinary newsprint. If the patient wears *corrective lenses,* the visual acuity should be checked *with* and *without* them.
5. Examine the pupils for *direct and indirect pupillary response.*
6. The III, IV, and VI (oculomotor, trochlear, and abducens) nerves are tested as a unit, since they all supply eye muscles for movement. The oculomotor nerve also supplies the muscles which constrict the pupils and those which elevate the eyelids.
   a. The range of *ocular movement is checked* by asking the patient to follow the movement of the examiner's fingers *in the cardinal directions of gaze* (see Chap. 19). If there is involvement of the oculomotor nerve, the patient will be unable to look up, down, or nasally with the affected eye, the pupil will be dilated, and ptosis will be present.
   b. If the affected nerve is the trochlear, the patient will be unable to look downward and laterally.
   c. If the abducens nerve is affected, the patient will be unable to look down laterally with the involved eye. In each of these positions (a, b, and c), the patient will complain of *diplopia.*
7. Observe for any signs of nystagmus when performing these tests.
8. To conduct a *visual field* test, the patient is asked to cover one eye and look at the examiner's nose. Using the confrontation method described in Chapter 5, ask the patient to identify the number of fingers shown in each quadrant of the visual field. This can be done verbally by the adult, or as a finger mimicking game with a child. Then move the fingers in from the periphery until they can be seen by the patient. The test is performed on each eye separately and can reveal gross defects.

   Visual field tests can reveal the normal blind spot in each eye as well as defects along the visual system (Fig. 18–4).

   A retinal lesion may produce a blind spot in the affected eye. An optic nerve lesion produces partial or complete blindness in the same eye. A chiasmal lesion causes a bitemporal hemianopsia, while a lesion of one optic tract or one lateral geniculate body results in blindness in the opposite half of both visual fields referred to as homonymous hemianopsia. An abnormality in the temporal lobe may produce blindness in the upper quadrant of both visual fields on the side opposite the lesion.

9. The neurological evaluation is not complete until a thorough *ophthalmoscopic examination* of the optic disc, vessels, and peripheral retina have been accomplished. Small pupils may hamper this examination for the nurse, and pupils will definitely have to be dilated at the conclusion of the *neurological examination* if fundoscopy is performed. Documentation of the nature of the cycloplegic eyedrop is mandatory.

10. Slitlamp examination by the physician will complete this examination.

REFERENCES

1. Bajandas, FJ: Neuro-ophthalmology Board Review Manual. Thorofare, N.J.: Slack, 1980, pp. 1–44
2. Glaser JS: Topical diagnosis: Prechiasmal visual pathways, in Duane TD, (Ed.): Clinical Ophthalmology. Hagerstown, Md.: Harper & Row, 1983, pp. 1–60

BIBLIOGRAPHY

Brown GC, Augsburger JJ: Congenital pits of the optic nerve head and retinochoroidal colobomas. Canadian Journal of Ophthalmology, 15:144–146, 1980

Brown GC, Shields JA: Tumors of the optic nerve head. Survey of Ophthalmology, 29(4): 239–264, 1985

Brown GC, Tasman W: Congenital Anomalies of the Optic Disc. New York: Grunes & Walton, 1983

Condi JK: Types and causes of nystagmus in the neurosurgical patient. J Neurosurg Nurs, 15(2): 56–64, 1983

Vaughan D, Asbury T: General Ophthalmology, 10th ed. Los Altos, Calif. Lange, 1983

Voke J: The visual pathway. Nurs Mirror, 156(9): 46–47, 1983

19
The Extraocular Muscles

NEW TERMS

Cycloductions: rotation of the eyeball around the anterior–posterior axis.
Esophoria: latent inward deviation of the eye.
Esotropia: manifest inward deviation of the eye.
Exophoria: latent outward deviation of the eye.
Exotropia: manifest outward deviation of the eye.
Hyperphoria: latent upward deviation of the eye.
Hypertropia: manifest upward deviation of the eye.
Hypophoria: latent downward deviation of the eye.
Hypotropia: manifest downward deviation of the eye.

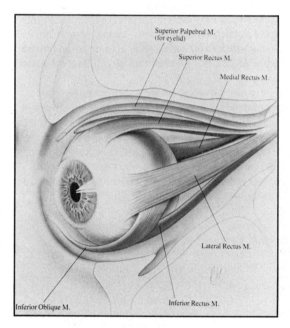

19–1. The extraocular muscles. (*From Friedman AH, Desmarest RJ, Westwood WB: The Optyl Atlas of the Human Eye. Norwood, N.J.: The Optyl Corporation, 1979, with permission.*)

The movement of an eye is produced by six extraocular muscles (Fig. 19–1). Four of these muscles are called *recti* and two are called *obliques*. The recti all originate from a cartilaginous ring at the apex of the orbit. The *superior rectus* muscle originates at the superior portion of the ring and runs over the top of the globe inserting anterior to the equator of the globe. The *inferior rectus* muscle originates from the inferior portion of the ring and inserts at the bottom of the globe anterior to the equator. The *lateral rectus* muscle originates from the lateral aspect of the ring at the apex of the orbit and inserts on the temporal side of the globe, in front of the equator. The *medial internal rectus* muscle attaches to the nasal side of the globe anterior to the equator.

The *superior oblique* muscle arises from the cartilaginous ring at the orbital apex between and above the origin of the superior rectus and the medial rectus muscles. It does not insert directly on the globe, but becomes a tendon as it approaches the superior nasal orbital rim where it passed through a cartilaginous ring known as the *trochlear*. Its direction is then reversed, and it courses backwards at about a 50-degree angle, to pass under the belly of the superior rectus, after which it inserts obliquely into the sclera just above the macula. The *inferior oblique* muscle originates on the nasal inferior orbital floor and passes beneath the belly of the inferior rectus to insert into the temporal sclera, behind the equator of the globe under the belly of the lateral rectus.

If one muscle contracts it will rotate the globe in the direction of pull. Some of the muscles will cause a twisting rotation movement of the globe which is known as *torsion*. The first type of pull is called *primary direction of rotation*. The torsional rotation is called *secondary rotation*. Table 19–1 identifies each extraocular muscle's primary and secondary action of rotation where there is one.

The superior and inferior recti have their greatest primary actions when the eye is turned temporally, and the obliques have their greatest primary action when the eye is turned nasally.

The muscles do not act independently, but must work with the muscle producing the opposite movement. When one contracts, the opposite or antagonist muscle must relax in order to produce a smooth movement (Table 19–2).

The six extraocular muscles are normally in a state of slight contracture. This gives the globe a stability even when at rest. All the extraocular muscles play a role in smooth eye movements either by contracting or relaxing. This muscle coordination is not only done with six extraocular muscles of one eye but in conjunction with the six extraocular muscles of the other eye (Fig. 19–2).

TABLE 19–1. ACTION OF SPECIFIC MUSCLES

Muscle	Primary Rotation	Secondary Rotation or Torsion
Lateral rectus	Toward the lateral side	None
Superior rectus	Upward	Toward the nose
Internal rectus	Toward the nose	None
Inferior rectus	Downward	Toward temporal side
Inferior oblique	Upward	Toward temporal side
Superior oblique	Downward	Toward the nose

TABLE 19–2. YOKE MUSCLES AND ANTAGONISTS

Yoke Muscles	Antagonists
Right medial rectus	Medial rectus—lateral rectus
Left lateral rectus	
Right lateral rectus	Superior rectus—inferior rectus
Left medial rectus	
Right superior rectus	Superior oblique—inferior oblique
Left inferior oblique	
Right inferior rectus	
Left superior oblique	
Right superior oblique	
Left inferior rectus	
Right inferior oblique	
Left superior rectus	

CARDINAL DIRECTIONS OF GAZE

The muscles in one eye are yoked to muscles in the opposite eye that produce the motion in the same direction. Cardinal directions of gaze enables the examiner to observe the actions of the extraocular muscles in six different positions. The schematic drawings demonstrate a pair of eyes looking in each cardinal direction. The dense black muscles represent muscles exerting major pull, while shaded muscles produce less pull. Muscles that are not shaded or blackened are not exerting any rotational power to the specific movement.

There are two other positions which can be tested. Upward gaze with superior recti of both eyes doing the major contracting and the obliques helping out. Downward gaze uses the inferior recti muscles with assistance from superior oblique muscles. The muscles must therefore produce motion in the same direction for both eyes (Figs. 19–3 and 19–4).

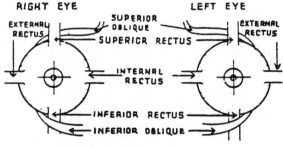

ALL MUSCLES RELAXED - EYES LOOKING STRAIGHT AHEAD

Figure 19–2. Schematic drawing of muscles with eyes looking straight ahead.

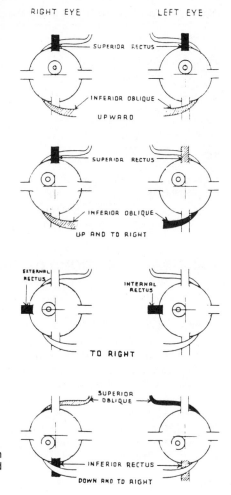

Figure 19-3. Extraocular muscles involved in each cardinal position of gaze with eyes turned to the right including upward gaze.

BINOCULAR VISION

Binocular vision is a term which means both eyes are functioning well with convergence of the line of sight, when an object is viewed within 20 feet and nearer. The *average pupillary distance is 63 mm for the adult;* therefore, the eyes converge in order to simultaneously look at a near object. *Accommodation* is another reflex associated with the convergence, and this necessitates the focusing of the eyes for near. The image is therefore kept in sharp focus on the same areas of the retinas. In convergence the eyes are also rotated downward and the internal recti and superior obliques of both eyes produce this complicated movement together so that their visual axis impinges on the identical object (Fig. 19-5). If superimposition of the objects seen can be accomplished in the brain, this is known as *single binocular*

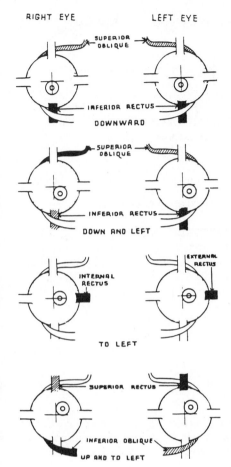

RIGHT EYE   LEFT EYE

Figure 19-4. Extraocular muscles involved in downward gaze and each cardinal position of gaze with eyes turned to the left.

vision. The degrees of fusional ability helps to hold single binocular vision. If fusion does not exist or is broken, the eyes tend to deviate outward or converge inward, and double vision (diplopia) may occur.

Methods of Testing for Extraocular Muscle Imbalances
Hirschberg Method. A flashlight is used as a fixation light, and the light reflex from the cornea is observed. *Normally, the light reflex is about 1 mm nasally from the center of each cornea.* If the reflex in one eye is temporal to the normal position this indicates that the eye is turning inward. This is called *esotropia* (ET) (Fig. 19–6). If the reflex is on the nasal side of the normal position which indicates the eye is turning outward, this is known as *exotropia* (XT) (Fig. 19–7). If the reflexes are located in a similar position on both corneas then a cover–uncover test may reveal a *latent deviation or phoria.*

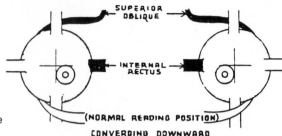

Figure 19–5. To accommodate the eyes, converge downward.

Cover–Uncover Test. To perform the cover–uncover test follow these steps:

1. First, cover one eye and have the patient fixate with the other eye.
2. Switch the cover to the fixating eye.
   a. If the uncovered eye has deviated, then it is important to *note the direction it moves* when it again picks up the fixation light.
   b. If the eye moves toward the nose then it is an outward deviation or an *exophoria*.
   c. If the globe moves from the nasal corner outward to pick up fixation, then it is called an *esophoria*.
3. The evaluation of extraocular muscle action can be performed with just a flashlight.
4. Determination of the amount of deviation is done by measuring with prisms.

STRABISMUS

Strabismus or *squint* is a condition in which the visual axis of both eyes do not fixate on the object being observed. There are two types of strabismus, *paralytic* and *nonparalytic*. Strabismus due to paralysis or paresis of one or more extraocular

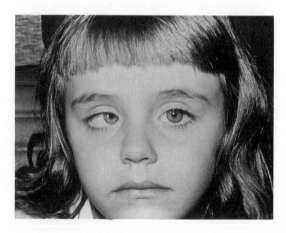

Figure 19–6. Right esotropia.

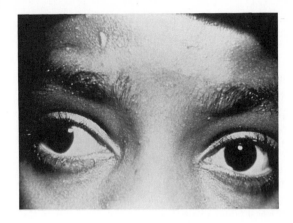

Figure 19-7. Right exotropia.

muscles, may have resulted from the weakening of the muscle or a lesion in the nerve nuclei or in the muscle itself. Both types can be either congenital or acquired.

Nonparetic causes are *inadequate fusion, overative accommodative convergence reflex,* and *refractive errors* which may be unequal or equal. All three, or any combination of the nonparetic causes, may influence the final muscle imbalance. Nonparalytic squints are described as being:

- Intermittent—when they are not present all the time.
- Variable—when the amount of squint varies from time to time or at different times during the day.
- Alternating—when the eyes alternate fixation, and the nonfixing eye deviates.

Congenital anomalies of extraocular muscles such as fibrosis, hypertrophy, and aberrant insertions of the muscles may cause squint. Other causes of squint are intraocular tumors, cataracts (which can be congenital, secondary, and/or senile), and optic atrophy.

Results of Strabismus

Head tilt can occur if the vertical corneal meridians are not parallel. By tilting the head, the posteral and fusional reflexes attempt to produce parallelism by rotating the eyes around the anterior–posterior axis. This type of rotation is known as *cycloduction*. The oblique muscles are the major muscles producing cycloduction. Sometimes a patient will tilt his or her head to avoid diplopia.

Amblyopia exanopsia is the decrease in vision of a normal eye due to nonfixation because of deviation. The treatment of this condition is to correct any refractive error and then occlude the good fixing eye, thus forcing the nonfixing eye to begin to fixate. In order for this to be successful, it must be carried out before a child is 6 or 7 years old.

Occlusion can be achieved by using an orthoptic eye patch applied to the closed eye or by patching the lens of the glasses, using a frosted lens or coats of clear nail polish. Proper and prolonged patching can restore useful vision. Muscle surgery is then used to correct the deviation and with good and equal vision, the eyes will maintain normal adjustment.

Muscle Surgery

Corrective extraocular muscle surgery for squint falls into three main categories:

1. *Strengthening* of a muscle by shortening the muscle or tendon.
2. *Weakening* of a muscle by lengthening the muscle.
3. *Transplanting* a muscle to improve the rotation of a paralyzed muscle.

Strengthening of the muscle can be accomplished in two ways. The muscle may be detached from its insertion and a portion *resected;* the muscle can then be reattached to the original site on the sclera or it can be advanced beyond the original insertion; or a tuck can be made in the belly of the muscle thus producing shortening of the muscle which will increase the amount of rotation obtained.

To weaken the muscle, the muscle may be detached from the globe and *recessed* to a more posterior location and then the muscle is reattached. This will weaken the action of the muscle. Partial marginal myotomies of the muscle belly will permit the muscle fibers to stretch and will weaken the action of the involved muscle.

In squint caused by muscular paralysis, the action may be implemented by transplanting a slip of another muscle to aid in the rotational movement of the eye.

Combinations of *resection* of one muscle with *recession* of the antagonist will produce greater correction than surgery on one muscle only. Recently, *adjustable sutures* have been employed which can be tightened or loosened the morning following surgery after the patient has recovered from anesthesia. This requires an overnight stay in the hospital and is done at the patient's bedside.

NURSING INTERVENTION

The cardinal directions of gaze are of value in assessing not only the extraocular muscles, but also the nerves which innervate them. Pupillary reaction is frequently used to assess neurological status.

In most instances muscle surgery is accomplished as a same-day surgical procedure, and the patient or parent of the patient will be contacted by telephone prior to admission to the surgical unit in order to offer preoperative instructions, and obtain pertinent health information.

PATIENT TEACHING

Following surgery, the eye(s) are not usually patched, but the parent of a child should be aware that the tears will appear serosanguianous for a little while. The cheek, rather than the eye should be mopped. Following surgery, a combination antibiotic–steroid eyedrop may be prescribed. The parent should be instructed with respect to instillation of this medication.

BIBLIOGRAPHY

Jay WM, Calvert JC: The child with strabismus. American Family Physician, 23(4): 156–62, 1981

Nelson LB: Pediatric Ophthalmology. Philadelphia: Saunders, 1984

Nelson LB, Wagner RS: Strabismus surgery. International Ophthalmol Clin, 25(4) 1–35, 1985

Scott WE, D'Agostino DD, Lennarson LW: Orthoptics and Ocular Examination Technique. Baltimore: Williams & Wilkins, 1983

Vaughan A, Asbury T: General Ophthalmology, 10th ed. Los Altos, Calif.: Lange, pp. 174–193, 1983

20

Glaucoma

NEW TERMS

Anterior synechia: adhesions between the iris and cornea.
Disc cupping: excavated and enlarged physiological cup.
Posterior synechia: adhesions between the iris and lens.
Rubeosis iridis: neovascularization of the iris.
Synechia: adhesions.

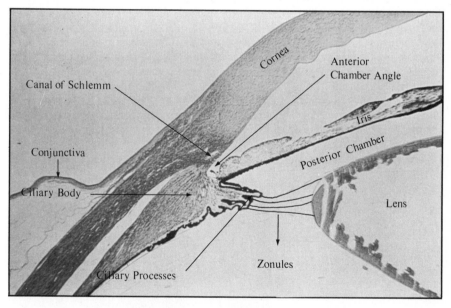

20–1. Histological section of the angle of a normal eye.

The anatomical iridocorneal junction forms an *angle* (Fig. 20–1) in which a sieve-like structure, called the *trabecular meshwork* is found. This meshwork of collecting channels is responsible for the constant drainage of aqueous humor first into a circular channel known as the *canal of Schlemm,* and then into the venous plexis.

Aqueous humor, made by ciliary body epithelial cells, bathes the anterior portion of the lens as it flows from the *posterior chamber,* through the pupil into the *anterior chamber,* and then out through the trabecular meshwork into the canal of Schlemm. This constant aqueous flow is responsible for maintaining the hydrostatic pressure of the eye, referred to as *intraocular pressure* (IOP). Normal IOP ranges from 12 to 21 mm Hg. A tonometer is used to measure the IOP or assess the tension in the eye. The angle when viewed with a Goldman-type goniolens (Fig. 20–2) is described as being wide or open, narrow, closed, or as having peripheral anterior synechia (PAS).

The importance of glaucoma as a leading cause of blindness in the United States cannot be overstressed. When the IOP is higher than the intraocular tissues and intraocular circulation can tolerate, destruction of the ganglion cells of the retina and atrophy of the optic nerve results from the increased pressure, and if this pressure is not relieved, blindness occurs.

The *primary glaucomas include congenital, chronic open angle and acute angle closure.*

CONGENITAL ANOMALIES

Congenital glaucoma is due to failure of the mesodermal tissue to develop into a functioning filtering meshwork so that the aqueous formation by the epithelium of the ciliary body cannot drain out of the eye through the canal of Schlemm. This developmental failure can begin in utero and the pressure can be excessive for a while before birth. The infant can be born with large eyes with edematous corneas. The eyes of all newborns should be checked, and if suspect they should be examined under anesthesia. Congenital glaucoma is bilateral in 75 percent of the cases.

Congenital glaucoma is a recessive hereditary trait with incomplete penetrance. Symptoms which should alert the health care personnel are epiphora, photophobia, and blepharospasm (Fig. 20–3). Other signs are large eyes with or without cloudy cornea.

When examination under general anesthesia is performed the intraocular pres-

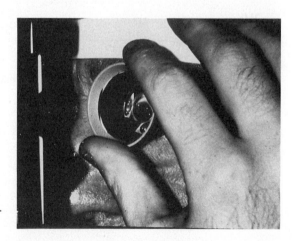

Figure 20–2. Goldman-like goni-olens on the eye.

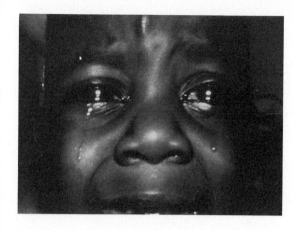

Figure 20–3. Constant tearing and photophobia may be symptoms of congenital glaucoma.

sure may change little during early stages of anesthesia but as the anesthesia progresses it may fall rapidly; the exception being ketamine anesthesia in which intraocular pressure may rise. Halothane plus ketamine anesthesia at our hospital is considered a good choice.

After the diagnosis of congenital glaucoma, treatment consists of goniotomy if the cornea is clear, and trabeculectomy if the cornea is cloudy.

NURSING INTERVENTION

Nursing intervention begins in the nursery. Since infants do not develop tears for the first couple of months of life, photophobia might be an early symptom. As the disease progresses, the larger than normal and occasionally cloudy cornea might become evident. Any young child who is constantly tearing, and tries to avoid the light should be referred to an ophthalmologist for evaluation.

ACQUIRED ANOMALIES

Chronic open angle glaucoma (COAG) or primary open angle glaucoma (POAG) is a painless, insidious elevation of intraocular pressure which over a span of years, may totally destroy the function of the retina and optic nerve and if left untreated, produces total blindness. The loss of peripheral vision is insidious, and may go unchecked through ignorance or neglect.

Primary open angle glaucoma is also a hereditary disease and genetically may be associated with diabetes. All patients with diabetes should therefore be checked for chronic open angle glaucoma and vice versa. A history of relatives with this disease is well documented, as is the fact that there are also optic nerve head cupping similarities in families. The normal physiological cup–disc ratio is about 0.3. As damage progresses, the cup–disc ratio increases (Fig. 20–4). Another interesting hereditary response is seen when steroid eyedrops are given to the

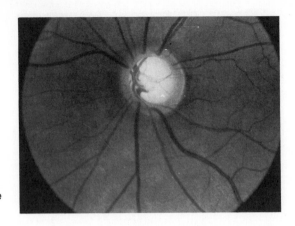

Figure 20–4. Cupping of the disc—about 0.7 cup–disc ratio.

patient. Of the general population, 5 percent will develop a rise in intraocular pressure when administering steroids locally to the eye, while in primary open angle glaucoma patients, 95 percent will demonstrate this response.

Chronic open angle glaucoma is seen with greater frequency in patients with diabetes mellitus, high myopia, retinal detachment, and central retinal vein occlusion. Because it is insidious and painless, it is important for patients to be checked for glaucoma at frequent intervals, especially after the age of 40.

The mechanisms for open angle glaucoma are that the trabecular spaces in the angle are not large enough, or the collector channels which drain the canal of Schlemm into the scleral and episcleral venous plexus are not large enough or numerous enough to drain the aqueous from inside the eye. While the formation of aqueous decreases with age, the outflow capacity may decrease faster and this discrepancy produces build up of intraocular pressure.

The symptoms are nonspecific eye problems, occasional browache, halos, or colored rings seen around lights. In the meantime, there is a slow, relentless peripheral vision loss.

Treatment of chronic open angle glaucoma is individually planned and closely followed by the ophthalmologist with intraocular pressure determination, visual fields, and disc photographs. The treatment is medical with a great number of drugs of varying percentage and actions. 0.25 percent or 0.5 percent Timoptic (timolol maleate) eyedrops, given b.i.d., is now the drug that is the most popular. Newer topical drugs, Betagan (levobunolol) and Betoptic (betaxolol), are now available alternatives. Pilocarpine drops are also used. The latter medication has a good track record with respect to the results and economy. Neptazane 50 mg q.i.d., is an oral pill which lowers intraocular pressure similar to Diamox, but has fewer side effects. Diamox can be given intravenously, which can be helpful in certain cases. Levoepinephrine or the prodrug, dipivifrin, are used for their antisecretory property, and in some cases, an irreversible anticholinesterase drug is also necessary. When maximum medical therapy is no longer well tolerated and the intraocular pressure is no longer controlled, then noninvasive laser trabeculoplasty or surgical trabeculectomy are measures to be considered.[1]

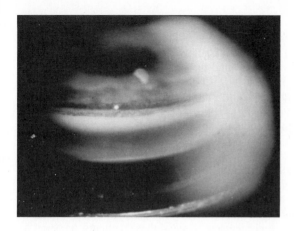

Figure 20–5. Laser trabeculo-plasty. The treatment will begin with an initial burn being placed at 6 o'clock, just anterior to the posterior trabecular meshwork (PTM). (*From Schwartz L, Spaeth GL, Brown GC: Laser Therapy of the Anterior Segment: A Practical Approach. Thorofare, N.J.: Slack, 1984, with permission.*)

Laser trabeculoplasty consists of small thermal burns on the meshwork which are made by aiming the laser beam through a Goldman-type goniolens into the angle. At present, it is felt that the scarring tightens the trabecular fibers and opens the intertercies, thus improving drainage (Fig. 20–5).

Surgical trabeculectomy is achieved by making a scleral flap and removing a piece of sclera containing the trabecular meshwork, an iridectomy is performed, then the flap is sutured in place under the conjunctiva. Aqueous is now able to drain directly from under the thin scleral flap covered by conjunctiva (Fig. 20–6).

NURSING INTERVENTION

Preoperatively, the trabeculoplasty or trabeculectomy patient will have the antiglaucoma drops instilled in the eyes. Usually the patient is using them in both eyes. Postoperatively, the surgical eye will be cyclopleged, and will also have steroid–antiobiotic medications instilled. There is an inherent danger here, and so patient teaching is important.

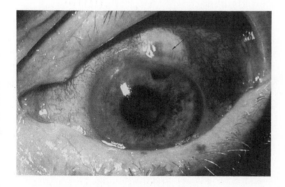

Figure 20–6. Trabeculectomy with functioning filtering bleb.

PATIENT TEACHING

After surgery, cycloplegic and combination steroid–antibiotic eyedrops will be prescribed t.i.d. If the patient cannot see well, these can be marked by placing a rubber band around the bottle, so that they can be identified by touch. Antiglaucoma drugs will continue to be instilled in the nonsurgical eye. The nurse should ensure that the patient does not inadvertently confuse the eyedrops, for if the wrong drops were placed in the nonsurgical eye, it might precipitate an acute attack of angle closure glaucoma.

Primary Acute Angle Closure Glaucoma

Primary acute angle closure glaucoma occurs less frequently than open angle glaucoma. The acute attack announces itself in a dramatic painful episode in and around the eye which occurs with decreased vision. The pupil is mid-dilated and the cornea hazy. Some patients are emergencies. Unless these patients respond to medical treatment or surgical treatment, irreversible damage to the optic nerve may occur. The fellow eye has an 80 percent chance of an acute attack.

The cause for acute angle closure glaucoma is blockage of the angle of the anterior chamber by iris tissue. The iris is usually pushed from behind as the ability of the aqueous to flow through the pupil is reduced. The pupillary block may be relative (usually) or absolute, in any case the iris bulges forward occluding the trabecular drain. The lens becomes larger with age and this can cause the pupillary block mechanism. This can be aggravated by the anterior position of the lens, as there is less room in the anterior chamber in hypermetropic than in myopic patients.

Intraocular pressure rises dramatically and measurements may range between 50 to 70 mm Hg. Attempts to lower the acute angle closure glaucoma pressure with parasympathomimetic drugs are made. These may not always work. The nurse will medicate the patient to help break the acute attack, and the patient will then require an iridectomy. This can be accomplished by the noninvasive technique of laser iridectomy (Fig. 20–7) or a surgical peripheral iridectomy, in the acutely affected eye and at a later date, in the unaffected eye.

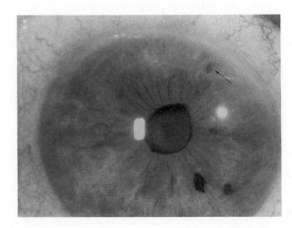

Figure 20–7. Laser iridectomy (*arrow*).

NURSING INTERVENTION

Usually this acute emergency patient presents holding one hand over the side of the face covering the eye that has the acute attack. The pain will be excruciating, and when the vision is checked it will be decreased. The pupil will be dilated and fixed, and the cornea may be hazy. After the physician has completed a Slitlamp examination of the patient, treatment will begin. This will consist of an I.V. push injection of 500 mg acetazolamide (Diamox); 2 percent pilocarpine eyedrops, given at frequent intervals of 10 to 15 minutes for four or five doses, will constrict the pupil and increase the outflow of aqueous; a drop of timolol maleate will also be given to reduce the pressure, and a unit or a measured amount of I.V. 20 percent mannitol may be given depending upon the weight of the patient. Once the acute attack has been broken, and the intraocular pressure reduced, either pilocarpine or timolol will be continued until a peripheral iridectomy can be performed.

Secondary Glaucoma

Secondary glaucoma can occur after inflammatory reaction, neovascular formation, lens induced reactions, trauma, or tumor.

Inflammatory reactions occur with iritis and the increased permeability of the blood aqueous barrier. Fibrin and protein escapes into the anterior chamber along with white blood cells, and in severe reactions red blood cells. This produces a secondary angle closure mechanism with the pupillary margin of the iris becoming adherent to the anterior lens capsule. As the pressure builds up behind the iris, the iris bulges into the anterior chamber (iris bombe) and blocks the angle. Organization of inflammatory debris and exudate makes the obstruction of the meshwork permanent.

Neovascular membranes may form on the anterior surface of the iris and corneal–iris angle blocking the filtering mechanism. This formation in the angle is seen following retinal vascular occlusion usually secondary to diabetes.

These secondary glaucomas are treated with cycloplegic drops, timolol maleate to reduce the pressure, and steroids to decrease the inflammatory response.

Lens-induced glaucoma may be due to lens swelling which leads to pupillary block and angle closure glaucoma. The other cause of lens induced glaucoma occurs when denatured lens protein leaks through intact lens capsule and stimulates a macrophagic reaction. These macrophages and protein can block trabecular meshwork causing an acute rise in pressure. Surgical lens removal is performed, once the IOP is reduced.

Traumatic glaucoma can follow contusion, anterior segment lacerations, hyphema, or traumatic cataract formation.

In contusion to the globe, the trabecular meshwork may be torn by the sudden displacement of the scleral spur which is the posterior insertion of the trabecular meshwork fibers. When this occurs, fibrosis takes place and the so-called contusion deformity gradually reduces outflow capacity and results in glaucoma.

Trauma to the anterior segment may be accidental, due to lacerations, or surgically-induced postoperative complications. In the accidental traumatic glaucoma, a subluxated or dislocated lens can lead to intermittent pupillary block. Blood and debris from laceration or foreign body penetration can cause angle blockage. This closure is made certain if the anterior chamber collapse is due to loss

or leaking aqueous. Corneal epithelial downgrowth can coat the trabecular meshwork with epithelial cells which block drainage through the meshwork to
Schlemm's canal. Hemorrhages beneath the choroid can cause shallowing of the
anterior chamber and result in iris blockage of the angle. Surgical insults to the eye
can cause all of the accidental injuries and add several others, such as those induced
by different drugs used in surgical procedures. For example, alphachymotrypsin
damages the endothelium of the meshwork, hyaluronic acid blocks the meshwork,
and topical corticosteroids can elevate pressure in steroid responders.

Glaucoma secondary to tumor is caused by the tumor cells in the debris
invading the angle or blocking the venous drainage of aqueous. Treatment is directed at the underlying cause.

Absolute glaucoma is the end-stage of glaucoma with a blind, hard eye which
may be enlarged, and the disc totally excavated. Prior to this stage being reached,
cyclocryotherapy is performed to decrease the production of aqueous. When the eye
becomes too painful, has no vision, and causes the patient constant distress, the
final surgical choice which is made by the patient is to have the blind, painful eye
enucleated.

DIAGNOSTIC EVALUATION

There must always be a high index of suspicion. In congenital glaucoma, large eyes
with large corneas which may or may not be clouded must be examined under
anesthesia. At this time, determination of the intraocular pressure and a complete
fundus examination must be performed. Other signs such as a port-wine birthmark
which includes both lids suggests Sturge-Weber syndrome (Fig. 20–8); while neurofibromatosis and aniridia should excite interest into the possibility of a secondary
glaucoma.

In open angle chronic glaucoma, a complete examination must be performed
which includes intraocular pressure determination and fundus examination. Beside
the visual acuity, central visual fields should be done, preferably with the newer,
more sensitive automated computerized field analyzer. Color vision determination
and steriofundus photography of optic nerve heads are methods of documentation
which can be used for comparison at a later date.

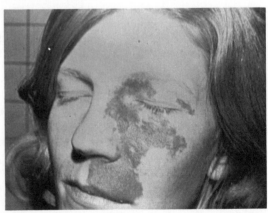

Figure 20–8. Sturge-Weber syndrome showing the port-wine birth
mark involving both lids.

If all the signs of chronic glaucoma are present except elevated intraocular pressure, a diagnosis of *low tension glaucoma* should be considered. A CAT scan should be considered for the outside chance of a tumor causing the changes.

Gonioscopy facilitates in differentiating the diagnosis of acute angle closure glaucoma from acute iritis with secondary pressure rise.

Tonometry
There are several methods by which the IOP can be measured. Although the Schiøtz method is an older method, it is still used in the operating room and when patients are unable to be helped up to the Slitlamp for applanation tonometry. The tonometer must be clean, and the plunger must move freely. Before use it should be checked, on the little button which resembles the cornea's shape, to ensure that it is calibrated. Applanation tonometry is the most frequently used method of measuring the IOP, but it requires that a Slitlamp be available because it attaches directly to this equipment. Various other instruments are available, and these include the pneumatonometer and an "air puff" tonometer, which is sometimes used in industry. However, the disadvantage of this equipment is that it is expensive and, therefore, is not in wide use.

Schiøtz Tonometry
The following technique may be used for measuring the intraocular pressure using a Schiøtz tonometer:

1. Have the patient lie down or sit in a chair that can be tilted to a reclining position.
2. Check that the patient who wears contact lenses has removed them.
3. Place one drop of topical anesthetic (proparacaine) in the conjunctival cul-de-sac, and as the patient closes the eyes, gently blot the outer canthus. Request that the patient not rub the eyes for the next 30 minutes.
4. Ask the patient to hold a hand up, so that the gaze can be fixed on the thumb.
5. Gently part the eyelids with one hand, and approach the cornea from the outer canthus, then gently rest the foot plate of the tonometer on the cornea (Fig. 20–9).
6. The stilette pointer will oscillate on the scale for a moment and then become stationary. Take the scale reading to the nearest half gradation.
7. Remove the tonometer from the eye, and ask the patient to close the eyes gently.
8. The scale reading now has to be translated using a standard conversion chart which will express the reading in millimeters of mercury.
9. To document the tension reading, identify the eye, identify the weight used on the tonometer, convert the scale reading to an IOP reading in mm Hg.
10. Example: O.D. has a Schiøtz tonometry reading of 6.5 with a 5.5 g weight. Using the conversion scale, the IOP is 13 mm Hg.

Applanation Tonometry. Applanation tonometry is the most accurate method of testing intraocular pressure (Fig. 20–10). It is performed by flattening the cornea with the small end of a truncated plastic cone, after anesthetic and fluorescein drops have been placed in the eyes. The cone is part of the Slitlamp which is attached to a

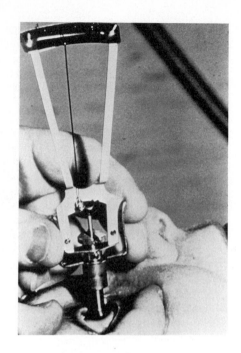

Figure 20–9. Schiøtz tonometry.

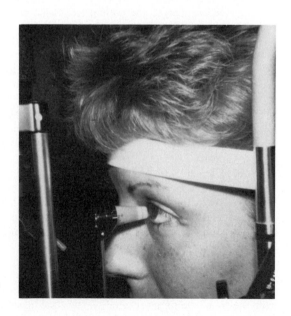

Figure 20–10. Applanation to-nometry.

calibrated wheel by a thin rod. Turning the wheel will move the cone forward or backward exerting more or less pressure upon the cornea. The plastic cone is aligned in front of an ocular and objective of the Slitlamp microscope with the visual axis passing through the scope and center of the cone. The light source from the Slitlamp is passed through a cobalt blue filter, and is focused on the cone from an angle of aboue 30 degrees.

When the flat surface of the cone flattens the cornea the rim will appear as a green ring. In order to make an accurate and consistent reading, the plastic cone has prisms incorporated in it which splits the green ring in half and moves the edges so that a half rim is seen through the ocular above and half below. These fluorescein rims are displaced laterally and as the calibrated wheel is turned and pressure on the cornea is increased or decreased, the half rings move toward or away from each other. When the inside edges of the fluorescein rings touch, the calibration is read off the wheel and is recorded as the intraocular pressure.

REFERENCES

1. Boyd-Monk H, Starita RJ: Surgical intervention to stop glaucoma. Journal of Ophthalmic Nursing and Technology, 4(3): 12–15, 30, 1985

BIBLIOGRAPHY

Boyd-Monk H: Screening for glaucoma. Nursing 79, 9(8): 42–45, 1979

Chandler PA: Chandler and Grant's Glaucoma, 2nd ed. Philadelphia: Lea & Febiger, 1986

Horowitz J: Laser light on glaucoma: The therapeutic burn. Sightsaving, 51(2): 12–15, 22, 1982

National Society to Prevent Blindness. Medical advisory panel on glaucoma: Questions and answers about glaucoma. Sightsaving, 53(1): 14–20, 1984

Spaeth GL: Glaucoma surgery, in Spaeth GL, (Ed.): Ophthalmic Surgery Principles and Practice. Philadelphia: Saunders, 1982

Appendix

SYSTEMIC DISEASES WITH OCULAR MANIFESTATIONS

Systemic Disease	Ocular Manifestations
Vascular	
Atherosclerosis and arteriosclerosis	*Retina*
	Retinal artery and vein occlusions
	Hypertensive retinopathy
	Diabetic retinopathy
	Optic nerve
	Ischemic optic neuropathy
	Extraocular muscles
	Palsies, i.e., sixth nerve palsy, etc.
Hematologic	
Leukemia	*Cornea*
	Corneal infiltrates
	Retina
	Infiltrates and hemorrhages
	Vascular occlusions
	Eyelids, conjunctiva, and orbit
	Tumor formation
Sickle-cell Disease	*Retina*
	Retinopathy
	Vascular occlusions of retinal vessels
	Exudates around retinal vessels
Metabolic	
Diabetes Mellitus	*Lens*
	Refractive error changes
	Cataracts
	Retina
	Retinopathy and vascular occlusions
	Vitreous
	Vitreous hemorrhage
	Iris and angle
	Neovascularization of the iris, leading to seondary glaucoma
	Extraocular muscles
	Nerve palsies, i.e., third and sixth nerve palsy
Endocrine	
Thyroid Gland Disorders:	
1. Graves' Disease	*Eyelids*
	Exophthalmos
	Lid lag
	Extraocular muscles
	Muscle palsies, resulting in diplopia
	Optic nerve
	Optic atrophy, secondary to compression
	Cornea
	Exposure keratitis and ulcer formation, secondary to exophthalmos
2. Myxedema	Edematous eyelids
Infectious diseases	
Rubella	*Lens*
	Congenital cataracts
	Retina
	Retinitis
Varicella	*Eyelids*
	Pocked lids

Systemic Disease	Ocular Manifestations
	Cornea
	Corneal scarring
	Uveal tract
	Iritis, anterior uveitis
	Retina
	Retinitis
	Trigeminal nerve
	Neuralgia
Cytomegalic Inclusion Disease	*Retina*
	Retinitis with retinal necrosis
Collagen	
Lupus Erythematosus	*Cornea and conjunctiva*
	Keratoconjunctivitis sicca
	Sclera
	Scleritis
	Retina
	Retinopathy
Rheumatoid Arthritis	*Cornea and conjunctiva*
	Keratoconjunctivitis sicca
	Sclera
	Scleritis
	Uveal tract
	Anterior uveitis
Connective Tissue	
Marfans's Syndrome	*Eyeball*
	Myopia
	Lens
	Dislocated lenses
	Retina
	Retinal detachment
	Cornea
	Keratoconus
Marchesani's Syndrome	*Eyeball*
	Hypermetropia
	Lens
	Cataract, dislocated lenses
	Glaucoma
	Retina
	Retinal detachment
Osteogenesis Imperfecta	*Sclera*
	Blue sclera because it is so thin
	Cornea
	Thin cornea
	Lens
	Cataract
	Optic nerve
	Atrophy due to bony compression due to thickening of bones of the optic canal.
Inborn Errors of Metabolism	
Albinism	*Uveal tract*
	Photophobia due to decreased pigment in iris, choroid, and retina
	Eyelids
	Sunburn easily because of decreased pigmentation

(continued)

Systemic Disease	Ocular Manifestations
Homocystinuria	*Cornea*
	Corneal opacities
	Lens
	Dislocated lenses
Galactosemia	*Cataract*
Miscellaneous Systemic Diseases	
Vogt-Koyanagi-Harada Syndrome	*Uveal tract*
	Anterior uveitis and posterior uveitis
	Lens
	Cataract
	Retina
	Bilateral retinal detachments
	Skin, lashes, and hair
	Vitiligo, poliosis, and alopecia
Stevens-Johnson Syndrome	*Conjunctiva and cornea*
	Conjunctival lesions, corneal scarring
	Optic nerve
	Atrophy
Pemphigus	*Conjunctiva and cornea*
	Corneal and conjunctival scarring

Index

Italic letters following page numbers refer to tables *(t)* and figures *(f)*.

Sclerosing pseudotumor, of orbit,
  chronic, 132
Scotoma, 7, 299
  testing for, 59, 61
Scrubbing time, 110
Sebaceous cysts, of eyelid, 167–168
Seborrheic keratosis, 168
Seizure disorders, history of, 50
Self-administration
  of lid hygiene, 22
  of warm compresses, 31
Self-medication
  with eyedrops, 28–29
  teaching about, 41, 47
Semilunar folds, 176
Senile cataracts, 241–242
Senile keratosis, 168
Senile macular degeneration, 293–294
  atrophic type, 293–294
  exudative type, 293, 294
Sensitivity testing, 35
Shield, 31, 32–33
  bubble, 149, 150f
Shigellae bacillus, 182
Sickle cell disease, 285, 286, 334
Siderosis, 251, 253, 268
Silicone oil, 121, 122
Sinuses
  cavernous, thrombosis of, 131–132
  ethmoid, 128, 130, 170
  frontal, 128, 130
  maxillary, 128, 130
  orbital abscess and, 131
  orbital cellulitis and, 131
  paranasal, 130
  periostitis and, 130
  sphenoid, 128
Sjögren's syndrome, 147
Skin
  assessment of, 51
  grafting, in exenteration, 134
Slitlamp, 8, 196–197
  examination, 46, 196–197
Smears, 35, 36
Smoking, 47
Snellen Eye Chart, 8, 53, 54f, 58
Soft contact lenses. See also Contact
    lenses
  aphakic continuous wear, 241
  for astigmatism, 71
  care of, 74, 76
  for corneal ulcers, 203
  extended wear, 74

HTLV-III prevention and, 76
  insertion of, 74
  removal of, 74
Solar burns, 235, 293
Sphenoid bone
  greater wing of, 128
  lesser wing of, 128
Sphenoid sinuses, 129
Spherical lenses, 69, 73, 74
  concave, 69
  convex, 69
Spherocylinder lenses, 70
Spherophakia, 239
Spots before eyes, 46
Squamous cell carcinoma, of eyelid, 168
Squamous cell epithelioma, of cornea,
    209, 210f
Squint. See Strabismus
Staphylococci phlyctenular disease, 188
Staphylococcus, 200, 203
  aureus, 142, 157, 178, 180, 188, 200
  epidermidis, 180, 200
Staphyloma, 7, 215
Sterile technique, 110
Steroids, topical, 96t–99t
  cataracts caused by, 188
  glaucoma caused by, 188
Stevens-Johnson syndrome, 147, 187,
    212
Strabismus, 6, 155, 315, 316–318
  acquired, 317
  congenital, 317
  convergent. See Esotropia
  divergent. See Exotropia
  nonparalytic, 316, 317
  paralytic, 316–317
  results of, 317–318
  surgery for, 123f, 124, 318
Streak, primitive, 11
Streptococcus, 180, 182
  beta-hemolytic, 142
  pneumoniae, 144, 200
  viridans, 200
Stress, decreasing, 39–41
Stroma, corneal, 196
  dystrophies, 198
Struge-Weber syndrome, 177, 328
Sty. See Hordeolum
Subconjunctival hemorrhage, 7, 177,
    178f, 191
Subconjunctival injection, 29
Subcutaneous emphysema, 170
Subretinal fluid, 286

Ulcers
  corneal. *See* Corneal ulcers in infectious blepharitis, 157
Ultrasonic cleaning
  of microsurgical instruments, 111
  of ophthalmic instruments, 109–110
Ultrasonography, 137, 269, 270*f*, 282
  A-scan, 269, 270*f*, 271
  B-scan, 269, 270*f*, 271
  M-mode, 269
Uveal tract, 4, 219–236. *See also*
    Choroid; Ciliary body; Iris
  acquired anomalies of, 7, 225–235
  anatomy of, 219–220
  benign tumors of, 229, 232
  congenital anomalies of, 220–225, 227
  malignant tumors of, 230–231, 232
  metastatic tumors of, 232
  trauma, 233–235
Uveitis, 7, 225–229
  anterior, 45, 225–226, 242
  granulomatous and nongranulomatous,
    differentiation of, 225–226
  posterior, 225, 226–228, 286
  sympathetic, 7, 228–229
  toxoplasmic, 225, 226–228

Van Lint akinesia, 112
Varicella, 334–335
Vein. *See specific name*
Venous dilation, irregular, 278
Venous plexus, 16
Venous thrombosis, 284–285
Vernal catarrh, 187, 188
Vessels, ghost, 204
Viral conjunctivitis, 182–185
Viral ulcers, 200–201
Viruses. *See also specific name; type;*
    Antiviral agents
  endophthalmitis caused by, 256
  macula infections caused by, 293
  uveitis caused by, 225
Vision
  binocular, 314–315, 316*f*
  blurred, 46
  color. *See* Color vision
  double. *See* Diplopia
  functional, 50, 51, 57
  loss of, sudden, 44, 253, 282
Visual axes
  in adult, 11, 13*f*

at birth, 11, 13*f*
  embryology of, 11, 13*f*
Visual acuity
  assessment of, 46
  documentation of, 44, 53
  recording, 54, 55*t*
  testing. *See* Visual acuity testing
Visual acuity testing, 8, 44, 46, 53–66
  charts for, 53–54, 55*f*, 56, 57
Visual field(s)
  central, 8, 53, 58
  defects, 303, 304*f*. *See also specific
    defect*
  normal, 58, 62*f*
  peripheral, 8, 53, 58
  testing, 8, 46, 58–64, 65*f*, 309
Visual pathways, 299, 305–307
Visual purple, 262–263
Visual screening methods, 53–67. *See
    also specific method*
Vitamin A deficiency, 147, 199, 269
Vitamin E, for retinopathy of prematurity, 274
Vitrectomy, 9, 109, 118, 121, 225, 252,
    253, 256, 257, 274, 279, 285
  technique, 121–121, 257–259
Vitreoretinal adhesions, 121, 251
Vitreous, 4, 251–259
  acquired anomalies of, 252–259
  anatomy of, 251
  base, 251
  congenital anomalies of, 252
  detachment, posterior, 254
  embryology of, 16, 17
  hemorrhage, 252–253, 269, 278, 279,
    284, 285
  loss, 117, 118
  opacities, 254
  primary, 16, 17
  secondary, 17
  tap, 9
  tertiary, 17
  trauma, 252, 253, 254–255
Vitreous-retinal surgery, 118*f*, 119*f*, 120–
    122. *See also specific procedure*
Vogt-Koyanagi-Harada syndrome, 336
Vortex veins, 214

Wall-eye. *See Exotropia*
Weill-Marchesani's syndrome. *See*
    Marchesani's syndrome